MEN'S HEALTH TODAY 2004

MEN'S HEALTH TODAY

2004

YOUR BLUEPRINT FOR A BETTER BODY

Edited by Deanna Portz, Men'sHealth. Books

RODALE

© 2004 by Rodale Inc.

All rights reserved. No part of this publication may be reproduced or transmitted in any form or by any means, electronic or mechanical, including photocopying, recording, or any other information storage and retrieval system, without the written permission of the publisher.

Men's Health is a registered trademark of Rodale Inc.

Printed in the United States of America
Rodale Inc. makes every effort to use acid-free ∞, recycled paper ♲.

"Are You a Sex Addict?" on page 57 reprinted with permission from Patrick Carnes, Ph.D.

"A Royal Pain in the Gut" on page 97 reprinted by permission of International Creative Management, Inc. Copyright © 2002 by Michael Perry.

"Meet Ralph" on page 106 reprinted by permision of International Creative Management, Inc. Copyright © 2003 by Michael Perry.

Book design by Drew Frantzen

ISBN 1–57954–873–3 hardcover

2   4   6   8   10   9   7   5   3   1   hardcover

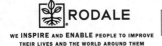

WE **INSPIRE** AND **ENABLE** PEOPLE TO IMPROVE
THEIR LIVES AND THE WORLD AROUND THEM

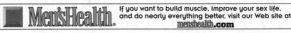

If you want to build muscle, improve your sex life, and do nearly everything better, visit our Web site at menshealth**.com**

EDITOR: Deanna Portz

CONTRIBUTING WRITERS: Fred Abatemarco, Don Alessi, Jamie Beckman, Sheri de Borchgrave, Brian Boyé, Steve Calechman, Adam Campbell, Kevin Cook, Alwyn Cosgrove, Shannon Davis, Webster Donovan, Ron Geraci, Bill Gifford, Brian Good, Bill Gottlieb, John Hyduk, Lisa Jones, Joe Kita, Jonathan Kantor, Susan M. Kleiner, Chris Lawson, Matt Marion, Robert Maurer, Christopher McDougall, Sarah Miller, Christian Millman, Hugh O'Neill, Michael Perry, Stephen Rae, Harold Ramis, Brian Reid, Bruce Schoenfeld, Lou Schuler, Ted Spiker, Laurence Roy Stains, Bill Stieg, Bill Stump, Zachary Veilleux, Jonathan Wander, Mike Zimmerman, Tom Zoellner

INTERIOR AND COVER DESIGNERS: Drew Frantzen, Joanna Williams

PHOTO EDITOR: Darleen Malkames

RESEARCH EDITOR: Bernadette Sukley

PROJECT EDITOR: Kathryn C. LeSage

COPY EDITORS: Anne Winthrop Esposito, Alan Lovell

LAYOUT DESIGNER: Donna G. Bellis

PRODUCT SPECIALIST: Brenda Miller

Rodale Men's Health Group

PRESIDENT, MANAGING DIRECTOR: Tom Beusse

VICE PRESIDENT, *MEN'S HEALTH* EDITOR-IN-CHIEF: David Zinczenko

MEN'S HEALTH AND SPORTS BOOKS EXECUTIVE EDITOR: Jeremy Katz

SENIOR MANAGING EDITOR: Chris Krogermeier

VICE PRESIDENT OF ART & DESIGN: Andy Carpenter

MANAGING ART DIRECTOR: Darlene Schneck

VICE PRESIDENT, PUBLISHER OF DIRECT RESPONSE BOOKS: Gregg Michaelson

SENIOR DIRECTOR DIRECT RESPONSE MARKETING: Janine Slaughter

ASSOCIATE CUSTOMER MARKETING MANAGER: Matthew Neumaier

CONTENT ASSEMBLY MANAGER: Robert V. Anderson Jr.

ASSOCIATE CONTENT ASSEMBLY MANAGER: Patricia Brown

CONTRACTS COORDINATOR: Jessica Nagle

ADMINISTRATIVE ASSISTANT: Pamela Brinar

Contents

Introduction ix

PART ONE: GET LEAN AND STRONG

Game Show:

Who Will Build the Best Abs? 3

Must Reads

How Sweet It Isn't 6

When the Urge Strikes 9

Supersize Your Muscles 12

Small Muscles, Big Results 17

Fit for Life 21

Know This 26

Down the Pike 29

Game Plan: Join a Gym without

Dropping a Bundle 31

Take Action 33

Any Questions? 38

PART TWO: TURBOCHARGE YOUR SEX LIFE

Game Show:

Who Will Have the Most Sex

This Year? 45

Must Reads

Keep Your Eye on the Balls 48

Playing the Odds 53

Too Much of a Good Thing 55

Surefire Seduction 63

Give Yourself a Big Hand 67

Know This 71

Down the Pike 73

Game Plan: A Weekend Away 74

Take Action 75

Any Questions? 78

PART THREE: SAVE YOUR SICK DAYS

Game Show:

Who Will Beat Back Pain First? 83

Must Reads

Treat Yourself 86

Stop the Bleeding 94

A Royal Pain in the Gut 97

Show Your Back Who's Boss 102

Meet Ralph 106

Know This 111

Down the Pike 113

Game Plan: Survive Your Visit

to the Drill Sergeant 115

Take Action 117

Any Questions? 121

PART FOUR: FEND OFF THE MEN KILLERS

Game Show:

Who Will Get Colon Cancer? 127

Must Reads

Healthiest Homes for Men 130

Survive a Heart Attack 139

Is Your Heart Sending Out an SOS? 146

Don't Blow Your Mind 149

This Is a Stick Up 152

The Wonder Drug 157

Know This 160

Down the Pike 162

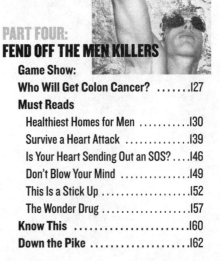

Game Plan: When You're a
    Guest Star on ER 164
Take Action 165
Any Questions? 169

PART FIVE: BEAT THE HEALTH CARE SYSTEM

Game Show:
Who Will Lower His Cholesterol
    for Good? .175
Must Reads
  Critical Condition 178
  Pushed to the Limit 187
  Just Say "No" to Drugs 197
  Scan Artists 202
  Time to Play Doctor 205
Know This 208
Down the Pike 211
Game Plan: Manage Your Care 213
Take Action .215
Any Questions? 220

PART SIX: MEND YOUR MIND

Game Show:
Who Will Get Alzheimer's? 225
Must Reads
  Mind over Matter 228
  Shrink Rap 233

  Fear Not 237
  Lighten Up 240
  Turn Your Luck Around 243
Know This 246
Down the Pike 248
Game Plan: Face-to-Face with 40 . .249
Take Action .250
Any Questions? 253

PART SEVEN: MAKE AN IMPRESSION

Game Show:
Who Will Win Her Over? 257
Must Reads
  Rebound like the Best of 'em 260
  Shake on It 266
  Stand and Deliver 269
  There's a Price on Your Head 272
  Saving Face 280
Know This 285
Down the Pike 288
Game Plan: Make a Big Deal
    over Dinner 289
Take Action .290
Any Questions? 292

Index 295
Photo Credits 310

Introduction

Home Improvement

You can learn a valuable lesson from the expression "Home is where you hang your hat." Think about it: The place you most likely hang your headgear is, well, on your head. So you could say that the structure housing your brain, muscles, and vital organs—your body—is the ultimate home, sweet home.

With this notion in mind, we compiled this book—this blueprint, if you will, for building a better body. No matter which area of your life has room for improvement—your waistline, your workout, your sex life, or your overall health—*Men's Health Today 2004* gives you the tools and know-how to fix it fast. Need a little help in the waist-management department? Discover the ingredient in food that may be making you fat. Find out what your food cravings mean and when it's okay to indulge in that bowl of Ben & Jerry's (and when it's not). Plus, learn why the fat from your gut is the last to go—and how you can lose it with two easy tricks.

Strengthen your structure in less time with the "super" workouts starting on page 12. If aches, pains, or sports injuries are stopping you, find a sport that'll be right for you over the long haul.

Home alone? Use the strategies on pages 63 and 258 to bring some lucky lady home with you *tonight*. But before you head out the door, evict any pimples or pustules from that prime real estate in the mirror, with the tips on page 280.

Home sick? *Men's Health Today 2004* makes house calls. Whatever it is that's cramping your style, we've got a do-it-yourself plan for you. Not to mention the ultimate home remedy: a drug in your medicine cabinet that prevents everything from cancer to heart disease to Alzheimer's. We've even included some help for your home economics—money-saving strategies for when you do get sick or end up in the hospital.

Got a, um, plumbing problem? This book is chock-full of information to help you make a diagnosis, plus tons of tips on fixing your pipes. Are cobwebs cluttering your, shall we say, "attic"? Turn to part six for some free counsel and personal housecleaning clues to make you happier, less stressed, and more productive.

You spend a lot of time and money maintaining and improving your castle. It's about time you put a little effort into that other place you call home—your body. Now put down the miter saw (careful!) and read on.

—**Deanna Portz, Editor**

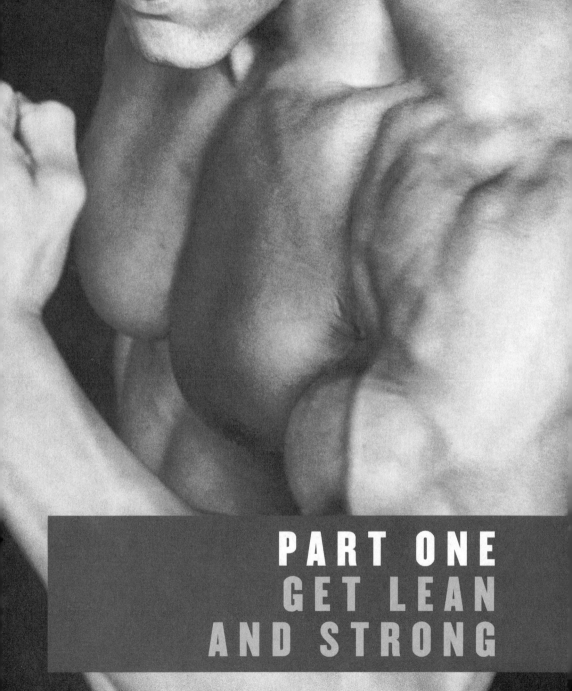

PART ONE
GET LEAN
AND STRONG

GAME SHOW

Who Will Build the Best Abs?
One of these identical triplets—or you?

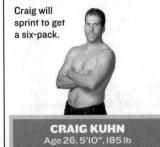

Craig will sprint to get a six-pack.

Chris will crunch in great numbers.

Curt will sweat his flab into abs.

CRAIG KUHN
Age 26, 5'10", 185 lb
Sign language teacher,
Jacksonville, IL

CHRIS KUHN
Age 26, 5'10", 185 lb
Career specialist,
Jacksonville, IL

CURT KUHN
Age 26, 5'10", 185 lb
Supervisor,
Jacksonville, IL

HIS PLAN
• A mix of cardiovascular and strength training three times a week for 8 weeks. The cardio: running intervals, beginning with three 30-second sprints in week 1 and working up to eight 45-second sprints from week 6 on. The weights: one set of eight repetitions of the squat, Romanian deadlift, bench press, lat pulldown, and shoulder press.

ADVANTAGES
• High-intensity interval training burns more calories than lower-intensity continuous exercise.

• Doing low reps (fewer than eight) with heavier weights works the abdominal muscles by default; it can do as much good as 50 crunches.

• His body-fat level is a low 13 percent.

• Building muscle raises metabolism and burns even more fat.

DISADVANTAGES
• Craig isn't doing any ab-specific exercises. And will a few sprints really burn enough fat to make his abs pop?

• An already overflowing schedule could make it difficult for Craig to hit the gym.

HIS PLAN
• Eight weeks of crunches and light weight lifting. He'll begin with three sets of 50 crunches every day for 2 weeks, then jump to 100 per set. After another 2 weeks, he'll add three sets of 25 Swiss-ball crunches. He'll also do squats, hamstring curls, bench presses, lat pulldowns, and shoulder presses (one set of 15 apiece, 3 days a week).

ADVANTAGES
• All those crunches will target the area he's trying to build.

• Weight training indirectly works the abdominal muscles and helps raise metabolism to new fat-burning levels.

DISADVANTAGES
• In some cases, endurance-based training actually shrinks the targeted muscles so they can perform better over longer periods.

• Doing crunches every day doesn't allow the muscles time to recover.

• This workout won't burn much body fat, and Chris is at 15 percent, higher than ideal, to begin with.

• Having a baby daughter means more time demands. Will Chris stick to his program?

HIS PLAN
• Pure cardiovascular training: 8 weeks of running three times a week. He'll start with 30 minutes per session and work his way up to 45 minutes at a time. No weight training or targeted ab exercises.

ADVANTAGES
• Of all the traditional cardiovascular exercises, running burns the most calories per hour. It's a great way to get lean fast and reveal hidden abs.

• Curt's body fat is an already low 13 percent.

DISADVANTAGES
• Running is a great workout, but Curt will burn only 300 to 400 calories per session, which may not be enough heat to further shrink that favorable body fat percentage.

• He's doing nothing to build muscle mass. This lack of weight training may reduce his overall fat-burning potential.

• Curt works the night shift and is married. His odd hours and home life demands could make it more difficult for him to adhere to his program.

And the Winner Is . . .
Craig Kuhn

Craig Ballantyne, C.S.C.S., a strength coach in Toronto, helped us design the quiz on the opposite page to find out which contestant has the best shot at causing a ripple above his navel. Take it yourself to see if you'll ever get a six-pack.

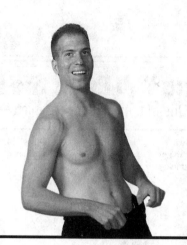

FINAL ANALYSIS

Here's the really, really good news: Every man has abs. But on most guys, they're hidden by a thick layer of belly fat, which is like wearing a parka over an Armani suit. To bring them out, you have to remember one thing: He who eliminates the most fat will see the most muscle.

The Kuhn triplets presented an irresistible testing opportunity: Take three men of the same age, height, weight, and genes, and see which ab program gives the best results. It's downright scientific. But here's the catch: While all three Kuhn brothers are trying to burn fat, their individual programs sealed their fates before they even started.

With the highest intensity of all three workouts, Craig, quite simply, is doing the most to combust fat. "With a combination of weight training and intervals, he's getting the most out of his workout time," says Ballantyne. "The weight lifting also helps maintain muscle mass."

Blasting the abdominals as Chris is doing is a long-standing six-pack myth. "It just isn't going to work," says Ballantyne. "Targeting the abdominal muscles doesn't reduce body fat. People persist because when they do 50 crunches, their abs burn—and they associate that with results. The abs may eventually get in better shape, but the fat covering them isn't going anywhere."

Curt's cardiovascular regimen is a good start on addressing that fat layer, says Ballantyne, but it's only a start. "Cardio is the way many guys think they'll get abs because of the calorie burn. That helps overweight men, but once you're fairly lean, your body doesn't respond as dramatically to burning a few hundred calories in 30 minutes." Additional weight training, along with some occasional high-intensity sprint workouts, would make a big difference for Curt.

BELLY BAROMETER

FACTOR	POINT VALUE	CRAIG	CHRIS	CURT	YOU
AGE Your metabolism slows with age. The older you get, the less fat you burn at rest.	Younger than 25? +2 25–35? +1 Older than 35? −1	+1	+1	+1	
BODY FAT The higher your fat level, the longer it'll take to see your abs.	Below 10%? +2 10–15%? +1 Higher than 15%? −1	+1	+1	+1	
MOTIVATION If you skip workouts, you'll skip the progress, too.	Consistently work out 4 or more times per week? +2 3 times per week? +1 Fewer than 3 times per week? −1	+1	+1	+1	
DIET If you want to lose the fat, avoid chewing it.	Less than 30% of daily calories from fat? +1 30% or more of daily calories from fat? −1	+1	−1	+1	
WEIGHT LIFTING Moving iron is proven to help raise your metabolism and build muscle mass, including the rectus abdominis.	Heavy weights 3 or more times per week? +2 Light weights 3 or more times per week? +1 No weight training? −1	+2	+1	−1	
CARDIOVASCULAR EXERCISE Aerobic exercise—running, stairclimbing, elliptical training— is an excellent fat burner.	Cardio 3 or more times per week? +1 No cardio? −1	+1	−1	+1	
INTERVAL TRAINING Sprinting is a high-intensity workout, burning more calories and raising metabolism.	At least one interval session per week? +2 No intervals? 0	+2	0	0	
STRESS High levels of the stress hormone cortisol may make you pack on abdominal fat.	Low stress? +1 Some stress? 0 High stress? −1	−1	−1	−1	
CRUNCHES It's the classic ab exercise, but doing too many too often can work against you.	3 crunch sessions per week? +1 Crunch infrequently? 0 No crunching? −1 More than 3 sessions per week? −1	−1	−1	−1	
TOTALS		7	0	2	

▶ IF YOUR SCORE IS 6 OR HIGHER: Look out! It's the abdominal showman!

▶ IF YOUR SCORE IS 2–5: You may be a gutless wonder, but you're probably abless, too.

▶ IF YOUR SCORE IS 1 OR LOWER: Cancel the Club Med reservation.

MUST READS

How Sweet It Isn't

Food companies are adding an evil ingredient to their products that may turn your body into a fat-storing machine

By Susan M. Kleiner, Ph.D., R.D.

During my first semester in graduate school, I took a course called food science, the study of ingredients in foods. It was 1980. "High-fructose corn syrup has recently been introduced into the food supply," my professor told us. "It's a very inexpensive sweetener and will likely replace sugar in most processed foods." I could tell she wasn't happy about that. She went on to explain that our understanding of how fructose works in the body was very limited, and we had no idea how it would affect the population.

Now we know.

High-fructose corn syrup is making America fat. How? By shutting off the switches that control appetite. It's more easily turned into fat than any other carbohydrate. And it's everywhere, from the obvious places, like Coke and Mountain Dew, to barbecue sauce and canned soup.

Consider this: In 1970, Americans ate about ½ pound of high-fructose corn syrup (HFCS) per person per year. By 1997, we were consuming up to 62½ pounds each, according to a study published in the *American Journal of Clinical Nutrition*. That's 228 calories per person per day, and the figure is based on 6-year-old numbers; consumption has almost certainly risen since then. And over the same period, the obesity rate has more than doubled.

HFCS is different from other sugars and sweeteners, which can make you fat indirectly, over time. HFCS makes you fat by the straightest possible metabolic path. Let's look at where this stuff comes from, what it does to your body, and—most important—how to get as much of it as possible out of your diet.

FRUCTOSE CAN MAKE YOU FAT

The problem with HFCS is the fructose—a sugar that occurs naturally in fruit and honey—rather than the corn syrup. Corn syrup is primarily made up of a sugar called glucose, which can be burned up as a source of immediate energy, stored in your liver and muscles for use later, or, as a last resort, turned into fat. But corn syrup isn't as sweet as other sugars, which is why the food-processing industry fell head over heels in love with high-fructose corn syrup, a cheap and doubly sweet chemical derivative.

But what's good for Coca-Cola's profit margins isn't that great for your health. That's because your body doesn't necessarily use fructose as an immediate source of energy. "Fructose is more readily metabolized into fat," says Peter Havel, Ph.D., a nutrition researcher at the University of California at Davis. Havel is among a growing number of scientists who suspect that there's a connection between fructose and America's skyrocketing rates of obesity and diabetes.

We should mention that we aren't saying that the small amounts of fructose you get through fruit or honey will make you fat. Fruit is packed with vitamins, minerals, and fiber, all of which are components of a healthy diet.

HFCS, though, delivers—mostly through soft drinks—amounts of fructose that are unprecedented in human history. "Soda consumption has doubled, from 25 to 50 gallons per person (per year) from 1975 to 2000," says Greg Critser, a journalist and author of *Fat Land,* which fingers fructose as one of the major culprits in the obesity epidemic.

Critser says that HFCS is about 20 percent cheaper than cane sugar. Both contain a combination of fructose and glucose, but the low cost of HFCS has made it easier for manufacturers to supersize their portions. "The serving size of sodas has almost doubled, from about 10 ounces to about 18 ounces," because of HFCS, Critser says.

WHERE THE FRUCTOSE IS HIDING

Foods High in HFCS or Fructose	Replace With . . .
Regular soft drinks	Unsweetened sparkling water or diet soda
Commercial candy (jelly beans and others)	Chocolate candy (check the label, though—some chocolate candy bars may use HFCS as an ingredient)
Apple juice (typically about 60% fructose)	Unrefined 100% apple juice, grape juice, orange juice, or (here's a shocker) whole fruit
Pancake syrup	Real maple syrup
Popsicles	Frozen-fruit bars (always check the label; some brands may have added HFCS)
Frozen yogurt	Ice cream
Fruit-flavored yogurt	Artificially sweetened or sugar-sweetened yogurt
Ketchup	Mustard
Highly sweetened cereals	Sugar-free or low-sugar cereals
Pasta sauce (especially Ragu)	Sugar-free pasta sauce
Canned soup	Organic, all-natural, or sugar-free soups (check the label— an HFCS-free soup won't list any sugar)

This wouldn't be a huge problem if we simply ate less of everything else to compensate for the fact that we're consuming more fructose. But we don't; average Americans now eat about 200 more calories per day than we did in the 1970s.

FRUCTOSE MESSES WITH YOUR HORMONES

Normally, when you eat a food that contains glucose or starch—or any other carbohydrate—your body releases insulin, a hormone that does a series of important jobs to regulate your body weight: First, it tries to push the carbs into your muscle cells to be used as energy and facilitates carb storage in the liver for later use. Then it suppresses your appetite—telling your body, in effect, that you're full and it's time to stop eating. Finally, it stimulates production of another hormone, leptin.

Leptin is manufactured in your fat cells and acts as a nutrition traffic cop of sorts. It helps regulate storage of body fat and helps increase your metabolism when needed to keep your weight in check.

"Fructose doesn't stimulate insulin and therefore doesn't increase the production of leptin," says Havel. This is the most important part of the case against fructose in general and HFCS in particular: Without insulin and leptin, your appetite has no shutoff mechanism. You can drink a six-pack of Mountain Dew or eat a half gallon of frozen yogurt, and your body will hardly acknowledge that you've consumed any calories at all. Eat the equivalent number of calories in the form of a Thanksgiving dinner and you feel stuffed.

A study published in 2002 in the *American Journal of Clinical Nutrition* looked at whether soda itself, or the high-fructose corn syrup in soda, was the problem. The study took two groups of overweight people and had one group drink regular soft drinks while the other drank diet soda for 10 weeks. The regular-soda group gained weight and increased their body fat—not surprising, given that they consumed 28 percent more calories than normal while on the soda regimen. Worse, they also saw an increase in their blood pressures.

The diet-soda group, on the other hand, consumed fewer calories than they normally would, lost weight, reduced body fat, and lowered blood pressure.

So now the Diet Coke drinkers of the world have reason to celebrate.

AVERAGE NUMBER OF
CALORIES FROM SWEETENERS
AMERICANS CONSUMED A DAY IN 1999: 686

HOW MUCH OF THE RECOMMENDED
2,250-CALORIE DIET
THAT REPRESENTS: MORE THAN A QUARTER

HOW TO FIND FRUCTOSE AND AVOID IT

Soft drinks are a major source of HFCS, but it's everywhere, even in hamburger buns.

Your first line of defense: Avoid regular soda. Next, read nutrition labels. Start with the ingredients. If a label says "sugar" or "cane sugar," the product contains sucrose, which is a 50-50 blend of fructose and glucose. That doesn't seem to be as much of a problem. If HFCS is listed first or second, look at the chart that accompanies the ingredients to see how much sugar is in the food. If it's just a gram or two, don't sweat it. But if you see a food that has 8 or more grams of sugar, and HFCS is prominent on the list of ingredients, buy something else. Remember that your body can deal with a little of anything, but a lot of fructose is a one-way ticket to Fat City.

My professor was right when she said that messing with the food supply is a deal with the devil. The money the food industry saved by using a cheap but unstudied sweetener was deposited on your waistline, and it's time to close the fructose account.

When the Urge Strikes

To lose that gut, you have to outlast your cravings. Use these strategies and you'll take temptation in stride

By Brian Good

Researchers define a craving as an intense desire to consume a particular food that is difficult to resist. But you're probably more familiar with the feeling in layman's terms: *I want a Mars bar, and I want it* NOW.

Cravings may be tough to withstand, but they're even harder to figure out. "You'd like to think that a craving is your body's way of telling you something, and that if you give in, everything will be okay. But that's not always the case," says Adam Drewnowski, Ph.D., director of the nutritional sciences program at the University of Washington in Seattle. "Cravings can have different triggers—stress, depression, hormones—and while there are some cravings you can indulge, there are others that you shouldn't."

So what's a man to do about his, uh, urges? Here's a cheat sheet for when to fight and when to fold.

8:00 A.M. YOU'RE CRAVING: THE WHOLE BOX OF CAP'N CRUNCH

Why? A big appetite in the morning is your body's way of coming out of starvation mode after hours of not eating. Going without food triggers your brain to release a substance called neuropeptide Y that helps to increase your appetite, says Janine Whiteson, M.Sc., a New York City nutritionist and author of *Get a Real Food Life*. The longer you've gone without food, the greater your hunger when you wake up.

Give in or fight it? Give in—just don't go overboard. "It's fine to eat a doughnut or a bowl of sweetened cereal in the morning, as long as you also eat some high-protein food with it," says Laura A. Lees, Psy.D., a Wisconsin-based eating disorders specialist. Studies show that protein keeps your appetite in check longer than carbohydrates or fat can. So go ahead and eat a bowl of Cap'n Crunch, but combine it with a couple of slices of Canadian bacon or a small block of cheese.

8:45 A.M. YOU'RE CRAVING: A JELLY DOUGHNUT

Why? You probably didn't eat enough at breakfast. "It's normal for cravings to pop up every 2 to 3 hours," says Heidi Skolnik, M.S., a sports nutritionist for the New York Giants and a contributing editor to *Men's Health*. That's roughly how long it takes for your body to break down the sugars in the food you eat, release them into your bloodstream, and convert them into energy, she explains.

Give in or fight it? Fight it. Instead of sugar, you need something that's high in fiber—it will fill you up now but won't interfere with snack time later. "Mid-morning snacks are great, but this isn't mid-morning, and you don't want to break out your big snack too early," says Skolnik. Instead of the doughnut, reach for dried fruit, a handful of nuts, or an energy bar. "Eat enough to satisfy your craving, but not enough to keep you from being hungry an hour or two later," she says.

10:30 A.M. YOU'RE CRAVING: A COKE

Why? You could be craving the caffeine. The coffee or soda you drank on the way to work is wearing off, and you want another hit to get your energy level back up to what feels like normal.

Give in or fight it? Fight it. Swear off the regular soda and opt for the caffeine-free diet variety. "Caffeine gives you a false sense of energy because it doesn't give your body any real fuel to burn," says Lynn Grieger, R.D., C.D.E., a Vermont-based nutritionist. If you switch to caffeine-free soda, not only will you break the caffeine/craving connection, but you probably won't even notice a difference in the taste. In a study from Johns Hopkins University, researchers found that fewer than 10 percent of people were able to tell the difference between regular and caffeine-free soft drinks.

12:00 NOON. YOU'RE CRAVING: MACARONI AND CHEESE

Why? You're stressed-out about your boss, your dog's dying, your boss's dog's dying—something—and that craving is your body's attempt to make you feel better. "Carbs trigger the production of a feel-good hormone called sero-nin, which helps to boost your mood and temporarily relieve your stress," says John Foreyt, Ph.D., director of the behavioral medicine research center at the Baylor College of Medicine in Houston.

Give in or fight it? Give in—occasionally. "Using food for temporary relief from a problem is fine, as long as you don't do it all the time," says Lees. A better alternative: Trick your mind into thinking about something else. "Use your lunch break to go running or lift weights," says Skolnik. "Or try to outthink your craving. When the urge to eat strikes, rate your hunger on a scale of one to 10. "Unless you're at a level of seven or eight, don't allow yourself to eat."

Still hungry? Go ahead and eat, but opt for a very small portion and eat it along with a high-protein food like steak, chicken, or tuna salad. "The last thing you want for lunch when you're working is something like macaroni and cheese," says Deborah Gleason, Ph.D., a psychotherapist in Rochester Hills, Michigan. A few carbs may boost your mood, but too many can leave you sluggish and tired, she says.

2:45 P.M. YOU'RE CRAVING: CHOCOLATE CHIP COOKIES

Why? You might not be getting enough magnesium. Semisweet chocolate chips are one of the top sources of magnesium, and according to one theory, having too little of the mineral in your system could generate a desire to eat chocolate. Or, if you eat chocolate all the time, maybe you're a chocoholic. Spanish researchers found that chocolate and cocoa contain some of the same potentially mood-altering compounds found in alcohol.

Give in or fight it? Give in. "If you have an intense craving for a bit of a very specific food like chocolate, it's best to go ahead and eat it," says Skolnik. "If you don't, your craving is going to get more intense until you eventually give in anyway, and you'll have eaten a lot of unnecessary calories in an attempt to make it go away." Make sure you keep your portions under control—meaning take two or three cookies at most—and then put the rest away. You may feel as if you want more, but according to a study from Pennsylvania State University, people who were served the smallest portions of a food felt just as full and satisfied after eating as people who were given unlimited helpings of the same food.

8:30 P.M. YOU'RE CRAVING: POTATO CHIPS

Why? You want to relax. In this case, the craving is less about the food and more about what the food signifies. "A lot of guys feel stressed-out and tired all day, and when they get home, they just want to relax and forget about their day with a bag of chips and the remote control," says Skolnik. "They feel like they've been in control and used restraint all day, and the chips are part of their reward for that good behavior."

Give in or fight it? Fight it. You're eating for the wrong reason. "It might not seem so bad in the short term, but over time, this kind of emotionally driven eating is one of the primary reasons men gain weight," says Skolnik.

To break the habit, go cold turkey: no food while the TV's on. "Even healthy snacks won't help break the association between food and relaxing," says Gleason. To make the process easier, rearrange your living room furniture or watch your favorite show in a room where you typically spend less time. Studies from Brookhaven National Laboratory suggest that hanging out in a spot where you've indulged past cravings can help trigger future ones.

11:00 P.M. YOU'RE CRAVING: ICE CREAM

Why? You want to watch Letterman, but your body wants you to go to bed. Men may crave foods like ice cream and crackers late at night because carbohydrates help to boost levels of a sleep-inducing compound called tryptophan. As tryptophan levels in your brain increase, you naturally become sleepier, say researchers at the Massachusetts Institute of Technology.

Give in or fight it? Give in. "Hunger can keep you awake at night, so you're better off eating something than eating nothing at all," says Lees. Her advice: Keep the serving small and pick a regular, full-fat ice cream, not the fat-free kind. According to a study from Purdue, taste buds can detect fat, and that may be why fat-free foods aren't as satisfying as full-fat foods.

Supersize Your Muscles

Cut your gym time and add muscle with our new superset solutions

By Alwyn Cosgrove, C.S.C.S.

Supersets are the extra-value meals of exercise: more of what you want, at a lower cost. They can give you more muscle in less time, with less energy expenditure and even less boredom.

I own a small training facility in Newhall, California, and if it weren't for supersets, I'd have to own a large training facility. I use supersets about 90 percent of the time with my clients, who range from teen athletes to porn stars. (Luckily, it's hard to tell a porn star from any other client when they're running on treadmills.)

You probably know the basic idea behind supersets: You alternate between sets of different exercises with little rest in between, rather than knock out all your sets of one exercise before moving on to the next.

Here's a quick example of why supersets are, for lack of a better word, super. Say you want to do four sets each of bench presses and seated cable rows, 10 repetitions per set, with 2 minutes' rest between sets. Let's assume each repetition takes 6 seconds, so a complete set takes 60 seconds. With straight sets, it takes 24 minutes.

CROWD CONTROL

We could wait for the calls or letters, or we could acknowledge right here that about half of you are looking at our suggested exercise combinations and saying, "Superset bench presses and deadlifts? At my gym? At 6 P.M. on a Monday?"

So here are a few examples of supersets you can do in the same space, with the same equipment.

For Fat Loss

Do 10 repetitions of each exercise without pausing, then rest 60 seconds; repeat three times.

- Using a barbell: Good morning, bent-over row; or stiff-legged deadlift, shrug
- Using a chinup bar: Hanging leg raise, chinup

For Bigger Arms

Do 10 repetitions of each exercise without pausing, then rest 60 seconds; repeat once.

- Using a single dumbbell: Left-arm biceps curl, right-arm overhead triceps extension, left-arm overhead triceps extension, right-arm biceps curl

For Strength and Power

Do five repetitions of the first exercise, then five to 10 repetitions of the second.

- Using a barbell bench-press station and mat: Bench press, plyometric pushup

Now, let's superset these two exercises and take 90 seconds' rest after each exercise. So you'll do a set of bench presses, rest 90 seconds, do a set of rows, rest 90 seconds, and repeat.

This time, you complete the same program in 20 minutes, which is nice. But the key difference is that you take a full 4 minutes to recover between one set of bench presses and the next, and between sets of rows. This means you can use more weight for these exercises and, as a result, get more total work done in less time.

With some creativity, you can use supersets to build more muscle, burn fat, and get stronger. So strap on your cape and get ready to supersize your workouts.

SUPERSETS FOR BIGGER MUSCLES

Your muscles have two types of fibers. The smaller, slow-twitch fibers are used primarily for endurance activities, and the bigger, fast-twitch fibers come into play mostly when you need to move a heavy object, or move a light object fast. But all the fibers—big and small, fast and slow—have the potential to get larger. So it makes sense to work them all if you want the biggest muscles possible.

The plan: Do 10 repetitions of one exercise, then 20 repetitions of a different exercise for the same muscle group, without rest. Then rest 60 seconds and repeat. Doing two or three of the following supersets is plenty.

Builds Chest, Triceps, Front Shoulders

INCLINE DUMBBELL BENCH PRESS

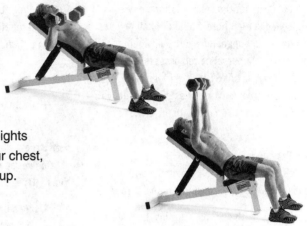

(10 repetitions) Set an incline bench to about 30 degrees. Hold the weights just above the top of your chest, then push them straight up.

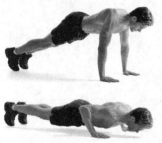

PUSHUP

(20 repetitions) Get on the floor with your back straight, your body weight resting on your palms and toes. Lower yourself to the floor, then push back up.

Builds Lats, Biceps

CLOSE-GRIP CHINUP (Not Shown)

(10 repetitions) Grab a chinup bar with an underhand grip, your hands 6 to 12 inches apart. Hang at arm's length, then pull your chin up over the bar, pause, and lower yourself.

WIDE-GRIP LAT PULLDOWN (Not Shown)

(20 repetitions) Grab the bar with the widest-possible overhand grip. Pull the bar down to your chest, pause, then return to the starting position.

SUPERSETS FOR STRENGTH AND POWER

Most of us use the words "strength" and "power" interchangeably, but they're actually two separate qualities. Strength is measured by the amount of weight you can move, at any speed. Power is weight times speed, or the ability to knock an inanimate object into the next ZIP code. Both qualities are important for sports performance. And the strength/power combo allows you to work with heavier weights in the gym, which means you build muscle faster.

The plan: Do a five-repetition set of a heavy-duty strength exercise, followed by five to 10 repetitions of a power exercise—something that involves moving your body as fast as possible while holding a lighter load.

**Builds Entire Lower Body,
Improves Vertical Jump**

SQUAT

(5 repetitions) Hold a barbell across your upper back and stand with your feet shoulder-width apart. Squat until your thighs are parallel to the floor, pause, then stand back up.

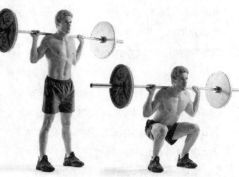

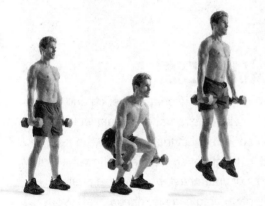

DUMBBELL SQUAT JUMP

(5 to 10 repetitions) Stand holding a pair of dumbbells at arm's length at your sides. Squat about halfway down, then immediately jump as high as you can. Bend your knees as you land. Regain your balance, then repeat.

SUPERSETS FOR FAT LOSS

Pure weight loss can be accomplished with something as simple and sedentary as having your lips stapled shut. But along with fat, you'll lose muscle. If that's your goal, be my guest. But if you want to lose only fat, you have to do intensive muscle-building exercises that require so much energy that your body suffers a massive caloric deficit.

The plan: Do 10 repetitions of one exercise for your lower body, then, without resting, do 10 repetitions of an upper-body exercise. Make sure both lifts tap the largest muscle groups possible. Rest 60 seconds and repeat. Do a total of four supersets of each exercise pair.

Works Entire Lower Body (Particularly Gluteals and Back of Thighs), Trapezius, Chest, Shoulders, Arms

DEADLIFT

(10 repetitions) Roll a barbell to your shins and squat over it with your feet shoulder-width apart. Grab the bar overhand with your hands just outside your legs. Straighten your back and lift your chest and head, then stand, keeping the weight against your legs at all times. Slowly lower it, sliding it along your legs. Let it touch the floor before you start the next repetition.

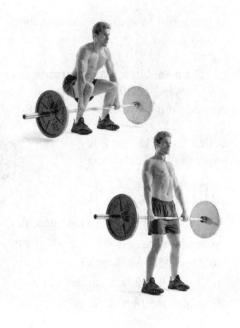

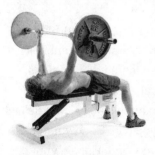

BENCH PRESS

(10 repetitions) Lie on a flat bench and grab a barbell with an overhand grip just wider than shoulder width. Lift the barbell off the rack and hold it straight over your chest. Lower it to the middle of your chest, pause, then push it straight up. You can use dumbbells, if you prefer.

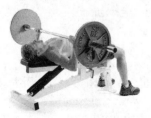

Small Muscles, Big Results

Build this supporting cast and your physique will be the star of the show

Let's start with a very safe assumption: You care a lot about your prime-time muscles—your biceps, pectorals, abs, quads. You know how to pump them up, show them off, make them perform party tricks.

But a star is only as good as his supporting cast, as anyone who's suffered with Ted Danson through a few episodes of *Becker* can attest. And the stars of your physique would look and perform a lot better if you spent a little more time developing the bit parts.

Take your serratus anterior, a set of fingerlike muscles on both sides of your rib cage. When developed, these muscles create the illusion that your chest and torso are wider than they really are. They transform your abs from a lonely six-pack into a full liquor cabinet. They prevent your arms from quivering during sex, and even help you get the barbell off your chest during a bench press.

Not a bad set of benefits from a muscle you've never heard of.

Keep reading and we'll tell you how to build the serratus, along with four other muscles that you won't hear mentioned during sweeps week. Make them a strong ensemble cast and these five bit players can take your body from the bottom of the Nielsens to the top of the charts.

SERRATUS ANTERIOR

What it is: Strips of muscle on both sides of your torso, stretching from the inside ridges of your shoulder blades to your ribs.

What it does: The serratus helps when you push heavy objects off your chest at various angles, controls the separation of your shoulder blades, and assists in lifting your shoulders.

Why it looks cool: If you're very lean and muscular, your serratus and external obliques (described on pages 18 to 19) form a crosshatch pattern, which lends credibility to your claim that you moonlight as an underwear model.

How to Build It: Crunch with a Plus

Grab a light barbell with a shoulder-width, overhand grip and lie on your back, knees bent and feet flat on the floor. Start with your arms straight and the bar directly above your eyes. Flatten your lower back against the floor.

Now use your abs to flex your trunk forward, as you would in a typical crunch. At the same time, push the barbell up toward the ceiling,

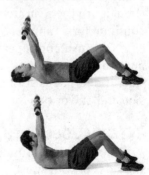

pulling your shoulder blades as far apart as you can. Pause, then slowly return to the starting position. Instead of counting repetitions, aim for 1-minute sets. (You'll probably want to start with 30-second sets.) Increase the weight when you can do three to five 1-minute sets.

LEVATOR SCAPULAE

What they are: Diagonal ropes of muscle that run from the top of the neck to the top of the shoulder blades.

What they do: As the name implies, they help lift your shoulder blades (scapulae), along with the trapezius.

Why they look cool: Visually, their impact isn't huge, although they do help fill out your shirt collar. Mostly, they need to be strong and flexible to help correct the neck-kinking rigors of modern desk life (e.g., trying to hold a phone between ear and shoulder, jot down notes, and gawk at the new receptionist simultaneously).

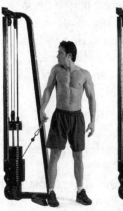 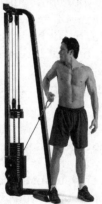

How to Build Them: Bent-arm Cable Shrug

Most right-handed men will find that their levator scapulae are stronger and tighter on the right side. These guys should start with the left (weaker) side. Lefties will probably want to start with the right side (as shown and described here).

Attach a stirrup handle to a low pulley and grab it with your right hand. Stand with your right side to the machine and turn your head so you're looking over your right shoulder. Slowly elevate your right shoulder as high as you can. Now, keeping your shoulder up, bend your right elbow slightly, pull your shoulder blades together in back, and rotate your right shoulder to the rear. Reverse the steps to return to the starting position, and continue for 1 minute.

Now turn and repeat with your left arm. If you find that your two sides are equally strong, you can either stop at one set or do one more set for each side. If one side is stronger than the other, do three to five sets for the weak side and one or two for the strong side until your strength equalizes.

EXTERNAL OBLIQUES

What they are: Muscles that start on the ribs and extend diagonally down the sides of your waist.

What they do: If a movement happens at your waist, the external obliques are involved. The torso rotation that's key to golf, tennis, and hockey is mostly a function of the external obliques. Even the basic crunching motion, attributed to the rectus abdominis (the six-pack muscle), wouldn't be possible without a strong contraction of the external obliques to stabilize the torso.

Why they look cool: Not only do well-developed obliques make your waist tighter, but their diagonal orientation also creates a virtual signpost that says, "Check out what I have down here!"

How to Build Them: Swimmer's Backstroke

Lie faceup on the floor, knees bent and feet flat. Flatten your lower back against the floor. Now do a crunch to flex your trunk forward and lift your shoulder blades as high off the floor as you possibly can.

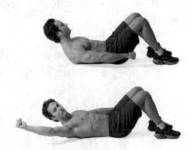

This is when the fun begins: Keeping your chest high, perform a backstroke with one arm at a time, allowing your torso to twist toward the arm that's reaching back. Work up to five sets of 45 seconds each, alternating arms on each repetition. The higher you lift your chest off the floor, the better the exercise will work. Add light dumbbells when the move becomes easy.

TRICEPS LONG HEAD

What it is: The biggest and strongest part of the triceps muscle, covering the inside and back of your upper arm.

What it does: Along with the other two parts of the triceps, it straightens your elbow and also assists your lats and lower chest in pulling your upper arm down to your side when it's above or out to the side of your body. (Picture a swimmer pulling his arm through the water at the end of his stroke.)

Why it looks cool: When the long head is built up, it fills in the gap between your rear deltoids and lats, providing the finishing touch for a perfectly V-shaped upper torso.

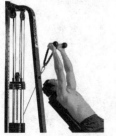
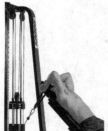

How to Build It: Cable Incline Triceps Extension with Rope Attachment

Set an incline bench at a 45-degree angle and place it in front of a low cable pulley. Hold your arms straight up above your eyes, slowly bend your elbows as far as you can, pause, then straighten them. Continue for 20 seconds. Rest 60 seconds and repeat. Do six to 10 sets. You want your muscles to feel exhausted at the end of each set.

GLUTEUS MEDIUS

What it is: A wedge of muscle on the side of each hip.

What it does: The gluteus medius lifts your leg straight out to the side and stabilizes your pelvis while you walk or run. You use this muscle most directly in martial arts and soccer, when you kick out to the side. The stabilization function makes it crucial in skating and skiing, which involve side-to-side hip action.

Why it looks cool: Men don't tend to carry much fat around their hips and upper thighs, so when the medius is well developed, it creates a dimple effect on the side of the hip joint.

How to Build It: Cable Side Stepup

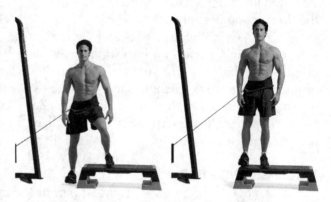

Set a step or bench near the low cable. Attach the pulley to a belt around your waist. Start with your left leg, if you're left-handed. Place your left foot on the step and raise the front of your right foot so your weight is on the heel. (This keeps the right foot from doing all the work.)

Now push down with your left foot and lift yourself up on the step. Make sure you're completely upright at the end of the repetition. Lower yourself until your right heel touches the floor, then repeat for 1 minute.

Turn around and repeat with your right foot on the step. Do a second 1-minute set with whichever proved to be the weaker leg. In subsequent workouts, do three to five 1-minute sets for the weaker leg and one or none for the leg that's stronger.

Fit for Life

A strong, flexible body makes everything in your life better, from running a 10-K to starting a business to catching her eye. But if you're working out the same old way, you've got to change

By Bill Stump

I've been using the same workout for 20 years, and I have the results to show for it: two prematurely arthritic shoulders, bursitis in my left hip, and a sacroiliac that threatens to immobilize me every time I engage in such death-defying moves as getting out of a car or drying my hair with a towel.

Doctors tell me that continuing to use the same weight-lifting program I started at age 18 to bulk up for college football (at a bladelike 6'1" and 155 pounds, I was so skinny my coach was afraid I'd cut somebody) is partly to blame for the problems I'm having now.

The rest is wear and tear from 2 decades of pummeling myself with long-distance running, basketball, and softball, with little—okay, no—thought given to the fact that I'd have to live the rest of my life in this same body.

But I'm starting to think now. (And my wife is encouraged by that recent trend.) I like playing basketball too much to give it up because my hip hurts. I don't want to have to buy a pitching machine to have a catch with my son when he's 10 because my throwing shoulder is shot. I want to stay active and fit to avoid health problems like heart disease and diabetes that are—wake-up call!—starting to show up in some of my friends.

The good news is that it's not too late for me—or you. Experts say I can stop my decline and even reverse some of the damage by doing a few simple things. For me, that means less heavy bench-pressing to take the stress off my shoulders and back, 10-minute warmups before I run or play ball, and stretching every day to keep the bursitis at bay and prevent injuries.

The payoff: I can work out and play harder than ever, and I get out of bed the next morning without an Advil IV-drip.

Below, we've corralled experts for their best tips to enhance your performance pain-free in a half dozen of your favorite sports. We also offer some new challenges you can try that take advantage of the skills you've spent years developing. So get ready; the new you is waiting.

RUNNING

Problem: Pounding the pavement erodes your body's natural shock absorbers—the cartilage, tendons, muscles, and ligaments that bundle your knees and ankles into functioning joints. Each step exerts a force of up to five times your weight and encourages these body parts to protest through inflammation, pain, and even rupture.

Solution: Walk as well as run, says Amby Burfoot, the 56-year-old executive editor of *Runner's World* magazine and the winner of the 1968 Boston Marathon.

If walking sounds soft, call it interval training, as Olympic runners do. Varying intensity within a workout is a tactic successful runners use to get faster or go longer. Even if you're not looking to set a personal record, walking burns the same number of calories as running and reduces common overuse injuries, such as shin splints, Burfoot says.

He suggests using a 1-to-1 ratio if you're getting into shape after a layoff, and then gradually ratcheting up the run portion. Your target should be to walk 1 mile for every 4 you run.

Alternative sport: Triathlons. These events are filled with former distance runners looking for a new rush and a way to take some strain off their battered bones, says Alwyn Cosgrove, C.S.C.S., a fitness expert in Santa Clarita, California. Triathlon training also allows a marathoner to use health benefits gained from years of long-distance training: increased lung capacity and an abundance of slow-twitch muscle fibers, which enhance aerobic endurance. And don't worry: Triathlon sponsors give out free T-shirts, too.

To get started, contact the International Triathlon Union at (604) 926-7250 or www.triathlon.org.

BASKETBALL

Problem: A game of hoops offers a great overall workout, but it beats up an unprepared body.

The sudden starts and stops place tremendous lateral force on your ankles and knees, and the jumping—actually, the landing—sends injury-causing shock waves throughout your body.

Solution: Break a sweat before you start playing. One guy we know hits the hot tub for 10 minutes before playing to make sure he's warm. No tub at your club? This simple 10-minute warmup will drastically reduce your chances of getting hurt, says Peter Bruno, M.D., an internist for the New York Knicks. Do each of these the length of the floor and back while windmilling your arms; then stretch as usual: Jog, skip, shuffle (continually slide one leg to meet the other without crossing them; don't forget to bend your knees), karaoke (run sideways, continually crossing one leg in front of and then behind the other), run backward, and skip as high as you can.

HOW LONG YOU HAVE TO ICE YOUR KNEES AFTER A RUN TO PREVENT OSTEOARTHRITIS: 10 MINUTES

Alternative sport: Volleyball. This activity incorporates the same lateral movement and quick-jumping ability you've developed while playing hoops, but it doesn't require you to cover as much ground, says Nicholas A. DiNubile, M.D., an orthopedic consultant for the Philadelphia 76ers. "It's still competitive, and you'll get all the great benefits of being on a team and working together."

SOFTBALL

Problem: Playing softball or baseball does little to improve your overall fitness—the only six-packs we see at games are in an ice chest—so you have to put in time away from the diamond if you want to avoid career enders such as rotator cuff tears and elbow or shoulder tendinitis.

Solution: Lift weights. It will strengthen your rotator cuff and surrounding muscles to protect you from suffering a tear the next time you try to make like Griffey and gun someone out at second, says Dennis Wilson, Ed.D., head of the department of health and human performance at Auburn University in Alabama. The best moves: lateral raises (daily, with light weights) and lat pull-downs and lat rows (every other day, with heavier weights). Also, stretch your shoulders before the first pitch by raising your throwing arm straight above your head, bending it at the elbow, then gently pushing it down and toward your spine with your other hand. Repeat with the opposite arm. (Best tip: Stay warm between innings by jogging and throwing. In a routine game, players can go 30 minutes between all-out efforts, giving their muscles ample opportunity to prepare for a pull.)

Alternative sport: Golf. "People who are good at baseball also tend to be good at golf," says Dr. DiNubile, because of their above-par hand–eye coordination and their ability to connect with a ball while rotating their hips.

Golf is easier on your body because you don't have the sudden starts and stops, and the swings aren't as violent. And since the ball isn't moving, you don't have to reach at odd angles to hit it, which can cause muscle strains. Golf is also better for your heart and gobbles up plenty of calories as long as you don't ride a cart—golfers cover about 5 miles during a typical round.

SWIMMING

Problem: Because swimming is non-weight-bearing—the water holds you up and keeps you from jarring your joints—injuries are few. When swimmers do get hurt, they tend to suffer from overuse injuries in their shoulders and knees.

Solution: Have a coach analyze your stroke each year for glitches so you don't fall into injury-inducing bad habits. Mix breaststroke, backstroke, or butterfly in with your freestyle every fourth lap to reduce your risk of hurting a shoulder joint, suggests Kevin Polansky, a Masters national and world champ from Loveland, Colorado.

Also, "strength training is extremely important for swimmers to help balance their musculature and to strengthen bones and tendons that don't get trained in the pool," says Cosgrove. The most important lifts: bench press for balance and squats for push-off and kicking.

Alternative sport: Single-scull rowing. The knock against swimming is that it can become torturously boring. Scull rowing will capitalize on the endurance and pain tolerance you've built over the years while still allowing you to compete *mano a mano* on the water, using your arms and legs to pull you through. Log on to www.usrowing.com for tips on how to get started.

CYCLING

Problem: Way to go—you've picked a great sport. It's easy on the knees, builds endurance and strength in your legs, gets you outside, and allows you to wear brightly colored tight clothes and cool sunglasses without feeling silly.

But cyclists do suffer injuries. Wrecks cause most of them—damn truck drivers—but repeating the same motion again and again (and again) while sitting hunched over the handlebar also puts stress on the vertebrae in your lower back, which causes pain.

Solution: Simply changing the angle of your bike seat could save your back, according to researchers from the Chaim Sheba Medical Center in Israel, who tested 40 cyclists with back pain. Six months after adjusting their seat angles, 75 percent of the cyclists felt better. The researchers believe that back pain in cyclists is caused when the angle between the pelvis and the lower end of the spinal column is overextended. Tilting the seat forward 10 to 15 degrees reduces the strain on the muscles and realigns the bones.

Most important: Spin, don't strain, by using higher gears. Lower gears can make you feel like you're working much harder, but a faster cadence is easier on your body and more efficient, says Jim Hagberg, Ph.D., an exercise physiologist at the University of Maryland in College Park.

Alternative sport: Soccer. You've spent years building endurance and Lance-like quads. Now use them on the soccer field, where both qualities will give you a leg up on the competition, and the wide variety of movements you'll deploy will round out your fitness better than riding a bike can. You'll also play on grass, which is heaven for joints and muscles.

Don't worry if the soccer boom arrived after you were in high school—local leagues are filled with latecomers like you.

TENNIS

Problem: Nearly half of all tennis players suffer from "tennis elbow," which is how country clubbers say "elbow tendinitis." Lower-back strains and shoulder and ankle injuries are also common. Playing a lot of tennis also weakens your shoulder blade muscles by repeatedly stretching and fatiguing

CHANGE THINGS UP

If you're lifting weights the same way you did when John Madden was a football coach, it's time for a change, hoss. Forget the vanity muscles. Think strength and cardiovascular fitness. Your new goal: roughly 50 percent cardiovascular exercise (including warmup), 40 percent weights, and 10 percent stretching. Susie Kania, an exercise physiologist at the Cooper Wellness Program in Dallas, suggests the following program.

Monday

10 minutes of aerobic exercise (running, jumping rope, tennis, cycling, or swimming) at a comfortable pace (60 to 70 percent of your maximum heart rate).

20 minutes of upper-body strength training. Do two sets of eight to 12 reps of the following: bench press, military press, lat pulldown, biceps curl, and triceps extension.

15 minutes of aerobic exercise at a slightly more intense pace (70 to 85 percent of your maximum heart rate).

5 minutes of stretching. Pay attention to back and hamstring muscles. Hit both areas with a simple two-step stretch: Lie on your back and draw your knees to your chest. Hold for 60 seconds. This stretches the lower back. Now put both feet flat on the floor, knees bent, and raise your left leg straight up toward the sky. Hold for 60 seconds; then repeat with the right leg. Do three reps of each stretch.

Wednesday

45 minutes of circuit weight training. Do three circuits, hitting the lifts from both the Monday and Friday workouts. Do eight to 12 repetitions of each lift, moving quickly between sets.

Friday

Same as Monday, except your 20 minutes of strength training will target the lower body. Do two sets of eight to 12 reps of the following: leg extension (quadriceps), leg curl (hamstrings), and abdominal crunch.

the tissues there, says Robert Nirschl, M.D., medical director at the Virginia Sports Medicine Institute in Arlington.

Solution: The good news is, tennis is a terrific lifelong sport—if you keep your strength and flexibility by doing, not surprisingly, strength training and stretching. "Tennis involves a lot of short, explosive moves," says Cosgrove. "You're essentially using your entire body."

To get the great workout without the elbow or shoulder problems, do military presses. While sitting on a bench or chair, raise a pair of dumbbells to shoulder height. Press the weights overhead. Do 10 to 12 repetitions. Repeat.

Alternative sport: Martial arts. "One of the martial arts, such as tae kwon do or kickboxing, can enhance the abilities you've developed in tennis—total-body movement, quick reactions—while adding the missing factor of flexibility," says Cosgrove. You can also take out your aggression on a real person, instead of your racket, while eliminating the repetitive motion that causes injuries in tennis.

KNOW THIS

Sleep It Off

May we suggest you turn off Letterman, put down the Cheetos, and go to bed? Research shows that not getting enough sleep can increase your appetite and slow down your metabolism, making you pack on pounds. "Sleep deprivation appears to increase your production of cortisol, a hormone that helps regulate your appetite," says Michael Thorpy, M.D., a sleep expert at Montefiore Medical Center in the Bronx. Insufficient sleep may also interfere with the body's ability to burn off carbohydrates, causing spikes in your blood sugar level and putting your body into fat-storage mode, he says. What's enough? Seven to 8 hours a night.

Family Feast

Blame your folks next time you have trouble passing up a piece of candy. A study from the University of Maryland reports that having an uncontrollable urge to eat may be a genetic trait passed on from one generation to the next. In a study of 624 Amish adults, researchers found that the people who had the hardest time resisting food often shared common bits of DNA.

The Skinny on Fat Blockers

A University of California at Davis study offers further proof that the shrimp shell extract chitosan won't help you lose weight. Ads for the popular dietary supplement claim that chitosan can help block the absorption of up to 120 grams of fat each day. To test these claims, UC researchers analyzed stool samples from a group of men on a high-fat diet who also took chitosan supplements six times a day. Samples from men who were taking the supplement didn't have a higher fat content, which suggests chitosan doesn't block fat absorption, the study authors report.

Choose Your Surgeon Wisely

Each year, an estimated 65,000 men undergo gastric bypass surgery. This invasive procedure essentially involves stapling your stomach to make it less than half the size it originally was. Afterward, you are forced to eat less, so you lose a significant amount of weight.

A new UCLA study reports that men are more than twice as likely as women to experience life-threatening complications during gastric bypass surgery. To boost your chances of a successful operation, choose a surgeon who's done at least 75 bypasses. Reports show that after 75 to 100 surgeries, the complication rates go down.

Lift for Longevity

Another good reason to invest in dumbbells: An 8-year study of nearly 8,000 men conducted at Erasmus Medical Center in the Netherlands found that men with high testosterone levels are less likely to have strokes, the third leading cause of death in the United States. Researchers discovered that men who had strokes during the course of the study had significantly lower testosterone levels than the men who remained stroke-free, leading the scientists to believe that having high levels of the male hormone may offer some protection. You can boost your testosterone levels drug-free by weight lifting. Resistance training is the number-one way to help your body naturally produce more testosterone.

Outrun the Reaper

One more reason to lace up the running shoes: A recent study from West Texas A&M University in Canyon found that running 20 to 40 minutes a day three to five times a week may reduce your chances of dying of cancer by up

HOW OFTEN YOU HAVE TO WEIGHT TRAIN TO LOWER YOUR HEART DISEASE RISK BY 23 PERCENT: 30 MINUTES A WEEK

HOW OFTEN YOU HAVE TO LIFT WEIGHTS TO HELP PREVENT DIABETES: 3 DAYS A WEEK

to 66 percent. "Exercise appears to boost the effectiveness of your immune system, reducing the concentration of carcinogens in the airways and inhibiting tumor formation," says Chong Do Lee, Ph.D., the study author. Further research is needed, however, to determine whether exercise actually prevents cancer or simply improves your chances of surviving it.

Clean Up Your Act

You may burn calories doing housework, but according to a new U.K. study, cleaning up around the house doesn't have nearly the same cardiovascular health benefits as do other forms of physical activity. One surefire way cleaning *can* help your heart: Dust off that treadmill and start using it for more than just a clothes rack.

DOWN THE PIKE

Keep Your Cool

The secret to improving your game may be as simple as staying cool. The reason: The lower your body temperature is, the longer you can work out, and the better your athletic skills become. To test the theory, Stanford researchers have developed a glovelike gadget that cools your blood so you can train harder and longer. The device uses steel plates to chill the blood in your hands. That cooled blood then circulates throughout the body, lowering your core temperature in minutes, says Craig Heller, Ph.D., the product's inventor. The Stanford football and tennis teams and the San Francisco 49ers are already using versions of the device. Portable models are in development and could be available within a few years.

Become a Beanpole

Researchers at UCLA believe a new pill made from white-kidney-bean extract may help people lose weight. The product—called Phase 2—works by deactivating the stomach enzyme alpha amylase before it converts carbohydrates into a form of sugar that the body stores as fat. In trials, people taking Phase 2 lost $\frac{1}{2}$ pound a week, twice the amount lost by people taking a placebo. The drug needs to undergo further testing before it becomes available.

Help from a Hunger Hormone

Researchers at Imperial College of London found that people who were injected with an experimental hormone ate one-third less food while visiting a buffet than people who hadn't gotten the injection. The substance—nicknamed the "third-helping hormone"—is secreted by cells in the intestine

PERCENTAGE OF AMERICANS WHO SAY
THEY WILL TRY ANY FAD DIET THEY THINK MIGHT WORK: 8

when you eat. "The injections fooled people's brains into thinking they'd already eaten," says Steve Bloom, Ph.D., the study author. A weight-loss drug containing the hormone is in development.

Hi-Tech Stomach Surgery

Stomach stapling to control obesity is becoming such a popular surgery that doctors are looking to robots to lend a claw. A robot named Zeus recently performed one of the first machine-assisted gastric bypass surgeries in the United States at Cedars-Sinai Hospital in Los Angeles. A live M.D. controlled the robotic device using video-game-like joysticks and voice commands, but the machine did the dirty work. Doctors say robot-assisted surgeries are safer and quicker than operations conducted by human surgeons because the machines make much more precise movements and don't get tired during long procedures.

Shock Till You Drop

There soon may be a new weight-loss option for overweight men who don't want to resort to gastric bypass or stomach stapling. A company called Transneuronix is developing a small pacemaker-like device called the Implantable Gastric Stimulator (IGS), which can be attached to the wall of the stomach. Once in place, the IGS sends out a series of tiny electrical shocks. Although patients don't feel anything, the shocks stimulate muscles in the stomach, leaving patients feeling more satisfied after eating. In a small trial, people fitted with an IGS lost an average of 35 pounds in just 9 months. More testing needs to be done, however, before the implant becomes widely available.

GAME PLAN

Join a Gym without Dropping a Bundle

How to find a good health club where you can drop pounds—not cash

You have two options when you're tired of grunting and sweating alone: Get married or join a gym. If you're considering the second option, or if you're ready to dump your current club for a new one, these tips can save you buckets of cash and hassles.

Inspect the showers. To be sure the staff keeps the gym clean, give the locker room a good looking over. Check the corners of each shower stall. If the corners are clean, the gym is clean. If they're dirty, you'll probably pick up a case of athlete's foot.

Ask about extras. Some gyms make money through hidden costs, such as towel fees and locker rentals. If stashing your trousers in a locker costs an extra $28.50 per month, figure that into the yearly fee.

Make sure he's qualified. A full-time trainer should have N.S.C.A., N.A.S.M., A.C.E., A.C.S.M., C.S.C.S., or N.A.F.C. qualifications and be certified in emergency first aid. "For minor injuries, a trainer can save you a doctor's visit," says Brian Sharkey, Ph.D., former president of the American College of Sports Medicine. But don't let him repair your hernia.

Think nationally. If you travel often, consider joining a national club, such as Gold's Gym, Bally, or the YMCA. When the hotel gym is god-awful, you can exercise for free, or for about $5, at the closest affiliated gym. If you move out of the area, transferring your membership to another branch will probably prove easier than wangling a partial refund of your membership fee.

THE CITY WHERE PEOPLE ARE MOST LIKELY TO EXERCISE: MADISON, WISCONSIN

THE CITY DWELLERS LEAST LIKELY TO GET OFF THEIR DUFFS: OKLAHOMA CITY

Check the equipment. "Good clubs buy some new equipment at least once a year," says Liz Neporent, C.S.C.S., a corporate fitness consultant in New York City. Ask what their newest piece of equipment is, and if you spy a few "Sorry, I'm Busted" signs, forget the place.

Dicker over the price. Say you're comparing clubs and won't be signing up today, says Neporent. Return in a few days and tell the club's rep that the gym across town undercut his price by $100, so how about striking that $99 "initiation fee"? Then try for a half-price yearlong membership for your wife or girlfriend.

Remember your pals. Your buddy is more likely to join you for a workout if he doesn't have to drop $15, so ask for a handful of free guest passes. They're easy to come by now; they'll be a lot scarcer once you're a member.

TAKE ACTION

More often than not, when men are faced with a challenge, we do what it takes to rise to the occasion. Well, here's a challenge of epidemic proportion: Across the globe, we're fatter than ever, and we're suffering the consequences in record numbers—soaring cases of heart disease, stroke, cancer, and diabetes. In response to this, uh, growing problem, men around the world have taken up *Men's Health*'s challenge to lose a combined 1 million pounds. Do your part and join them by going to www.mhmillion.com. We'll even help get you started with the following get-fit strategies.

I. Grab a morning meal. The quickest way to jump-start a weight-loss plan is to wake up and eat. Breakfast revs up your metabolism by putting your body into fuel-burning mode, says Julie Burns, M.S., R.D., founder of the nutrition consulting firm SportFuel. "Breakfast skippers tend to be heavier and unhealthier," she says.

You're not a breakfast eater? Ease into it. Breakfast should be relatively light. Skipping late-night snacks will help you feel hungry in the morning.

The processed carbohydrates found in the typical breakfast of sugary cereal, milk, and juice can leave you feeling hungry later. A protein source (an egg, cottage cheese) and healthy fats (a handful of nuts) will keep you satisfied.

2. Go nuts. Speaking of nuts, if you eat a bunch of almonds before dinner, *you will lose weight*. A Purdue University study showed that people who ate nuts high in monounsaturated fat felt full an hour and a half longer than the sissies who ate rice cakes. "With 9 grams of monounsaturated fat, an ounce of almonds is enough to keep most guys from going ballistic at dinner, the time when they're most likely to overeat," says Elizabeth Ward, R.D., a nutritional consultant in Massachusetts.

And odds are the weight you lose will stay off. Researchers found that of two groups of people who lost weight, those eating a diet high in monos were still slim after 18 months, while those going low-fat quickly porked up again.

For best results, wash down 24 almonds with 8 ounces of water. "The fluid expands the fiber in the nuts to help you feel fuller," says Ward.

3. Snack on chicken. Another great weight-loss food is chicken. Protein makes an especially great snack because it keeps you full. So stock up on pre-cooked chicken, like Perdue Short Cuts Chicken Strips. They're white meat, already roasted and ready to eat. Healthier than wings, easier than driving to KFC. Eat them cold, or zapped, by themselves, on a salad, or wrapped in a tortilla. Lots of protein, little fat.

4. Spoon your way to a slimmer waist. An 8-ounce yogurt (the light kind) contains 400 milligrams of calcium, almost half of the 900 milligrams research shows you need to eat each day to keep the obesity gene turned off. "If you don't get enough calcium, the body stores fat more readily," says Susan Kleiner, Ph.D., R.D., a nutritionist and author of *Power Eating*. Plus, yogurt has 8 to 10 grams of protein, which, according to Kleiner, helps suppress appetite and may boost the activity of leptin, a hormone that plays a key role in calorie burning.

5. Control your appetite. Ask your doctor about the antidepressant bupropion. In a study published in the journal *Obesity Research*, overweight people who took 400 milligrams of the drug daily while dieting and exercising lost 8.6 percent of their weight after 48 weeks, versus 5 percent for those who had taken a placebo. Researchers believe bupropion helps to control appetite by regulating neurotransmitters in the brain.

6. Munch on raisins. To lose the most fat while preserving muscle, your best bet is to combine diet *and* exercise. On your way to the gym, grab a handful of raisins. Strenuous exercise can leave your body swimming in free radicals—compounds that damage your cells, making it harder to recover from a workout. However, a study presented at the American College of Nutrition's annual meeting suggests that eating raisins before or during a workout can lower levels of free radicals in your body. Researchers studied eight triathletes who competed in races 2 weeks apart. In one race, the group ate raisins. In the other, they didn't. "The raisins significantly reduced the amount of free radical damage the racers experienced," says Gene Spiller, Ph.D., of the Sphera Foundation in Los Altos, California, the study author.

7. Track your flab. When we lined up five body fat monitors in our offices, everyone from the scrawny runners to the beefy lifters wanted to see his readings. Buy one. It may provide better motivation than a traditional scale does "because a monitor increases your awareness of the fat you need to lose," says John Foreyt, Ph.D., director of the behavioral medicine research center at the Baylor College of Medicine in Houston. Our favorite monitor, for reliability

THE PERFECT BODY FAT PERCENTAGE FOR MEN: **11**

and ease of use, is the Tanita BF662 Family Model ($100, www.tanita.com). Shoot for 16 percent body fat or less.

8. Make a date with your dumbbells. Grab one of those extra calendars that show up this time of year. (No, not the Snap-on tool-girls calendar. That's special.) This will be your fitness log, your key to commitment. Planning your workouts and then recording exactly what you do "is a proven successful strategy," says Steve Edwards, Ph.D., professor of health and educational psychology at Oklahoma State University in Stillwater. "It's a form of contracting. When you get to the gym and meet those goals, it's self-sustaining." It works for running, lifting, weight control, you name it, says Edwards: "It firms up the commitment you've made."

9. Stay on track. When it's cold and wet outside, you can keep up your walking or running routine with a treadmill. Lace up and try different brands at the stores. But know that our brother mag, *Runner's World*, recently tested 12 models from the top companies and declared the True 540HRC ($3,800) the editors' choice for its quiet operation, stability, and adjustable cushioning. The magazine's best buy: the PaceMaster ProElite ($2,200), which is lighter than most and easier to move around.

10. Soothe sore feet. The key to weight loss is consistent exercise. But if you're in pain after a workout, you're more likely to skip the next one. To soothe sore feet after a run, lace up your shoes again; you may have plantar fasciitis, an overstretching of the tissue in your arches. "A lot of people think that walking without shoes is good for you, but it's a misconception," says Michael Robinson, D.P.M., a podiatrist in Brookline, Massachusetts. "Your feet need support, or the problem will get worse." That means not letting your dogs run naked, except when you hit the sack.

11. Sculpt your abs. As you lose weight, you'll want the abs to show for it. To build a strong midsection, exhale forcefully at the top of your crunches. It forces your abs to work harder, and hard work means more muscle.

In addition to crunches, try this move to make your abs pop: Grab a pair of light dumbbells (5 to 10 pounds) and lie faceup on the floor with your feet flat and your knees bent at about 90 degrees. With your elbows slightly bent, extend your arms straight back so that your biceps are next to your ears and the dumbbells are about an inch off the floor. Now, using your abdominals to keep your lower back pressed flat against the floor, slowly raise and lower the dumbbells about an inch. Repeat as many times as you can. This exercise will increase your abdominal strength as well as improve your posture, says Jolie Bookspan, Ph.D., author of *The Ab Revolution*. As the exercise becomes easier, do more reps.

12. Boost your bench press. Building muscle helps you lose weight, because muscle burns more calories than flab *all day long*. Here's a way to put on more muscle with the most common gym move—the bench press. During the last repetition in your last set, pay attention to the point in the bench press where you feel weakest. Got it? Okay, lower the weight, stand up, and adjust the rack so the barbell is resting at this sticking point.

Next step: Slide on more weight than you can possibly press. Now lie down and grab the bar as if you were going to try to raise it, but instead do five to 10 contractions against the weight—push, relax, repeat. Do this once a week. "You'll train the muscles and joints at the specific angle at which you're weakest," says Richard Kreider, Ph.D., professor of human performance at Baylor University in Houston. Eliminate your weakest link and you'll be able to press more.

13. Get stronger. "The pullup is the perfect exercise to gauge your strength because it forces you to lift your entire body," says Michael Mejia, C.S.C.S., exercise advisor to *Men's Health*. A fit man who weighs between 170 and 200 pounds should be able to do six pullups. (If you're lighter, it's 10. Heavier? Four.) "Men who can do this many shouldn't really encounter too many situations that they can't physically accomplish."

But six means six *perfect* pullups. Keep your hands shoulder-width apart, palms facing out, and legs together. When your chin completely clears the bar, pause for a count of two, then slowly lower yourself and repeat.

Not quite there yet? Place a bench under the bar and do negative pullups. Stand on the bench, grasp the bar, and then bend your legs so your feet hang free. Take 5 seconds to lower yourself until your arms are straight. Step back on the bench and repeat three more times. Do two to three sets twice a week. "These will develop your muscles enough so that you'll eventually be able to lift yourself," says Mejia.

14. Get a leg up. For stronger legs, try this stepup variation from Alwyn Cosgrove, C.S.C.S., owner of Cosgrove Results Training, in Santa Clarita, California; it works one leg at a time, intensely. With a dumbbell in your left hand, stand facing a step that's about 15 inches high. Place your left foot on the step and push yourself up onto it; don't let your right foot touch the step at any time. Step back down with your right leg while keeping your left foot on the step, and repeat until you complete your set. Using one heavy dumbbell in

PERCENTAGE OF MEN
WHO MAKE A NEW YEAR'S RESOLUTION: 41

THE TYPICAL RESOLUTION: TO LOSE THE GUT

NUMBER WHO STICK TO THEIR
RESOLUTIONS FOR AT LEAST A MONTH: 1 IN 2

one hand instead of light dumbbells in both hands focuses the weight on your working leg, stressing its muscle fibers more intensely. As you improve in strength, increase the height of the step.

15. Make your butt a chick magnet. Your glutes are the largest muscles of your body, and it turns out that women like men with buns of steel. Galvanize yours with this tweak to the classic deadlift. Instead of the large, 45-pound weight plates you usually load onto the bar, use 25-pound plates (but still the same total weight you'd normally lift). The smaller-diameter weight plates will allow the bar to go closer to the floor, forcing you to extend your range of motion during your deadlifts. "This not only makes you move the weight a greater distance—which builds more muscle—it builds strength at the bottom part of the move, where guys are usually weakest," says Cosgrove.

ANY QUESTIONS?

Beer Belly Blues

When I exercise, I lose weight but not my beer gut. Why?

—H.G., Lantana, Florida

It's not just your MGDs, but your DNA as well. "Men with beer guts are genetically programmed to store more fat in their abdominal area than lean guys or women," says Claude Bouchard, Ph.D., executive director of the Pennington Biomedical Researcher Center at Louisiana State University in Shreveport. That means your gut is the easiest place to gain fat—and the most difficult place to lose it. The cause: An enemy enzyme is allowing fatty acids to enter and be stored in your fat cells, so your body is storing fat in your gut at a higher rate than normal.

These same men also have a more sluggish lipolysis—the process the body uses to release fat for energy. Combine the two and you have a recipe for a gut that rises like Visa debt. But don't give up: All of this can be reversed with diet and exercise. As your results from your weight-loss program start to wane, cut back an additional 100 calories from your diet (less than what's in a light beer). Then add another 10 minutes of daily physical activity—running, cycling, lifting weights—to put the pressure on your gut to disappear.

Burning Question

Is it true that it takes 20 minutes of exercise before you start burning fat?

—D.P., Flagler Beach, Florida

Not necessarily. Your body starts tapping fat as fuel the moment it creates an energy deficit. If you exercise regularly and cut back on your calories (thus creating energy deficits), you can burn flab all day long.

PERCENTAGE OF MEN WHO SKIP OR POSTPONE EXERCISE WHEN FEELING TOO STRESSED OR BUSY: 54

Get It Off Your Chest

I'm gaining fat—in my chest. How can I stop before I have breasts?

—T.Y., Soquel, California

The clinical term for "man breasts" is gynecomastia, and up to 36 percent of men have it at any given time. There are four ways you may have flipped on your headlamps:

1. You "juiced" at the gym (two more reasons to avoid steroids).
2. You smoke too much pot, which can give you a chest like Cheech's.
3. Medication—such as some antidepressants—is messing with your hormone levels. (Your doctor can prescribe something to counteract the breast effects.)
4. The most likely scenario: You're too fat.

Brian Windle, M.D., a cosmetic surgeon in Cleveland, proposes ultrasonic liposuction; sound waves rupture the fat cells, making the junk easier to extract. We propose that you join the Million-Pound Challenge at www.mhmillion.com and drop 20. Lose the weight, lose the man breasts, too.

Running Strong

I'm a running fool (four times a week), but I've never lifted a weight in my life. Am I missing something important?

—L.Z., Minneapolis

You mean besides chiseled abs, hard arms, bulging glutes, and callused hands? Absolutely. After the age of 30, men who don't lift lose an average of 7 pounds of muscle per decade. This reduction in muscle is a recipe for packing on fat. For example, say you weigh 180 pounds and have 20 percent body fat at age 30. This means you have roughly 144 pounds of muscle, bone, and soft tissue, and about 36 pounds of fat. If you simply lose 7 pounds of muscle by the time you're 40 but maintain your overall weight, you've just increased your body fat percentage to 24, the upper limit of the safe range for men. Next stop: diabetes, heart disease, or—worse—plumber's crack.

But you can save your muscle. In a 2001 study at Louisiana State University, researchers found that older men, ages 60 to 84, who ran three times a week for 30 minutes a day increased their strength by 21 to 44 percent when they added a simple 10-minute, eight-exercise circuit to their workouts. Each study participant performed only one set of each exercise—leg press, leg curl, seated row, chest press, lateral raise, seated dip, and biceps curl—with a weight he could lift eight to 12 times.

No Pain, No Gain

Why do my muscles feel sore after a tough workout? Do I need to let the pain subside before I lift again?

—D.J., Newton, Massachusetts

No get-out-of-workout-free card here. Exercise causes damage to some muscle fibers, and soreness is part of the natural repair process that is important to growth. Sore now, huge later. So keep at it.

But you can limit the aches in two ways, according to Priscilla M. Clarkson, Ph.D., professor of exercise science at the University of Massachusetts in Amherst: by lightening up on the so-called eccentric portion of the lift (normally the "down" part) during early training, or by starting out slowly, at a very low intensity (more repetitions, low weight), and gradually increasing your workouts. But if you can't extend your arms or walk comfortably down a flight of stairs, take a break. "You're likely to be weaker, so you won't be able to do as much anyway," Clarkson says.

A third option is to take your medicine early: Start your rebound with a very high intensity workout and lift until your muscles are exhausted. You'll be in more pain initially, but less later.

Don't Be a Failure

A guy tells me I need to train to failure on every set to build muscle. Is he a prophet or a lost cause?

—E.C., Nyack, New York

The idea of training to failure—lifting weights until your muscles can't complete another repetition—is pushed with religious zeal in some circles. But if it were such a good idea, they wouldn't need to push it so hard.

A 1997 study in the *Journal of Strength and Conditioning Research* showed that guys not working to failure in multiple sets gained 50 percent more strength in the squat than guys who were doing a single all-out set.

On the other hand, none of the subjects gained muscle or lost fat, even though they all got stronger. You'd think that the men who got the strongest would've gotten bigger, too. But the study didn't show this after 14 weeks.

Strength gains usually result from a good training program, but muscle gains come from the combination of the right program and the right diet. Or even the wrong program and the right diet.

If you aren't eating enough food, you won't gain muscle, no matter how good your program is.

Sick Days

What kinds of exercise can I do when I've got a cold?

—B.V., Scranton, Pennsylvania

Hard, intense exercise temporarily weakens your immune system, which is the last thing you want when you're already threatening the nation's strategic Kleenex reserve. But a Japanese study found that moderate exercise preserves levels of CD8+ T cells, an important part of your internal illness-fighting apparatus. Grant yourself immunity: Forget about sniffling through a high-intensity workout. Go for slow, easy cycling, jogging, tennis, golf, or anything else you enjoy. When your head clears, you can go back to the hard stuff.

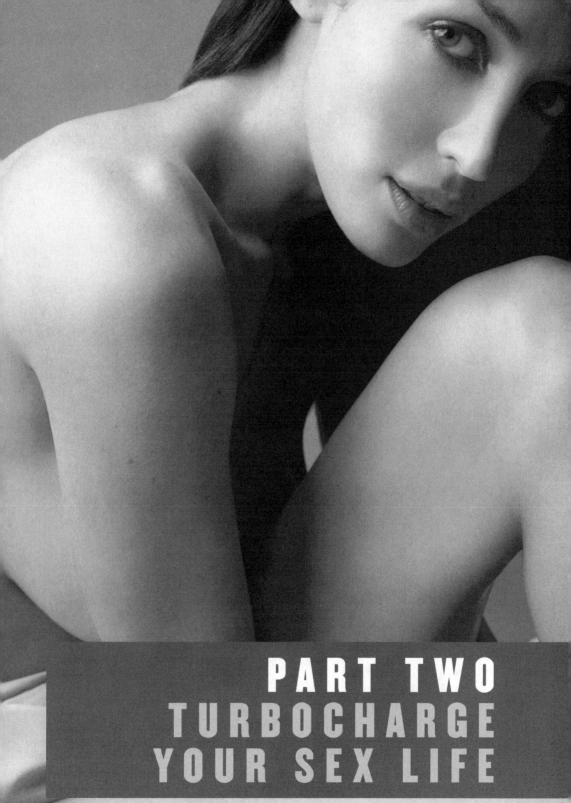

PART TWO
TURBOCHARGE
YOUR SEX LIFE

GAME SHOW

Who Will Have the Most Sex This Year?
One of these hot-blooded single guys? Or you?

The looks . . .

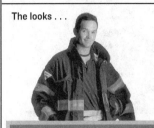

TIM SULLIVAN
Age 25, 5'11", 170 lb
Firefighter,
Yonkers, New York

The loot . . .

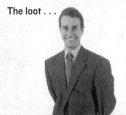

KYLE VOLLUZ
Age 34, 6'0", 170 lb
Corporate attorney,
Dallas

The laughs . . .

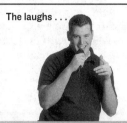

KEVIN MCDONOUGH
Age 25, 6'4", 230 lb
Comedian/law student,
Hoboken, New Jersey

HIS STATS
- Cash: Makes a comfortable living
- Car: '98 Pathfinder (and that fire truck)
- Crib: Lives with parents
- Clothes: Casual with edge, mostly Guess? and Express for Men

HIS APPEAL
- Looks: Most women find Sullivan very handsome. Plus, his job as a firefighter gives him status, which is a high-ranking factor in sexual attraction.

DISADVANTAGES
- Living with his folks might indicate a lack of independence and could potentially cramp his style when inviting women back to his place.

- He can carry a woman out of a burning building, but only 20 percent of women in a recent global survey listed physical strength as the most sexually attractive characteristic.

- In the same survey, 65 percent of women named intelligence as the most desirable male trait. Although Sullivan is a college graduate, his blue-collar job may keep him from being perceived as scholarly.

HIS STATS
- Cash: Earns about $170,000 annually
- Car: '02 Mercedes SUV
- Crib: Owns a house
- Clothes: Business casual, Cole Haan and Hickey Freeman

HIS APPEAL
- Money/success: Volluz will significantly increase his salary and become a partner in his law firm within 4 years. Besides his law degree, he also has an M.B.A. Plus, he's fit (he ran three marathons in the past year) and a bit older (which may be perceived as "distinguished"—another chick magnet).

DISADVANTAGES
- He's required to bill 2,000 to 2,500 hours per year. So much time working means less time (and energy) for circulating.

- Women are attracted to a man who seems likely to commit, research shows. Volluz is 34 and hasn't been married yet. In fact, with the time he devotes to work and marathon training, meeting women doesn't seem to take precedence in his life.

HIS STATS
- Cash: Little to none
- Car: None
- Crib: Shares apartment with college roommate
- Clothes: Gap, J. Crew, Express for Men

HIS APPEAL
- Personality: McDonough is a popular guy with a knack for making people laugh, whether he's onstage or at a party. Sense of humor is one of the top traits women look for in men, as is confidence, which he obviously must have to do stand-up. Being in the spotlight at clubs every weekend gives him a chance to meet lots of women. Plus, he's tall, and one study shows that women select male partners based on height.

DISADVANTAGES
- Since he has little money, no wheels, and limited free time after work and school, women might find McDonough not worth the trouble.

- He has average looks and is slightly overweight.

And the Winner Is . . .
Tim Sullivan

Michael Cunningham, Ph.D., professor of psychology at the University of Louisville in Kentucky, helped us devise the quiz on the opposite page to gauge how well our contestants will fare with the ladies. Take it yourself and see how you'll do.

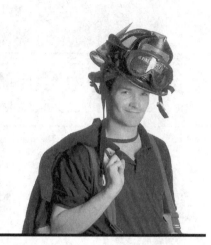

FINAL ANALYSIS

All three contestants did well, but Sullivan got the nod because he's a firefighter, and that's one hot profession right now. "It adds to his attractiveness," says Cunningham. "Firemen have always been popular, but since September 11, they're seen as particularly heroic."

Sullivan also has a chin up in another category, literally. "Bigger chins tend to be associated with being masculine," says Cunningham, who has researched how the size of certain facial features influences the opposite sex. He has found that a broad chin, medium-size nose, high cheekbones, thick eyebrows, and large eyes make men more attractive to women. "Sullivan is probably marginally more attractive than Volluz, who is marginally more attractive than McDonough," says Cunningham.

Volluz wins points for his stable job and high income. However, Cunningham notes, his long work hours could be a turnoff. "According to my research, women are looking for trade-offs," he says. "They're looking for a guy who makes above-average money, but they're also looking for a guy who has some availability and spare time."

McDonough wins the most points for dynamic personality. But humor can work both ways. "If a woman feels a guy is a little too good for her and he has self-deprecating humor, it makes her feel at ease," says Cunningham. "But if she thinks he's a bit of a loser and he uses self-deprecating humor, then she thinks he doesn't take himself seriously enough."

Like the other contestants, McDonough is intelligent. However, at present he ranks lowest in terms of status because he's still in school. "Starting law school is a long way from finishing law school," says Cunningham. "We're not talking about what his life might be like 3 years from now."

The Who-Will-Score-More Card

FACTOR	POINT VALUE	TIM	KYLE	KEVIN	YOU
SINCERITY Women are most attracted to men who seem genuinely interested in having a relationship.	A marrying man? +3 A one-night stand? +1 Somewhere in between? +2	 +2	 +2	 +2	
STYLE How you dress makes a big difference in whether she's initially impressed.	Sharp-dressed man? +3 Average dresser? +2 Account at Goodwill? −1	 +2	+3	 +2	
CIRCULATION The more women you meet, the greater the odds of getting one into bed.	Meet oodles of women? +3 Meet many women outside of work? +2 Meet few women outside work? +1	 +2	 +1	+3	
AVAILABILITY If you come across as very busy, women may assume you're too busy for them.	Lots of free time? +3 Little free time? −1	+3	 −1	 −1	
CAREER Women most desire men who are professionally successful, well-educated, financially secure, wise, and mature. (Score points for all that apply.)	College graduate? +1 Advanced graduate degree? +1 Salary above $60K? +1 Potential for large future success/earnings? +1	+1	+1 +1 +1 +1	+1 +1	
STATUS What you do for a living gives you a particular standing.	Heroic job? +3 Respectable position? +2 Job shows potential? +1 Doing hack work? −1	+3	 +2	 +1	
PHYSICAL ATTRACTIVENESS Women are drawn to fit, handsome men partly because they'll father cute, healthy children. (Score points for all that apply.)	Drop-dead handsome? +2 Likely to produce cute children? +1 Look physically fit? +1 The missing link? −1	+2 +1 +1	 +1 +1	 +1	
DYNAMIC PERSONALITY Being an all-around fun guy can often compensate for a lack of looks and money. (Score points for all that apply.)	Known for sense of humor? +3 Outgoing? +1 Popular? +1	 +1 +1	 +1	+3 +1 +1	
VITALITY AND HEALTH A man who takes care of himself is seen as a more competent protector.	Exercise regularly? +2 Job requires physical strength? +2 Healthful diet? +1 Overweight? −1	 +2	+2 +1	 −1	
TOTALS		21	17	14	

▶ **IF YOUR SCORE IS 16 OR MORE:** You're going to see more action than our armed forces. Call 1-800-NEW-MATTRESS.

▶ **IF YOUR SCORE IS 10 TO 15:** You're interesting, but not irresistible. You'll have a few flings.

▶ **IF YOUR SCORE IS 9 OR LESS:** Want to come over and play some foosball?

MUST READS

Keep Your Eye on the Balls

This disease can rob you of your manhood—and more. Here's the heads-up on what's down below

By Donovan Webster

For John Perez, life was good. It was December 2000, and after several years of grinding labor—working through cooking school and sautéing his way up the food chain of Manhattan's finest restaurants—he'd left his assistant chef job at a three-star eatery called Zoë to start his own catering house.

At 35 years old, the sturdy, dark-haired Perez was living the life he had dreamed of. Through the fall and winter of 2000, he spent his days jetting around the country, cooking up parties and meals for the famous and powerful, a group that included the fashion designer John Varvatos. Then, in mid-December, during the peak of his fledgling company's holiday rush, Perez's world suddenly became very small.

"I felt this little mass the size of a pea on my left testicle," he says. "I thought, 'What? That's new.' So after I got out of the shower, I told my wife, Marisa."

The following day, Perez consulted his urologist, who performed a series of blood tests. The results came back 90 minutes later. They were positive for a "marker compound" called beta human chorionic gonadotropin (beta hCG), which occurs naturally only in the blood of pregnant women and in people with certain cancers, testicular cancer among them.

After the positive beta hCG screen, Perez's doctor ordered a sonogram. The left testicle showed an unusual growth. ("When he found it, the technician shouted, 'Aha! There's your tumor!'" Perez now jokes.) But with positive findings from the most accurate tests for testicular cancer, the uncertainty Perez had felt for the past day now plummeted into dread.

"By 7 that night," he says, "I had cancer."

A SNEAK ATTACK

While testicular cancer ranks among the rarest forms of the disease— comprising only about 1 percent of all cancers in men—it's the most common cancer among men age 15 to 35. Last year, according to the National Cancer Institute, 7,600 American men were diagnosed with it, though those cases were far from equally distributed among the races: Testicular cancer is four times more prevalent in white men than in blacks of similar age, and two times more prevalent than in Asians.

Doctors may have identified the disease's target demographic, but they've yet to figure out its trigger. "All we know is this: If you had an undescended testicle as a child, your risk of testicular cancer rises 25- to 50-fold, though we don't know the reason," says Jerome P. Richie, M.D., professor of surgery at Harvard Medical School.

Some researchers believe abnormal growth of the testicles in childhood or a rare genetic condition called Kleinfelter's syndrome (a disorder in which males have two X chromosomes and one Y chromosome) may start the cancer, but Dr. Richie—one of the country's top testicular cancer specialists—discounts these theories as questionable. Instead, he reiterates that testicular cancer can occur in any young man, regardless of risk factors. "Even a seemingly healthy man can be afflicted with it."

Although we don't know much about what triggers testicular cancer, the prognosis for defeating it has become exceedingly positive. According to Craig Nichols, M.D., chairman of oncology at Oregon Health Sciences University in Portland, the past quarter century has seen the rate of cure skyrocket. "In the 1970s, only 10 percent to 20 percent of all men diagnosed with metastatic testicular cancer survived," he says. "Today we have about a 95 percent cure rate. A testicular cancer diagnosis isn't the death sentence it was 25 or 30 years ago."

CUT AND RUN

But before any patient can begin to hope for a cure, his doctor has to identify the type of testicular cancer he has. And, unfortunately, there's only one way to find out: Remove the testicle.

Using an outpatient procedure called an inguinal orchiectomy, the surgeon makes a small incision in the groin a few inches below the belt line and pulls the affected testicle up and out. (Picture a large, somewhat misshapen pearl onion.) "We need to take out not only the testicle but also its spermatic cord, which is how the cancer most often spreads to other parts of the body," says Dr. Richie. The good news: Because the cancer travels up the spermatic cord, there's no way for it to spread to the remaining testicle. And that sole survivor is all a man needs to retain normal fertility, sensitivity, and sex drive.

ESTIMATED NUMBER OF MEN WHO DIED LAST YEAR OF TESTICULAR CANCER: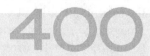

BE YOUR OWN PRIVATES INVESTIGATOR

Forget cleaning behind your ears; the only must-do during a shower is checking yourself for testicular cancer. Here's your refresher course: Gently roll each testicle between your fingers, feeling for any lumps, bumps, or other irregularities. Of course, coming up empty-handed is good, but it doesn't mean you're in the clear. "In the early stage of the disease, there often aren't lumps, so a vague heavy feeling or any difference in the size of a testicle should immediately be checked out by a urologist," says Lawrence Ross, M.D., head of urology at the University of Illinois in Chicago.

Perez underwent the procedure 3 weeks after his diagnosis. By this time, he had switched physicians, to specialists George Bosl, M.D., and Joel Sheinfeld, M.D., at Memorial Sloan-Kettering Cancer Center in New York City.

Perez had good reason to make the jump, says Dr. Sheinfeld—and not only because Sheinfeld got the business. With 7,400 testicular cancers diagnosed a year and roughly 8,000 urologists around the country, a doctor may see only one case a year. "And while an orchiectomy is a pretty straightforward surgical approach," Dr. Sheinfeld says, "the cancer management beyond that step becomes more difficult. You want somebody who has performed all of the treatments several—if not dozens or hundreds of—times."

Perez agreed. "I wanted treatment by the best. It's like my work as a chef. I do a better job filleting a salmon or preparing a chicken than somebody who does it once a year."

His orchiectomy was a success. (Some men will opt for a prosthetic testicle—saline-filled, like a breast implant—but not Perez. "Dressed, there's no difference. After a shower, when your testes are more pendulous, it becomes more apparent," he says. "I actually like the spare room.")

Dr. Sheinfeld's next step: Determine the type of cancer—seminoma or nonseminoma—and the stage.

The less aggressive of the two types, seminomas usually remain localized and spread slowly; they account for about 35 to 40 percent of all testicular cancers. Nonseminomas move quickly up the spermatic cord to the lymphatic system and comprise about 60 percent of all testicular cancers.

To help orient doctors toward the best treatment after an orchiectomy, more blood tests are performed. If the cancer is gone, existing blood markers usually drop off significantly or disappear. Doctors also use ultrasound or CT scan imaging to pinpoint other cancerous growths, and sometimes they do further biopsies. Finally, after reviewing all this data, they label, or categorize, the stage of the disease.

In stage I, the cancer is confined to the testicle; stage II cancers have spread to the lymph nodes located at the back of the abdominal cavity and below the diaphragm; and, finally, stage III cancers have spread beyond the lymph nodes and into other parts of the body, such as the lungs, liver, and brain. This type almost killed cycling great Lance Armstrong.

In Perez's case, his pathology report indicated that he had a form of cancer with both seminomas and nonseminomas in evidence. But it was stage I. "The plan," Perez says, "was just to do regular surveillance, just periodic checkups."

Life, after a distracting detour, was back on the main highway. "It was as if this strange bad dream was finally over," says Perez. "Then, a week after the surgery, I got a phone call. And, well, the bad dream was back."

It was the pathologist. After further review, the doctor discovered that he'd missed something. The nonseminoma cancer had spread and might have entered Perez's lymph nodes.

CHEMICAL WARFARE

For those men whose cancer has spread, depending on the type of tumor present, the majority of specialists prescribe a course of chemotherapy. While the particular "recipe" of cancer drugs varies, it always includes a medication called cisplatin.

Widely thought to be the magic bullet against testicular cancer, cisplatin—a platinum-based drug that attacks the DNA of the cancer itself—is the reason so many physicians now believe testicular cancer has become curable. "These days," says Dr. Nichols, "even patients with stage III cancers stand a very good chance of being cured, thanks to cisplatin."

There are, of course, drawbacks. Because chemotherapy attacks most of the rapidly growing cells in the body, any area where cells are dividing quickly may be damaged. In some men, this causes hair loss, gum sores, tinnitis (ringing in the ears), a compromised immune system, and a permanent decrease in sperm production in the remaining testicle. Still, because cisplatin-centered treatments are so successful, most doctors employ them as the first line of defense in nonseminoma cancers.

Localized radiation therapy is also an option, but only for men with the slower-moving seminomas. Finally, for aggressive nonseminomas that have spread to the lymphatic system or beyond, there remains a more absolute option: surgery. Specifically, it's called a retroperitoneal lymph node dissection, or RPLND, a procedure that saved comedian Tom Green and figure skater Scott Hamilton.

In this operation, which can take from 2 to 6 hours, an incision is made from just above the pubic bone to the sternum. Then surgeons examine the abdomen to remove all cancerous-looking lymph nodes and tissues throughout the area. Before surgery is over, the gastrointestinal tract's organs have been examined and moved out of the way since the abdominal lymph nodes are located deep inside, near the kidneys. Further complicating matters, there's a slight chance that the doctor may damage a hard-to-see nerve that controls ejaculation. Severing this nerve results in permanent retrograde ejaculation, a condition that causes ejaculate to go into the bladder instead of toward the penis.

"Most of the surgeons who do RPLND's are extremely familiar with nerve-sparing techniques," says Dr. Sheinfeld. "But even with the best surgeon, there will still be a period of local discomfort after the surgery, and for several months to up to 2 years, the patient may also be unable to ejaculate. Make no mistake; this is a big and involved surgery."

DISSECTING THE PROBLEM

Three weeks after receiving that fateful phone call, Perez was under Dr. Sheinfeld's knife for his own RPLND. His combination of seminoma and nonseminoma placed him in a small, rare group for whom this is the optimal treatment. And while his doctors advised him of all his options, Perez was in favor of the most radical therapy first.

"I just wanted to stay away from chemo and radiation," he says, "because, for me, the side effects were more frightening than the surgery. I also wanted my cancer gone the most 100 percent certain way."

Perez's surgery was over in 5 hours. "I checked in to the hospital and they put me under, split me open from crotch to craw, then looked around and fixed what they found."

It would be 3 weeks before Perez was finally back up and moving around normally. "I tell ya," he says, "for days after the surgery, every time I stood up, I felt like my guts were gonna come tumbling out. Literally, they field-dressed me like a deer." He also recalls that for weeks after the surgery he could feel his innards "sloshing around" as they reattached and settled back inside his body. "It wasn't pretty," he adds. "But I also felt assured of this: The RPLND got all my cancer. After the surgery, I knew I was clean."

SPECIALIST DELIVERY

If there's a downside to the low rates of testicular cancer, it's that most urologists haven't seen enough of the disease to become experts at treating it. And the handful that have? You'll find their names at www.acor.org/TCRC/experts.html.

Continually updated by the Testicular Cancer Resource Center, this list includes the names of and contact information for the 30-some testicular cancer specialists in the country.

His doctors had, in fact, gotten it all. However, since there's a 15 percent chance that cancer will develop in the remaining testicle within the next 5 years, Perez must continue with his self-exams. Except for this, and that big scar down his belly, the unpleasant journey of John Perez's testicular cancer is now behind him.

And he already knows what lies ahead: Only 7 months after the surgery, Perez's ability to ejaculate returned and Marisa became pregnant with their first child.

"We did it naturally and everything," he says. "We had a baby girl in June."

Playing the Odds

Each time you have unprotected sex, you're taking a gamble

By Zachary Veilleux

In Vegas, home of showgirls and brothels, men have been known to stake their entire fortunes on a game of chance with a simple spin of the roulette wheel. But the game you're playing is more like the Russian version every time you take a new woman home. It's estimated that one in three women in the United States has a sexually transmitted disease. Your risk of disease from one bout of unprotected sex with a beautiful stranger? About 33 percent. Here's how it breaks down.

HERPES: I IN 9

It's one of the most widespread STDs—45 million Americans are infected. This bug won't kill you, and outbreaks are treatable, but if you get it, you'll have it forever and women will turn down sex with you forever.

Scary fact: Condoms might not help, because any infected skin-to-skin contact beyond the reach of the latex can result in transmission.

Protect yourself: Don't have sex with a partner while she's having an outbreak.

HUMAN PAPILLOMAVIRUS (HPV): I IN I2

Most women who carry one of the viruses that cause genital warts don't even know they're infected. For many women, infections appear to be temporary, and the immune system clears the virus before it can cause medical complications (such as cervical cancer).

Scary fact: As many as 46 percent of women under age 25 are HPV-positive at any given time.

Protect yourself: Condoms help, but, as with herpes, they protect only what they cover.

CHLAMYDIA: 1 IN 18

It's on a rampage. The Centers for Disease Control and Prevention estimates that half of all sexually active women will have been infected with chlamydia by the time they reach age 30.

Scary fact: Three-quarters of women (and half of all men) with chlamydia have no symptoms and never seek treatment—but if you pass it on to your partner, you could render her infertile.

Protect yourself: Use condoms.

GONORRHEA: <1 IN 36

This one hasn't gotten much attention since World War II, but it's still around, and it still makes it burn when you pee. It's most common in women in their teens and early twenties.

Scary fact: In men, gonorrhea has been linked to epididymitis—a painful disease of the testicles—and prostate problems.

Protect yourself: If you're infected, the antibiotic Cipro (remember the anthrax scare of 2001?) is effective at clearing it up.

SYPHILIS: <1 IN 36

There's a national plan to eliminate syphilis from the United States by 2005. The disease is not very widespread, is easily detectable, and can be cured with a single dose of penicillin if treated within 1 year.

Scary fact: Rates of syphilis are about five times higher in the Deep South.

Protect yourself: Use condoms.

HIV: <1 IN 36

Roughly 40,000 women are infected with HIV, and another 140,000 have AIDS.

Scary fact: There's still no cure.

Protect yourself: Condoms are the best way to avoid getting HIV, but you have to use them during oral sex, too.

HEPATITIS B VIRUS: <1 IN 36

If you catch it, spin another wheel: About 6 percent of those infected develop chronic infections, and of those, 25 percent die of liver disease.

Scary fact: If she's infected, the virus is present in nearly all of her bodily fluids—you could potentially get this deadly liver disease simply by sharing a toothbrush.

Protect yourself: Go to your family doctor for a vaccination. It wasn't routinely given to infants until 1991, when you were too old for shots.

OTHER BUGS

They don't make the news, but there are 18 other diseases that are spread primarily through sex. Trichomoniasis, for example—a parasite that causes penile irritation and discharge and may increase risk of HIV—infects about 5 million people each year.

Too Much of a Good Thing

This is my sex life. It might seem like the stuff of your dreams. But for me, it's been nothing but a nightmare

As told to Sarah Miller

I lost my virginity at age 13 on a playground in north Jersey. Since then, I've slept with so many women I've lost count. People ask, Is it over 100? I laugh. It's way over 100.

You might think that you'd like to be me. However, if my sexual history were still a source of pride, I wouldn't be telling you about it right now. I am what is known as a sex and love addict, and I've come to face a terrible reality: A man who does the things that I've done is not considered a good man.

I am trying to become a good man. Here's my story.

I came home from a business trip one day last winter to find my fiancée, Cathy, packing. Usually when I got home after a while away, she'd be waiting for me with wine and lingerie. This time, her blonde hair, which she usually wore down, was up in an I-mean-business—and don't-touch-me—scrunchie.

"I know everything," she said.

"Look," I said, hoping "everything" didn't really mean *everything*, "the thing with Karen is over."

Cathy's sardonic laugh let me know that she really did know everything. About the girl from the trip to Chicago, the woman she plays tennis with, et cetera. And in my case, at least, that is a very substantial et cetera.

She left.

THE MOST COMMON SEX ADDICTION, ACCORDING TO THE LEADING NATIONAL EXPERT ON SEX ADDICTION: MASTURBATION

WAKING UP

At first, I was furious at Cathy for ruining what we had. It literally took 3 weeks before I figured out, *Excuse me, dumb-ass, the problem isn't Cathy's finding out. The problem is you.*

I called a shrink.

TRUTH

The shrink asked me if I'd ever told myself I wasn't going to sleep with anyone but then done it anyway. He asked me if I felt that my sex life wasn't part of my life, but my whole life; if I ever had trouble concentrating because of sex; if I often slept with women I didn't even like. . . . I answered yes to 37 out of 40 questions. The easiest A of my life.

"You are a sex and love addict," he said. "You're addicted to the thrill of romance and sexual conquest. Do you feel this is true?"

"Sir, with all due respect, if there were a pussy on the other side of a brick wall, I would chew through it to get there."

I think he might have smiled a little.

The shrink told me I had a disease that's something like alcoholism. I was addicted to the conquest of women, and engaging in this pursuit created reactions in my brain—the release of dopamine and other pleasure-inducing agents similar to narcotics.

He told me that sex was almost harder to shake than drugs because drugs aren't part of normal life. Sex is. So not only would I have to learn to stop being addicted to sex; I'd have to learn how to enjoy it in a less insane way.

SAY HELLO TO YOURSELF, CRAZY!

March. I was supposed to be planning a wedding, but instead, I was in a church basement in midtown Manhattan at a Sex and Love Addicts meeting. Sex addicts are everything and everyone—fat, thin, tall, white, black, rich, poor. They—or, rather, we—come from every social and economic class, and dress in $3,000 suits, $100 suits, uniforms, and rags.

Someone told a story about squandering his house down payment on prostitutes. Another guy had slept with his brother's wife when his brother was overseas in the army. I was thinking, *Good thing I'm not like these guys!* Then the leader, about 50, in chinos and a golf shirt, stood up and said, "We are all men whose self-esteem is totally regulated by sex. We're men who relate to the world, and to ourselves, through sex." It's not exactly the way I've always dreamed of defining myself, but was it ever true.

FEARLESS MORAL INVENTORY

So once you find out you're a sex addict, it's not just a question of quitting and moving on. With the help of the 12-step program and the guidance

ARE YOU A SEX ADDICT?

1. Were you sexually abused as a child or adolescent?

2. Do you regularly purchase romance novels or sexually explicit magazines?

3. Have you stayed in romantic relationships after they became emotionally or physically abusive?

4. Do you often find yourself preoccupied with sexual thoughts or romantic daydreams?

5. Do you feel that your sexual behavior is normal?

6. Does your spouse (or significant other or others) ever worry or complain about your sexual behavior?

7. Do you have trouble stopping your sexual behavior when you know it's inappropriate?

8. Do you ever feel bad about your sexual behavior?

9. Has your sexual behavior ever created problems for you and your family?

10. Have you ever sought help for sexual behavior you did not like?

11. Have you ever worried about people finding out about your sexual activities?

12. Has anyone been hurt emotionally because of your sexual behavior?

13. Have you ever participated in sexual activity in exchange for money or gifts?

14. Do you have times when you act out sexually followed by periods of celibacy (no sex at all)?

15. Have you made efforts to quit a type of sexual activity and failed?

16. Do you hide some of your sexual behavior from others?

17. Do you find yourself having multiple romantic relationships at the same time?

18. Have you ever felt degraded by your sexual behavior?

19. Has sex or have romantic fantasies been a way for you to escape your problems?

20. When you have sex, do you feel depressed afterward?

21. Do you regularly engage in sadomasochistic behavior?

22. Has your sexual activity interfered with your family life?

23. Have you been sexual with minors?

24. Do you feel controlled by your sexual desire or fantasies of romance?

25. Do you ever think your sexual desire is stronger than you are?

Keeping score: This sex addiction screening test was created by Patrick Carnes, Ph.D., clinical director of sexual disorders services at The Meadows in Wickenburg, Arizona. He recommends having your results assessed by a therapist, especially if you answer yes to at least 13 questions. For a referral, call The Meadows at (800) 632-3697.

of the shrink, I worked on facing what (and whom) I had done. Then came the hard part. I had to apologize. In 12-step-speak, we call it making amends, and it is a big part of the cure. Fortunately, I had handy reference material.

One of the characteristics of sex addiction is keeping lists of your conquests. I'd had a black book since high school. It was detailed and scrupulous and extensive. Once I left it in a Boston gas station and drove back an hour from Rhode Island to get it. It was weird to remember being proud of that thing. Now I knew what I had to do. I copied down the name of every woman I thought I could find. Then I put the book in the fireplace, and it burned while I dialed numbers.

MEG

Meg was my main "booty call." I would call her when I was out at bars and hadn't succeeded in picking up anyone. She would always come to me. I convinced her that I was in love with her but that I was just afraid of intimacy, and at the time I actually believed this was true. She was a pretty girl, but a tiny bit overweight, and always wearing heels that were a little too high and lipstick that was a little too bright.

I found her number. She lived a few towns out, in New Jersey. "I have to talk to you," I said. "I know it's been a long time, but I have something I really want to say to you."

She said, "Why now?"

I told her I would tell her when I saw her. It turned out that she worked just a few blocks away from me, so we decided to meet at a bar near her building.

She looked great. The awkwardness, and the flesh, of her student days were gone. She was wearing an expensive suit, and her calf muscles twitched a little above her stacked-heel pumps. I blurted out, "You're so thin."

"I started working out constantly because you made me hate myself so much," she said.

Now was a good time to start apologizing. "It was my fault," I said. "I kept coming up with excuses why you weren't a lovable person, but I was the one who was crazy. I am so sorry if I made you feel bad about yourself. I'm so sorry that I would tell you I loved you and tell you that I didn't love you."

By then she was crying. "You don't know how long I've wanted to hear you say that. I'm married now, to a great guy. But my relationship with you, it was always this little dark spot . . . this piece of my soul that felt dirty."

She said, "I forgive you." I was crying, too. This is part of the therapy: to try to see women as total human beings, and to let them see me the same way. It felt great. I thought, Wow, this is easy. It had never occurred to me how much cheer I could spread just by admitting what an asshole I am.

BETSY

Betsy was my girlfriend in college. She was one of those small, compact blonde girls who are hot and also look as if they'd be great moms. The first night I met her, I told her I wanted to marry her. Betsy is low maintenance, but not so much so that she was willing to let it go that I slept with several of her closest friends. The night before her medical school boards, I called her up and told her I didn't think we were right for each other anymore. (She took me back after that. Twice. But hey, this isn't about what she did wrong.)

"Betsy?"

Silence. Then, "What do you want?"

"I've been thinking lately, and I have something I want to say to you."

She laughed. "I have something I want to say to you, too. Actually, just one thing. Go f— yourself."

She hung up.

For a minute I thought about how cute Betsy looked in a pair of jeans, and how I hadn't earned my right to see her take those Levis off as many times as I did.

MORGAN

Morgan was a woman from work. I'd told her she was the woman of my dreams and that loving her was the single greatest pleasure of my life. After 4 months, she really started to annoy me. She didn't actually do anything wrong, of course; it's just that when you think someone's perfect, they're bound to disappoint you. So what did I do? I met Cathy and decided, No, Cathy is really the perfect one. (Cathy would, naturally, also fall from this pedestal.)

Anyway, where did I break up with Morgan? In front of the copy machine, at 8:30 in the morning. She had to leave the company.

Morgan and I arranged to meet at the same bar where I'd had my talk with Meg. I called it the Reformed Male Slut Saloon.

Morgan is British and exudes chill. She looked so beautiful, long and lean in tailored pants and boots, that I had trouble concentrating on my apology. "I am sorry that I idealized you and then let you down. I'm sorry I made commitments to you that I did not keep. I'm sorry. . . . "

"Are you done?" she said. I said I guess so.

She tapped out a cigarette, and I lit it for her. "It's fine," she said. God bless the British and their lack of emotion, though I did enjoy the grand-finale catharsis with Meg.

We ordered drinks and talked about other things. She said quite warmly, "I'm sorry about your fiancée, and you look great." Suddenly I was leaning in. "You look really fantastic," I said. I leaned in closer, and I think she saw me smell her.

"Oh, my God, you think you're going to get laid!" she said. She leaned back with her cigarette and whirled it around. "I was just being nice. . . . You're going around the city half apologizing to girls and half hoping you can rope them in again." She laughed again—at me.

NINA

That night I went out to a bar and put my best rap on a 24-year-old design student. Nina. And she was ready to listen. "I love design," I said, even though

I know nothing about it. She had a drawing in her bag. "You are so talented," I said. I felt good.

Shyly she said, "Do you really think so?" She had that shaggy haircut all the young girls have, with sexy little orange tips. When I slipped my arm

SEXUAL HEALING

Sex addiction is not about getting laid a lot; it is about very extreme sexual behavior characterized by obsession, compulsion, and the inability, despite trying, to stop.

"When we talk about sex addicts, we're talking about a degree of interest in sex and sexual material that is way out of bounds," says Charlie Walker, a marriage and family therapist with the Meadows Institute in Wickenburg, Arizona. "We're talking about people engaged in behavior that they can't stop, that they have tried to stop, and that is inhibiting them from living normal lives."

Somewhere between 3 and 7 percent of the population show signs of sexual addiction, and the majority of sufferers are men. Just like alcoholics and drug addicts, sex addicts are hooked on a high. "When a sex addict is in pursuit of his prey—be it regular women, prostitutes, or pornography—he has a single-minded determination and an extreme level of excitement," says David O'Connell, Ph.D., of the Caron Foundation in Weenersville, Pennsylvania. It's this excitement, this rush, that the sex addict craves.

That said, despite his single-minded mission, the sex addict doesn't find sex satisfying. The only thing on his mind is, When will I get off again, and how, and what can I do, even at this very moment, to make that happen?

As with other addictive behaviors, there are risk factors in sex addiction. According to research conducted by Patrick Carnes, Ph.D., clinical director of sexual disorders services at the Meadows Institute, 72 percent of sex addicts were physically abused, 81 percent were sexually abused, and 97 percent were emotionally abused. Having parents who were addicted to something—whether it was booze, drugs, or sex—is a factor. So is having grown up in a very rigid, moralistic family with a repressed attitude toward sexuality. "Some sex addicts grew up feeling that sex was bad, dirty, or wrong. So it's no wonder they would have problems with it," says Carnes.

But while sex addiction has its own treatment protocol, its own 12-step process, it's a more complicated foe than other compulsions, like drugs or alcohol. Simply put, sex, in moderation, is a normal part of life. So the battle is to learn moderation, not abstention. Whether it's officially a 12-step program or not, recovery involves facing what you've done, apologizing to the people you've hurt, and struggling to keep from abusing the substance you're addicted to. "This is difficult because you can be having sex and tell yourself and everyone, 'I'm not really abusing it,' even if you know you are," says Walker. "Recovering from sex addiction begins when you've learned to look honestly at your behavior and realize there is little or no moderation in your sexual activities. Which is not so easy."

For an online self-test administered by Sex and Love Addicts Anonymous, go to www.slaafws.org/pamphlets/fortyquestions.html. You can also look in your local phone book under "Sex Addicts Anonymous." It's a nationwide nonprofit group similar in principle to AA. Not only is it anonymous; it's free.

around her waist, she didn't push it away. Back at her place, she let me do what I wanted. When she was in the bathroom, I left.

And then I had to apologize to her. I called her and said, "I'm sorry that in my pursuit of ego validation and sexual release I did not treat you as a person."

"That's cool," she said. "Whatcha doin' this weekend?"

"I'm going to be pretty busy," I said. "I'm trying to become a human being."

KAREN

I felt so lame after Nina that I knew I had to try to do something healthy. I needed psychological and behavioral salad, if you will, as opposed to pepperoni pizza. Cathy was still on vacation, and I was planning my amends to her when she returned. But before I apologized to Cathy, I had to talk to Karen.

She wouldn't speak to me, so I scheduled a meeting at work and put it into her electronic date book. Conniving creeps learn to do that kind of thing. As I booked the appointment, I thought of how I had initially been so impressed by Karen's meticulousness, her neat bun at the back of her head, her dark, serious look. Cathy's a lawyer, but she's more of a free spirit than Karen, and I had thought Karen's tough confidence would provide everything I was lacking in life. Of course, scratch the surface and she didn't turn out to be so tough or so confident, and even if she had been, I doubt the mere force of her personality could have saved me.

As soon as she got to the empty conference room, she figured out what I'd done. "I'm out of here," she snapped.

I begged her to stay and hear me out. She didn't sit down, but she didn't walk out, so I started to talk, fast.

"I want to apologize," I said. "I used your concerns about your last relationship to manipulate you. And in return, I used the love you gave me to fill the pathological need that I had. I had enough chances to break it off, but I could never bring myself to do it—the addiction was too great . . . the thrill was too much to pass up. And I'm sorry for not having the respect for either of our relationships to stop."

She sat down at the conference table.

She took a deep breath. She said, "I want to get back together with you, too."

"No, no, no!" I said. "Don't you see? I'm telling you that because of me the whole basis of our relationship was wrong, and I'm apologizing for not having the maturity to treat you the way. . . . "

Her eyes were filled with tears, and her voice shook. "That's your idea of an apology?" she said. "Telling me that you never loved me?" She stood up, snapped the white cuffs of her shirt around her wrists, and collected her face into that look of perfect composure that once had captivated me and now freaked me out. She paused at the door. It was amazing how she could collect herself so quickly; no one seeing her leave that room would have guessed at the emotion underneath her cool exterior. "Don't ever talk to me again," she said.

I called my sponsor. "I feel terrible," I said.

"Good," he said. "Feeling terrible is how you remember not to keep being the same person."

CATHY

Despite the fact that none of my amends—except for the first one, with Meg—had gone as well as I'd wanted them to, I did feel I had made significant progress. I was ready to face Cathy, to tell her I was sorry about everything I'd done, and to tell her about what I had already done to change my ways, and what I would do in the future to make sure I was a great husband to her.

She came over to the apartment that we used to share. I tried not to notice how good she looked, how tan and relaxed, because I knew if I did, I'd start trying to get her into bed and forget about trying to get her to forgive me. I owned up to every single stupid thing I'd ever done when I was with her. From Karen to the woman in Chicago, to the woman at the shore house, to the tennis woman, to all the women I'd kissed in bars. (I didn't tell her about Nina. Maybe this was lame. But I thought, Hey, I'm up against enough here.)

"I hate watching you as I tell you this stuff," I said, "because I know how much I hurt you, and I love you more than anything in the world, and I would do anything to get you back." I told her about my amends, about burning my black book, about the thinking I'd done, about how I grew up and how this might have caused my addiction.

Remember how I said I was too stupid to understand that what had happened was my fault? Well, this time I was too stupid to realize that she wasn't going to be thrilled by all the work I'd done, so much as shocked and repulsed that I'd had to do it.

She told me that when she thought about our life together, she felt sick. She told me, naturally, that it was over.

NOW

My father died when I was 12. Up until he died, I took accordion lessons— accordion lessons in north Jersey, in the 1980s—because he was screwing my accordion teacher. I remember his lying to my mother, and my sitting there thinking, This is how relationships work, right? I'm not blaming him; I guess I'm just giving you an idea of how someone could turn out like me.

Selfishness is the root of what's wrong with me. I got where I am because I've been unable to see beyond my own desires and urges. So it's not surprising that I thought all of my apologizing would result in seamless personal catharsis. It didn't occur to me that these women, who had had to make their own recovery from whatever I had done to them, might not be all that interested in hearing what I was going through.

Gradually, I've become less interested in the thrill of the chase and more interested in my ability to resist my impulses. Cathy is gone, and I can't do anything about that. For a while I was obsessed with getting her back, but the shrink told me to cut it out. "It's not about being obsessed with the right woman," he said. "It's about not being obsessed."

Alcoholics quit drinking. Sex and love addicts aren't expected to quit sex and love, but we do have to change entirely the way in which we operate.

For me, this means really getting to know women before I sleep with them, and coming to see them as whole people, not conquests to win and then forget, or goddesses who, once they reveal their true nature, I condemn for being mortals.

We all have urges, but even when I was young, really young, my urge felt as if it had a motor on it. Talking to girls, I was like, Wow, this is what I was made to do. It felt so right, so exhilarating to be so good at something. Nowadays, I have to pay attention to when I feel that rush, that buzz, that urgency, and ask myself whether I really feel a connection with the woman I'm talking to, or if I'm just desperate for her to say yes.

I told this whole story at one of my meetings. I spoke for a full hour and didn't leave out a single thing about what a jerk, a slut, a manipulative liar, and a con artist I've been for the past 20 years. I told a roomful of men exactly who I am and how I plan to become someone different. Afterward, I felt elated. Men twice my age came up to me and told me they'd been living like me their whole lives. "You have the time to turn this around," said a 60-year-old sports manager who had spent half his life savings at one Manhattan topless bar and the other half on prostitutes and porn. "You have a great opportunity to make a real life for yourself," he said.

If I don't, I will have to face him. I'll have to face more women. Worst of all, I'll have to face myself.

Surefire Seduction

You are now enrolled in Seduction: The Master Class. Pay attention. There will be a take-home test

By Sheri de Borchgrave

You can probably still picture her: your best friend's hot mother, your aunt with the mysterious (and frequently changing) boyfriends, your sexpot neighbor who was astonishingly careless with the Venetian blinds. They defined sex for you at an age when you couldn't even find it in the dictionary. They were the women who had accumulated a kind of experience no man can: the knowledge of what works, and what doesn't, through long, comparative experience of sex with a variety of partners.

It may seem presumptuous to say it, but I am such a woman. I have a sexual history in the Santayana sense: I have learned from it because I don't want to be doomed to repeat anything. Novelty, after all, is the only reliable aphrodisiac; I make sure that my partners have a ready supply. Perhaps that's why *Cosmopolitan* magazine asked me to be its online sex expert. In that capacity, I've given an entire generation of young women instruction in what to look for in a man—both dressed and un-. And if they're benefiting from my experience, why shouldn't you?

Below, you'll find my advice for men who seek to be the most satisfying lovers. Master these moves and you'll be the one she's been looking for all along—whether you've been together for 30 minutes or 30 years.

Check your ego at the door. Never ask a woman if you're the best she's ever had, or any version of that question. An honest answer may disappoint you. The key to quality lovemaking is to concentrate on being the best you've ever been. You'll be less self-conscious—and more effective.

Be presentable. Waitresses might still ogle the guy with the rumpled frat boy look, but that act gets old once a man hits his late twenties. To play in the big leagues, you need a pressed shirt, shined shoes, and an aroma of something other than stale beer. You may also want to sign up for Fine-Dining Etiquette 101. Women love a man who knows how to eat—even better if he can cook.

Find out in which direction she's looking. A quality woman will be turned on not by what you've done but by what you hope to accomplish. There's nothing quite so sexy as a young guy on the verge, with plans and dreams and elaborate schemes. If a woman seems more interested in your past and present than in your future, well then, the only future she's really invested in is her own.

Be hands-on. Your hands and fingers are great sex toys, but don't limit yourself to the three obvious places. Never leave your hands on just one spot of her—that's the hallmark of a dull lover. Instead, try these:

Hair. While you're making love from behind, tug her hair gently. It's an animalistic reaction.

Hands. Hold her hands above her head and kiss her underarms or neck. It's an intimate change of pace.

Face. Gently stroke her cheeks and temples. Move stray hairs from her face. Women like to feel taken care of during sex.

Neck. Cradle her nape, lightly. That will give her a feeling of trust and safety, what she needs to really surrender herself.

Butt. You're there already; I know. Now focus on the sensitive crease where her thighs meet her butt. Use varying motions to create different sensations.

G-spot. When in the missionary position, press gently just above her pubic bone. You're stimulating her G-spot from the inside with your penis and from the outside with your hands, and it just feels amazing.

Develop a signature move. To keep her coming back for more, learn to do at least one thing really, really well. Here are a few that I've encountered:

The precoital massage. As a warmup to the main event, start by massaging the length of her legs, from her upper thighs down to her ankles. Then focus on the feet, kneading her heels and all other points beneath. Then zero

TURN ONE DATE INTO 20 . . .

With these can't-go-wrong moves of the sophisticated lover.

• Always present yourself as a man with a plan. For dinner. For the weekend in Paris. For the urgent lunchtime rendezvous at your place.

• Buy your lover lingerie and ask her to wear it for you immediately.

• Feed your partner either before or after sex.

• Carry CDs with you to her place—take tunes that both inspire you to action and get her motor running.

• Keep sex a private matter. It's a pleasure conspiracy of two, and only two.

• Observe classic etiquette as if it's second nature, not a self-conscious attempt at chivalry. Open the car door for her. At a restaurant, give her the seat facing into the room, not the wall. Ask her what she'd like to eat, and then order for both of you.

• Use all available technology to rev up the flirtation when you're apart.

• Spare her the details of your past love affairs. Keep the recriminations to a minimum and simply synopsize in one line: "We weren't right for each other." Don't probe for specifics of her past affairs— especially not for sexual details or number of lovers.

• Undress with sensual ease. Be able to go from clothed to naked in seconds—but not in a frantic, clumsy sort of way. Remove your T-shirt with one fluid movement by putting one arm back and yanking the shirt from the collar.

• Know how to unlatch the trickiest bra or bikini bathing suit top, from the front-hook version (pull together and down) to the snap-back closing (push sides in opposite directions until they snap apart and lift off).

• Tell your lover with creative invention, and ardor, what you love about her body.

• Don't whine about using a condom.

• Constantly expand your sexual repertoire together as a couple. Make it a collaboration between equals in search of the ultimate.

• Engage in after play—spooning or light massage—that serves as foreplay.

• Observe proper morning etiquette: Get up and dressed and walk her to her car or flag her a cab, even if you're almost asleep. Pay for the cab or parking fee.

• Make the morning-after call, knowing this turns the corner from postcoital bliss to a renewed seduction.

in on the toes and stretch them individually. Of course, if her impeccable hygiene encourages you to suck on her toes, you'll have her in ecstasy.

The neck bite. By biting into a fleshy area along the top of her shoulders that flares out from the back of the neck, you will bring out the animal in her. Lie with her in a spooning position. Gently bite into the curve of flesh on either side of her neck, taking a generous amount of it into your mouth; alternate between pressure and suction. Writhing and cooing are good responses; screaming and threats mean you've taken the Cujo act too far.

The figure-eight tongue technique. When you're at her service down below, work the supersensitive area around her clitoris in a figure-eight pattern. Arouse her with gentle sucking until the little button swells, then carefully expose the area with your fingers. Use the slippery underside of your tongue to circle it to the left and then to the right. With the rougher, top side of the tongue, flick from right to left and then up and down. Finally, work up to figure eights, alternating between your tongue's smooth underside and the firmer tip. Constantly vary the degrees of pressure you use.

Latin-style thrusting. Latin lovers often thrust in a circular motion. Whether they got that from salsa dancing, or salsa got it from the thrusting pattern, we'll never know. Either way, it not only creates a good internal massage but provides the right friction on her hot spots as well as around the vaginal opening. Rotary motion also gives the woman a feeling of more volume—of truly being filled.

Time it right. Most women have memorized the two times that men want sex: when they're awake and when they're asleep. Anytime except during the game. Women are trickier. Flowers and dinners and foot rubs work. Sometimes. Then there are the times when her desire comes out of nowhere. Here are six occasions when her lustiness may take you by surprise.

When someone she cares about dies. Your squeeze is craving comfort and affirmation of life, and sex fills that bill. What better way than sex to celebrate being alive? It's the same reason there's so much food at funerals. Both sex and food are ways to reinforce vitality and appease the senses.

When her friend is going through a breakup. She's just heard every detail of her friend's war of the roses. She'll look at you and think about how lucky she is, and she may want sex to reinforce her own sense of security.

When it's that time of the month. She may be nervous as she awaits her period, especially if she's not craving motherhood. When she gets it, she'll feel relieved. This makes some women (warning: just some) feel sexy and adventurous. A woman is very aware of her sexuality at this time, and hormones are raging. And that's not always bad.

When she finishes a 70-hour week. She wants you to focus on her pleasure and needs. She might want the comfort of being near somebody who cares for her, who will understand that she wants sex but she might be too tired to do a lot of the work.

When she's just bought a killer pair of jeans. Trying on clothing often gets a woman in the mood for sex because she's turned on by enhancing herself—either by being happy with her body or just by buying an article of clothing she feels good about.

When you just broke up. She wants sex now, to make one last emotional connection with you and to show you what you'll be missing.

Give Yourself a Big Hand

How masturbation can improve your sex life, boost the quality of your sperm, and even make you look good at work

By Stephen Rae

Twice a week, Howard, a 34-year-old engineer, slips out of bed where his wife lies asleep, and creeps downstairs to watch porn videos and masturbate. "It's something I've done since I was single," he says. "When we first got married, I did it less because we had more sex. But we've been married for 6 years now and have two young kids, so things are different."

Once, he says, his wife walked in and caught him. "It was slightly embarrassing, but surprisingly she didn't make a big deal of it. Actually, I think she's half-glad: This way, I don't have to bother her when she's tired."

Twice a week is also the number of times Nick, a 32-year-old businessman, masturbates in the men's room at his office. That's about as often as he has sex with his girlfriend, but he says it serves a different purpose. "I suppose fantasizing is better, sometimes," he says. "It's a spur-of-the-moment thing." While he has gotten over his initial guilt about it, he still wouldn't dream of telling his girlfriend. "I don't feel I'm doing anything wrong," he says, "but it's a very private thing, and that gives it an extra kick."

NOTHING WASTED, NOTHING GAINED

Concerned you're "wasting" perfectly good sperm when you give yourself a hand? Don't be. The sperm produced during masturbation is very different from that produced during intercourse, explains Robin Baker, Ph.D., professor of zoology in Manchester, England, and coauthor of *Human Sperm Competition: Copulation, Masturbation and Infidelity.*

"Under the microscope, copulatory ejaculates look much more fertile than masturbatory ones," Baker says. "Since sperm for in-vitro fertilization is usually obtained through masturbation, this may explain the low success rate of the procedure," he points out.

According to sexologists, this kind of furtive behavior isn't unusual. In fact, masturbation is the most commonly kept sexual secret in relationships. So what's all the secrecy about? Why the taboo?

"Sadly, some men still view it as an issue of self-esteem or inadequacy," says New York City sexologist Betty Dodson, Ph.D., author of *Sex for One*. "They feel 'a real man doesn't do this' or 'I should be having sex.' Some men who write to me feel very positive about masturbation, though, because it allows them to be more in touch with their own sexual desires. But I doubt if they share that information with other men."

Our own—unscientific—survey of colleagues and friends yielded a variety of reasons men masturbate. Some were obvious, such as the lack of an available partner, but others were less expected.

"I tend to do it more when I'm anxious, if I'm really stressed at work, or if I'm trying to wrap up a big deal," one 29-year-old stockbroker confided.

Bernie Zilbergeld, Ph.D., a psychotherapist in Oakland, California, and author of *The New Male Sexuality*, considers this typical. "A lot of people use it to relax," he says. "Men say that having an orgasm before talks or an important business presentation relaxes them." Just remember not to masturbate *during* your presentation.

WHY WE GO IT ALONE

Many men claim that orgasms they have when masturbating are actually much better than the ones they have with their partners. "The buildup of sexual tension is more controllable and intense with masturbation," says Howard. "I find it more satisfying than intercourse in a curious way."

There's a good reason for this. "You are the best expert on your own body; you provide the best sensational experience that even a lover can't match," says therapist and sexologist Michael Perring.

Not having to concern yourself with a partner's needs allows for total immersion in fantasy, which can be as wild as you care to make it. "Sometimes the emotional input (of sex with a partner) can actually reduce the intensity of the orgasm; sometimes there's conflict between intimacy and sex," says sex therapist Martin Cole, Ph.D., of Birmingham, England. "For some people, sharing is crucial. But other people simply prefer this intense sexual, genital reward."

There may also be subtle physiological differences between coital and masturbatory arousal and orgasm. "The glands that secrete pre-ejaculative

**HOW OFTEN
THE AVERAGE GUY MASTURBATES:** ONCE A DAY

FOUR GOOD REASONS TO BUFF THE BANANA

It's normal. In one survey, 90 percent of men interviewed said they had masturbated at some time in their lives. And those who masturbate most often were between ages 25 and 34.

It's useful. Not only does masturbation allow us to discover our own sex triggers; it's also recommended by sex therapists for men suffering from impotence and premature ejaculation. Some therapists believe that masturbation without ejaculation an hour or so before sex can produce a firmer erection and better staying power.

It's a mark of intelligence. According to a 1994 survey, 80 percent of men with college degrees reported masturbating in the current year, as opposed to fewer than 50 percent of those without.

It may help get her pregnant. Masturbating actually may serve a purpose in human reproductive strategy, says Robin Baker, Ph.D., professor of zoology in Manchester, England, and coauthor of *Human Sperm Competition: Copulation, Masturbation and Infidelity.* "Sperm older than about 4 days are often dead or tend to be slower and have coiled tails," Baker says, "and they get in the way of the younger, healthier sperm."

If there is a long interval between acts of intercourse—say, 4 or more days—"then there is a reproductive advantage in shedding the sperm that are waiting, and replacing them with new stock."

fluid often aren't switched on in masturbation, but they are in kissing or sex play," Cole explains. "So you've got a different set of neural circuits working, and this will influence the nature and quality of the orgasm you experience."

LOCATION, LOCATION, LOCATION

We were surprised to find out *where* men masturbate—in the bedroom or bathroom at home, of course, but also at work. "One thing that's never been addressed is men who wank at work," says Neil. "I was out with a group of men and women, and we just started talking about wanking. After a few beers most of the men said they had done it in the office men's room. The women were horrified."

WHAT THE OTHER HALF THINK

Not all women are so outraged, though. "He'd better," says Vanessa, a legal secretary, when asked if her husband masturbates. "After an 18-hour day, all I'm thinking of is going to sleep, so he has to fend for himself." And Jane, a colleague who walked in on our conversation, said that when she found her first husband's porn magazines in the back of a wardrobe, she wasn't upset by the mags but rather by the fact that he was hiding them from her.

But some women react badly. Avodah Offit, M.D., a New York City–based psychiatrist and author of *Virtual Love,* once made an emergency, middle-of-the-night house call to calm a patient who was "disturbed and appalled" when she woke up to find that her husband was masturbating in bed. "Her naïveté was such that she believed her husband's sole sexual outlet was her," she recalls. "A lot of women see sexuality as something expressed by two people together rather than by one person on their own."

Most women aren't so upset about male masturbation so much as intrigued by it. "The problem I've always had with women in my life is that they want to know what I think about when I masturbate," Neil says. "They assume I must be fantasizing about them. In reality my imagination is a lot more adventurous than that."

The good news is that this kind of fantasy can be beneficial to your sex life. According to Michael Perelman, Ph.D., a sex and marital therapist in New York City, wives who see masturbation as a form of "mental adultery" aren't recognizing its value in maintaining monogamy by providing variety in thought rather than deed. "A woman who has the attitude 'He can think about whoever he wants, as long as he brings it home to me' is most likely to have the best sexual relationship."

SLOW HAND

A final question: When men masturbate, how long do they take? Not too long, claim our respondents. "I'm sure there are real artists out there who turn it into an entire evening," says Lloyd, who has it down to 90 seconds. "For me, it's very much a function, and I just want to get it over with."

To sexologist Betty Dodson, this kind of talk is anathema. We should all be setting aside 30 minutes to an hour to do the job properly, she insists. "It breaks my heart that men are doing it and not enjoying it as much as they could be."

KNOW THIS

Bar None

Looking for that special someone? Skip happy hour and head to Borders. Bookstores, independent record stores, libraries, and cool movie rental places all rate higher than bars for meeting potential girlfriends.

Don't Go There

Expecting a child? If so, you may want to avoid performing oral sex on your wife until after she gives birth. Researchers at the University of Michigan recently discovered that streptococcus bacteria can be spread easily during sexual activity, particularly oral sex. While the bacteria are harmless to most adults, they can be deadly to infants—causing pneumonia, sepsis, and meningitis. It's still perfectly safe for her to satisfy you, however.

Love Sick

Married couples may share more than home, car, bed, and bath. Try high blood pressure, depression, asthma, and ulcers. (Happy anniversary!) According to a new British study, people who live together are much more likely to develop the same diseases. In a study of 8,000 couples, researchers found that men whose partners suffered from asthma, depression, ulcers, high blood pressure, or high cholesterol were up to 70 percent likelier to develop the condition themselves.

Keep Your Blood Pressure in Check

A study of 220 men found that guys with normal blood pressure have sex 25 percent more often than men with high blood pressure. Why? Men with

PERCENTAGE DECREASE IN A MAN'S RISK
OF HAVING A HEART ATTACK OR STROKE
IF HE HAS SEX AT LEAST THREE TIMES A WEEK: 50

normal blood pressure have more testosterone, doctors say. That translates into better bloodflow to the penis—and firmer erections.

Know Your Blood Sugar

If you're having difficulty achieving and maintaining an erection, ask your doctor to give you a fasting blood sugar test. In a study published in the *British Journal of Urology*, researchers tested 129 men complaining of erectile dysfunction and found that diabetes was causing the impotence in 22 of them, six of whom didn't even know they had the disease.

Keep It Up

While Siberian ginseng is purported to be an erection booster, only the rarer red Korean kind has actually helped guys defy gravity. In a recent study of men with erectile dysfunction, researchers found that 60 percent of those who took 900 milligrams of Korean ginseng three times daily had improved erections, compared with only 20 percent of the placebo poppers. "It's known to have a positive effect on bloodflow," says Natan Bar-Chama, M.D., assistant professor of urology at Mount Sinai School of Medicine in New York City. "Theoretically, there may be a benefit for men with impotence." You can find red Korean ginseng in most health food stores.

DOWN THE PIKE

A Quicker Picker-Upper

It takes half an hour for a Viagra pill to work its magic. That's too long to wait, say researchers at Nastech Pharmaceutical who have developed a nasal spray that gives you an erection in less than 15 minutes. The spray's active ingredient, apomorphine, stimulates your brain's dopamine receptors—which are responsible for triggering arousal.

"Signals go from the brain through the spinal cord and right to the penis, so the effect is faster than swallowing a pill and waiting for it to enter your bloodstream," says Steven Quay, M.D., Ph.D., the product's developer. The apomorphine spray could be on the market sometime this year, pending FDA approval.

Measles May Help Stop AIDS

Researchers have discovered that measles may delay the growth of the HIV virus. In a study of African children with HIV, physicians found that viral levels of the disease were lower in children who also had the measles, compared with children with HIV alone. The discovery may advance development of an AIDS vaccine.

Just around the Bend

Peyronie's disease is a condition that occurs when scar tissue forms in the penis, causing your erection to curve at an odd angle during sex, making sex uncomfortable and even painful. The new injectable drug, Cordase, may dissolve scar tissue, helping to straighten curved penises. Clinical trials of Cordase—which was designed to help wounds heal faster—found that it also cures up to 50 percent of Peyronie's cases. Further clinical trials are under way.

CITY WITH THE HIGHEST IMPOTENCE RATE: ATLANTA

CITY WITH THE LOWEST IMPOTENCE RATE: ANCHORAGE

GAME PLAN

A Weekend Away
How to execute the perfect romantic escape

After a year of unspeakable child-rearing mayhem, you've decided to escape to a posh hotel sans kiddies for a weekend of intimacy, romance . . . hell, sex. Follow these tips to make the most of your weekend away.

Tip big. Always tip room service at least $5 after you sign the tab; it shows that you know the gratuity is in the bill, but you want to be generous.

Ask for the honeymoon package. Some hotel chains, such as Hilton and Hyatt, offer "romance packages" that may include champagne, breakfast, and late checkout. Always tell the hotel staff it's a special occasion beforehand, advises Matthias Sandner, director of the Towers at the New York Palace Hotel. You may snag a scenic view or other favors.

Bring some bubbly. "Champagne is the only way to go," says Ralph Hersom, wine director for Le Cirque 2000 in New York City. Bring your own and keep it on ice all weekend. Hersom's picks: Ruinart 1990 Brut or Perrier Jouet Brut NV ($35 to $60); Laurent-Perrier Brut NV or Veuve Clicquot Yellow Label Brut NV ($20 to $50).

Surprise her. If the hotel is less than an hour from home, "leave her a note with directions to the hotel—and a key to the room," says sex therapist Linda De Villers, Ph.D., author of *Love Skills: More Fun Than You've Ever Had with Sex, Intimacy and Communication.* The note should tell her to bring nothing—you've taken care of it all, says De Villers.

Don't forget flowers. Order flowers from a nearby shop (not the hotel) and have a bellhop bring them to the room. Red roses can't fail, but a mix of purple lilacs and yellow tulips near the bed, and white hyacinths next to the bathtub, scores points for ingenuity, says Jennifer Stone, co-owner of Stonekelly Florists in New York City.

Be prepared. Assemble a bag of tricks, advises Pepper Schwartz, Ph.D., coauthor of *The Great Sex Weekend.* Suggestions: scented candles, massage oil, scented bubble bath, body paint, lubricants, silk scarves, condoms, and some red lightbulbs—to help create a low-rent New Orleans decadent thing.

Remember to refuel. You'll be famished between rounds. Bring smoked salmon, fresh grapes and strawberries, olives, crusty French bread, a wheel of good Brie cheese, and Godiva chocolates, advises De Villers. Store perishables in the room refrigerator; you'll save about three million bucks in room service.

TAKE ACTION

Men, quite rightly, are known for their appreciation of tools, their proper maintenance, and their most effective use. Which makes it that much more shocking that we fail to properly maintain our own carnal implements, be they mini-drivers or 12-inch drill bits. From puberty onward, our tools suffer all kinds of self-abuse and outward abuse, from overexcitement in tight Levi's to weekend-long binges with women from whom we caught everything but their names. The result, long-term, can be a dulled edge, a balky ball bearing, a flexible extension for the wrench when only a rigid one will do the job.

Luckily these eight tool-saving tips will keep you sharp well into your master craftsman days. And you'd better pay heed: If you're not careful, the woman in your life just might invoke the inviolable rule of tools: "If you want something done right, hire a handyman."

1. Avoid penis shrinkers (a.k.a. cigarettes). In a study conducted at the University of Kentucky, researchers found that when asked to rate their sex lives on a scale of one to 10, men who smoked averaged about a five—a far cry from nonsmokers, who rated theirs at nine.

One reason, of course, is that smoking is a known cause of impotence. And there's some evidence that smoking affects erection size. In one study, researchers found that smokers' penises are significantly smaller than nonsmokers'. "In addition to damaging blood vessels, smoking may cause damage to penile tissue itself, making it less elastic and preventing it from stretching," says Irwin Goldstein, M.D., a urologist at the Boston University School of Medicine. We have yet to hear a better reason to quit.

2. Get a vasectomy. If you're finished producing offspring (or you're absolutely sure you don't want kids), consider investing in permanent renovations at the sperm factory. "The risk of a contraceptive failure can be a big source of anxiety for some men, especially those who've had a birth control disaster—or a scare—in the past," says Karen Donahey, Ph.D., director of the sex and marital therapy program at Northwestern University in Evanston, Illinois. That anxiety can in turn lead to erection problems—and cause the same vicious circle that makes performance anxiety such a mood killer. But if there's no sperm, the risk of pregnancy is beyond minuscule: A properly performed vasectomy has an effectiveness rate of 99.9 percent. And at $1,500, it's a bargain compared with college tuition.

3. Fire your mistress. It's common for men who start having affairs to stop having erections—so common, in fact, that doctors who treat erectile dysfunction often ask their patients if they're getting any action on the side. Unless your wife knows about, approves of, and participates in your new sex life—in which case, we'd like to meet her—you're bound to feel at least a little guilty about it when you're with her. Guilt can turn to anxiety, and that can kill an erection.

4. Lose your gut. Next to joining a monastery, having diabetes is the quickest route to a lifetime of celibacy. In fact, more than 50 percent of all men with diabetes are impotent. The disease hits the penis with a double whammy. It accelerates the process of arterial disease, and it slows the transmission of stimuli along nerves throughout your body. And trust us—a numb penis is not a happy penis.

Staying trim is the best way to avoid diabetes. If it's too late for that, be vigilant in checking your blood sugar (talk to your doctor about the best methods). Men who are sloppy about controlling their levels have 70 percent more erection problems than those who stay on top of it, according to an Italian study.

5. Avoid ramming your penis into hard objects. One vigorously misplaced thrust is all it takes to rupture the corposa cavernosa, the elongated "erectile chambers" that run the length of your penis. Don't believe us? Try aiming your erect penis at the trunk of a tree—it's roughly the same density as your partner's pubic bone. A complete rupture will require surgery within 24 hours to stanch internal bleeding and reduce the risk of permanent damage. A partial tear isn't as serious, but it may cause problems later on. As the lining of the corposa heals over with scar tissue, it loses its elasticity—leading to curvature, pain, and eventually impotence. By some estimates, more than a third of impotent men have a history of "penile trauma." To protect yourself, be careful when she's on top. That's the position most likely to cause damage.

6. Skip the taxi. Start walking. In one recent study, researchers found that men who walked just 2 miles a day had half the rate of erection problems of more sedentary men, says Dr. Goldstein. (Twenty minutes of jogging or 30 minutes of weight training will work, too.)

Deposits that clog or stiffen penile arteries can wilt an erection faster than a cold shower. "Guys tend to think of their arteries as simple pipes that can become clogged, but there's a lot more going on than that," says Laurence Levine, M.D., a urologist at Rush-Presbyterian Medical Center in Chicago. "The linings of those blood vessels are very biologically active areas where

NUMBER OF ORGASMS MEN SHOULD HAVE EVERY WEEK FOR OPTIMAL HEALTH, ACCORDING TO UROLOGISTS: TWO OR THREE

chemicals are being made and released into the bloodstream." The more you exercise, the healthier, cleaner, and more flexible those linings become.

7. Yawn a lot. As far as your body's concerned, yawning and getting an erection are practically the same thing. They're both controlled by a chemical called nitric oxide. Released in the brain, it can either travel to the neurons that control mouth opening and breathing, or go down the spinal cord to the blood vessels that feed the penis. Sometimes it does both (that's why a big yawn can cause a tremor down under). We don't recommend foreplay with your mouth hanging open. But allowing yourself to yawn now and then throughout the day may help prime the neurochemical pathways that lead to good, sturdy erections.

8. Fall asleep immediately after the last thrust. We know: You hate to give up on 1 minute of postcoital pillow talk, but ultimately you're going comatose for her. Your penis needs as much shut-eye as it can get.

Every night while you sleep, you have between three and five hour-long erections. You probably noticed this phenomenon the last time you had to pee at 4 A.M. Those erections are not there just to make life interesting for your bedmate. They work to recharge your penis—keeping it well-nourished with oxygenated blood. "Theoretically, the more nocturnal erections you have, the more flexible your erectile tissue will become. And that may help keep erections strong as the years wear on," explains Dr. Goldstein.

ANY QUESTIONS?

Toys in Babeland

My girlfriend wants to use a vibrator during sex. Is there something wrong with me?

—L.M., Arlington, Virginia

No, there's nothing wrong with you. In fact, just the opposite. "It shows that she trusts you, that you've built a great deal of intimacy together, and that she's not afraid to try new things with you," says Susan Crain Bakos, a sexologist and author of *Sexational Secrets*. "If she wasn't satisfied with your performance, she'd be faking her orgasms with you and using the vibrator behind your back."

A vibrator isn't stud service. It's simply value added. Check out the Sweet Heart Vibe ($40, www.babeland.com). This tiny, 2-inch, heart-shaped, battery-operated, jelly rubber vibrator can stimulate her clitoris (less work for you!) during foreplay while her hands—and yours—are free to roam. And what's the downside? She begs you for more?

I Got the Blues

Sometimes my girlfriend and I get interrupted, and if we don't resume, my testicles ache. Are "blue balls" dangerous?

—J.P., Detroit

No, but if you want to tell her that it's dangerous, we'll keep quiet. What you're feeling is called epididymitis. When you are in a state of arousal, the passage (called the epididymis) leading from each testicle to your penis fills with sperm, blood flows to the pelvic area, and reproductive fluids build up. If there's a shutdown, an inflammatory reaction occurs in the epididymis. This is the ache you feel. There's another version as well. If (as we suspect) you have an active sex life that goes on hiatus, you may get a similar feeling. An aspirin can ease the discomfort. So can your hand.

Too Hot to Handle

Can hot tubs really make a man sterile?

—D.T., Burlington, Vermont

Not if you have a normal sperm count, says Neil Baum, M.D., a urologist at the Tulane University School of Medicine in New Orleans. However, if your sperm count is low, a hot tub will help keep it there and also make your boys slow swimmers. The fix: Keep the water temp lower than scrotal temperature, about 97°F, and get out before your eggs are hard-boiled.

Down for the Count

After my wife and I have sex, I can't get another erection for hours. Am I becoming impotent?

—L.K., San Antonio

You're being way too hard on yourself. Every football game has a halftime, and after orgasm all men have a "refractory period," when they're more wet noodle than Norwegian wood. (Even porn stars can't spring back instantly, which is why there are film editors.) The purpose of your penile downtime: to restore your penis's supply of blood and ejaculatory fluids. The younger you are, the shorter your downtime, from 10 minutes (or less, remember?) for a teenager to hours, even days, for older men. But in any case, it's just a temporary letdown, not impotence, says Daniel S. Stein, M.D., author of *Passionate Sex: Discover the Special Power in You.* "There's nothing wrong, nothing broken," Dr. Stein says. "Don't worry; the erection will soon return, often stronger than before."

In the meantime, Dr. Stein suggests making the most of the one good orgasm you do have. To improve the quality of your erection and your ejaculatory control, practice the pelvic crunch exercise, similar to the exercise for women developed by the Los Angeles doctor Arnold Kegel, who remains one of our personal heroes. The exercise targets your pubococcygeus, or PC, muscle—the one you use to cut off your urine flow. "Squeeze, hold for a few

PERCENTAGE OF MEN WHO ARE AFFECTED BY A PMS-LIKE BEHAVIOR DISORDER CALLED IRRITABLE MALE SYNDROME, WHICH TRIGGERS A BAD TEMPER AND DROP IN LIBIDO: NEARLY 50

seconds, and relax those muscles. Do three sets of 20 repetitions while you're sitting at a stoplight, writing a report, anywhere. You'll soon become aware of your ability to control those muscles and delay orgasm until you choose," he says. Like when she screams, "NOW, NOW, NOW!"

Double Dribble

I take a leak, give it a shake, and then still dribble into my boxers. Never used to happen. I'm 35, not ready for Depends. What's up?

—B.L., Bismarck, North Dakota

It's called postvoid dribble. Most likely, urine is getting trapped in your urethra, either by an enlarged prostate or by scar tissue in the urethra from an old injury or infection. Spicy foods and caffeine can affect your prostate, too. Suspect infection if you feel slight burning at the tip, or discomfort after ejaculation—and get antibiotics.

Drugs like Flomax can improve urine flow. Saw palmetto works, too. (Buy ProstActive; it's got the best herb in it.) As for the enlarged prostate, try frequent ejaculations. (You can take it from here, yes?)

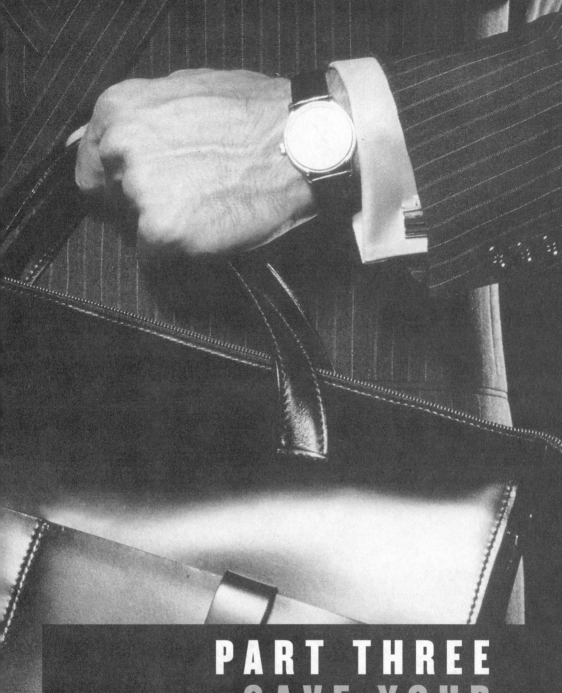

PART THREE
SAVE YOUR
SICK DAYS

Who Will Beat Back Pain First?

One of these spasm sufferers—or you?

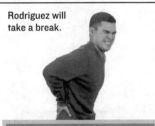

Rodriguez will take a break.

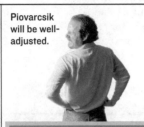

Piovarcsik will be well-adjusted.

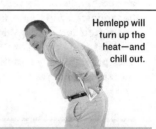

Hemlepp will turn up the heat—and chill out.

ABE RODRIGUEZ
Age 22, 5'6", 150 lb
Truck driver,
Denton, Texas

JOHN PIOVARCSIK
Age 36, 5'8", 170 lb
Record store owner,
Manteca, California

MIKE HEMLEPP
Age 37, 5'7", 215 lb
Prosecutor,
Winnsboro, South Carolina

HIS BACKBREAKER
• On the job, delivering beer.

HIS PLAN
• Rest on the couch for a few days while taking over-the-counter ibuprofen—200 milligrams every 4 to 6 hours, the dosage recommended on the label.

ADVANTAGES
• Rodriguez gets a break from his job. (As a deliveryman for a major brewery, he lifts roughly 300 cases of beer daily.)

• Ibuprofen is an anti-inflammatory that treats not just the symptoms but also the cause of pain, helping him heal.

• He's 22, and youth speeds healing.

DISADVANTAGES
• Too much rest can actually weaken the back. "The whole idea is to temper your activity, not stop it," says Ralph Rashbaum, M.D., cofounder of the Texas Back Institute, headquartered in Plano.

• Rodriguez may not be taking enough ibuprofen. "The label dose is good for a headache," says Dr. Rashbaum, but it may not touch a backache. He recommends 800 milligrams three or four times daily.

HIS BACKBREAKER
• Playing soccer.

HIS PLAN
• Visit a chiropractor once a week.

ADVANTAGES
• Piovarcsik is seeing a back specialist. This raises his recovery chances not just from treatment but also from the advice he'll get about preventing future back strain.

• According to Dr. Rashbaum, short-term chiropractic care—usually 4 to 6 weeks—can be effective in eliminating muscular lower-back pain.

• Daily stretching is a big help in rehab.

DISADVANTAGES
• Piovarcsik's job keeps him on his feet all day and requires some light lifting (10- to 30-pound boxes) and lots of bending.

• Except for what the chiropractor does to him, Piovarcsik isn't exercising as part of his rehab—another reinjury red flag.

• He's taking no medication to ease inflammation or pain.

• At 36, he has a spine that has seen better days. Age is a factor.

HIS BACKBREAKER
• Slept on an old sofa at a vacation house.

HIS PLAN
• Follow his doctor's advice to take ibuprofen (800 milligrams three or four times a day after meals), use hot and cold packs, and do gentle exercise and stretching.

ADVANTAGES
• Hemlepp is consulting his doctor.

• He's alternating ice (twice a day for 20 minutes) with a heating pad (twice a day for 20 minutes) for 24 to 36 hours.

• His plan of light weight training three times weekly and daily stretching of the lower back, abs, hamstrings, quads, hip flexors, and glutes is recommended.

DISADVANTAGES
• Hemlepp's aggressive personality—he's a prosecutor and a competitive powerlifter—could cause him to rush his comeback.

• His dosage of painkillers is higher, which could mask the pain and tempt him to exercise harder than he should.

• At 37, he's is the oldest contestant.

And the Winner Is . . .
Mike Hemlepp

Ralph Rashbaum, M.D., a spinal surgeon and cofounder of the Texas Back Institute, headquartered in Plano, helped us design our quiz to determine which contestant has the best chance of beating minor muscular back pain. Take it yourself and see if you, too, can be pain-free.

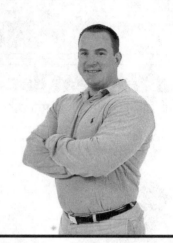

FINAL ANALYSIS

Back spasms, or what Dr. Rashbaum calls "weekend-warrior syndrome," can humble a grown man. He sees hundreds stagger into his clinic begging for mercy—and rightly so. If your back hurts, life sucks.

Hemlepp's doctor-recommended plan of medication, hot and cold packs, and gentle exercise (stretching and light weight lifting) is the best starting point—and usually the ending point—for any man with muscular back pain. "The majority of patients on this type of program respond in 72 hours," says Dr. Rashbaum. "After that, they just have to be careful doing what injured them in the first place."

As for Piovarcsik, the doctor says there's nothing wrong with his trip to the chiropractor, other than timing. Dr. Rashbaum and his colleagues at the Texas Back Institute usually reserve chiropractic treatment for those patients who don't respond to Hemlepp's style of treatment, which is the first line of offense. And why pay a chiropractor when the cheaper self-treatment usually works? That said, Dr. Rashbaum fully supports chiropractic care. "One knack chiropractors have is getting patients out of pain quickly," he says. "My only caveat is that if there's no improvement in 2 weeks, something else needs to be done." It could be physical therapy, or it could be a consultation with an orthopedic surgeon to see if the injury involves more than muscle.

Rodriguez's self-prescribed rest and ibuprofen could help him, Dr. Rashbaum says, but not nearly as quickly as ice, heat, and exercise would. And he's doing nothing to strengthen his back to ward off another injury, which is bound to happen in the beer delivery business. Bottom line: When back pain strikes, one of the things you don't do is nothing.

Spinal Map

FACTOR	POINT VALUE	ABE	JOHN	MIKE	YOU
AGE Your spine degenerates with age, increasing your risk of injury and your recovery time.	Under 30? +1 Over 30? −1	+1	−1	−1	
ACTIVITY LEVEL Sedentary people are less prone to back injury because of their lack of activity, but once hurt, they take the longest to recover.	Daily activity/exercise? +1 Some activity/exercise? 0 Couch potato? −1	+1	+1	+1	
HEAVY LIFTING AT WORK Shouldering big loads is a reinjury risk, and men injured on the job are less motivated to go back to the activity that hurt them.	No lifting? +1 Some lifting? 0 Lots of lifting? −2	−2	0	+1	
MOTIVATION TO RECOVER How aggressive your personality is will determine your reinjury risk. Slow and steady wins this race.	Gung-ho personality? −1 Everything at medium speed +1 Just plain lazy? −2	+1	+1	−1	
WEIGHT TRAINING Working the abs, lower back, glutes, hamstrings, quads, and hip flexors can help back pain.	Light weights 2 or 3 times a week? +1 No weight training? −1	−1	−1	+1	
STRETCHING Even mild work on those above-mentioned muscles can speed rehabilitation.	Stretch daily? +2 Stretch less than daily? +1 Do no stretching? −1	−1	+2	+2	
MEDICATIONS A high dosage of ibuprofen (800 milligrams 3 or 4 times a day after meals) can help heal muscular inflammation.	High dosage? +1 Moderate dosage? 0 Drug-free? −1	0	−1	+1	
HOT AND COLD PACKS Alternating icing and heating for the first 24 to 36 hours promotes healing.	Fire and ice? +1 No compresses? −1	−1	−1	+1	
DOCTOR A medical exam will provide the best advice—and determine if your problem is more than just a spasm.	Made the appointment? +1 Toughing it out? −1	−1	+1	+1	
MANIPULATION Short-term chiropractic care can be effective.	Getting chiropractic care? +1 Not seeing a chiropractor? −1	−1	+1	−1	
SMOKING There's a correlation between smoking and back injuries. (Chronic coughing can injure disks in the spine.)	Smoke-free? 0 Puffin' away? −2	0	0	0	
TOTALS		−4	2	5	

▶ IF YOUR SCORE IS 5 OR HIGHER: You'll be back in business in no time.

▶ IF YOUR SCORE IS 0 TO 4: You're on the road to recovery. Continue seeing that nurse.

▶ IF YOUR SCORE IS LESS THAN 0: Picture yourself in a brace.

MUST READS

Treat Yourself

When illness strikes, you can let your doctor wage war for you. Or—like these tough guys—you can take matters into your own hands

By Mike Zimmerman

We lead heroic lives. Then we get sick. Achilles had his heel problem. Superman, his allergy to kryptonite. Dylan, his pericarditis (and worse, no words that rhymed with it). And our reaction to sickness—be it interstitial or interstellar in nature—is not a battle cry, but denial, then some creative profanity, then surrender.

Well, fellas, that plan is obsolete. You can beat any ailment—actually hold it at arm's length while it snaps at the air like a baby bulldog in a *Tom and Jerry* short. We've assembled a group of men who have done just that to their worst health problems. The guys have one thing in common: They took control of their situations, got their own help, and found a way back. Are they medical miracles? Nope, just regular guys with great stories who want to show how you, too, can kick the tail of what ails you.

HIGH BLOOD PRESSURE
How he beat it: Tomato juice and cayenne pepper

Jerome Kotch, 55, stews in his share of daily stress as a bank examiner for the Federal Reserve (no, he doesn't know Alan). Fifteen years ago, the Berkeley Heights, New Jersey, resident was diagnosed with high blood pressure (147/95) during a routine physical. His doctor put him on a diuretic blood pressure pill, hydrochlorothiazide. Only problem: "It made me dizzy, and I'd feel like I was about to pass out," he says.

After follow-up blood work showed that the diuretic was lowering Kotch's potassium and magnesium levels, his doctor prescribed supplements to take with the medication. But Kotch still felt like a man without a floor under him. Fed up, he stopped all the pill popping and tried a natural remedy: tomato juice and cayenne pepper. "It's an acquired taste," says Kotch. But after only a month, the spicy new cocktail had lowered his blood pressure. Kotch now walks and bikes regularly, and his BP checks in at a robust 123/80.

Make it work for you: Before you agree to go on blood pressure medicines, ask your doctor if you can try Kotch's daily concoction: 8 ounces of low-sodium V8 juice with a teaspoon of cayenne (stirred well). "There are probably three reasons why it worked," says Joe D. Goldstrich, M.D., F.A.C.C., a cardiologist in Henderson, Nevada. First, cayenne delivers capsaicin—the "heat" in peppers—which has been found to have some positive effect on blood pressure. Also, the antioxidant punch of the lycopene in the tomatoes could knock out free radicals, an excess of which can raise blood pressure. And then there's the high potassium content of tomato juice. "Potassium tends to take the place of sodium in the body's tissues," says Dr. Goldstrich. Too much sodium can cause arterial walls to retain water, boosting BP.

CLAUSTROPHOBIA
How he beat it: His imagination

Wigging out is no picnic. Wigging out in high school, on a bus to a football game, coming this close to screaming "Stop the bus!" is excruciating. That was the moment when Terry Welch, now a 31-year-old communications specialist in Kansas City, Missouri, realized that his claustrophobia was beyond his control. But professional help wasn't wired into his thinking. "I grew up in a small town in Kansas," he says. "You didn't go to a psychologist for your problem. You rubbed some dirt on it and moved on."

One night while he was bathing—in a small bathroom with no windows—panic crept in again . . . and Welch decided to try something radical. He shut the lights off and stuffed a towel under the door, creating a pitch-black environment where, for 15 minutes at a clip, he could pretend he was in smaller and smaller rooms. If he started to wig, he flipped the light on, and the bathroom would seem like an auditorium. After 8 months of on-and-off "self-treatment," he started to feel better. The big test came when he joined the navy and had no trouble sleeping aboard the USS *Abraham Lincoln*—an aircraft carrier with three-deep "coffin racks."

Make it work for you: Working with a doctor is advisable, of course, but "if somebody practices control, he can get over his phobia," says Harold Levinson, M.D., a psychiatrist practicing in Great Neck, New York, and author of *Phobia Free*. According to Dr. Levinson, the key is training yourself to recognize and adapt to your anxiety triggers. That's what Welch did, albeit unknowingly. "Bathrooms and tubs are enclosed spaces. By turning off the light, he allowed his apprehensions to escalate. By concentrating on these apprehensions, he lessened his anxiety," says Dr. Levinson.

PET ALLERGY
How he beat it: Kitty tranquilizers

Tom Kasle couldn't be in the same room with the family cat—and it wasn't because he's a dog person. Sneezing, mucus, itching—Kasle had it all. "My allergist couldn't give me shots, so we had to get rid of our cat," says Kasle, a 49-year-old from Maumee, Ohio. "My wife and daughter were devastated."

Seeing this heartbreak—caused by a condition he couldn't control—made Kasle try a different strategy: Treat the cat, not the human. He'd heard about a diluted sedative you can add to your cat's food to help fight severe allergies. Playing the odds, Kasle adopted a new cat and doped its water daily. After 4 weeks, Kasle felt better. These days, he can sit near Puss with nary a sneeze.

Make it work for you: Hit up your vet for the animal tranquilizer acepromazine H_2O ($12 for a month's supply). "It changes the chemical composition of the cat's saliva, making its dander less allergenic," says William Lutz, D.V.M., a veterinarian in private practice in Whitehouse, Ohio. But won't Kitty become a stumbling junkie? Absolutely not, says Dr. Lutz. "The tranquilizer is so diluted that the cat's day-to-day activity and mood are unaffected." Unfortunately, however, acepromazine doesn't work with dogs. For them, try Allerpet D, a dry shampoo (no rinsing needed) available in most pet stores.

MIGRAINE HEADACHE
How he beat it: Cutting back on carbohydrates

Every afternoon, as the northern California shadows grew long, Matt Mitchell suffered. On good days, it felt as if a pro wrestler were sitting on his head. On bad days, the 24-year-old lay in a darkened room, waiting for the pain to stop. But almost every day, the migraines returned. His doctor ran tests (all with normal results), and eventually prescribed high-dosage Tylenol. It didn't help.

A year ago, the woman he was dating asked the 275-pound Mitchell to join her on a low-carb diet she wanted to try. Not cool—at first. "I love to cook Italian food," says Mitchell. "I knew what that meant." But he gave it a shot. After 2 weeks of pasta deprivation, the migraines disappeared. "I didn't put two and two together at first," he says. "Then one night I tried a piece of cheesecake. Bam. Migraine." A big bonus: Mitchell also ended up losing 70 pounds.

Make it work for you: Relax. You don't need to swear off carbohydrates, but you can't keep bingeing on them, either. Mitchell's bread-and-beer habit may

"Two roads diverged in a wood and I—I took the one less traveled by,
and that has made all the difference."   —Robert Frost

have triggered migraines by keeping his blood sugar on a perpetual roller-coaster ride, says Lisa K. Mannix, M.D., a neurologist in private practice in Cincinnati. "Migraines are a chronic disorder. If you have them, you'll always be susceptible. But consistency of lifestyle is a key to holding them off." In addition to dramatically fluctuating blood sugar levels, all those extra carbohydrates created another migraine trigger for Mitchell: obesity. Excess weight increases the risk of sleep apnea, a nighttime breathing disorder that causes daytime headaches. If you have migraines, try limiting your carbohydrate intake to no more than 300 grams per day.

HIGH CHOLESTEROL
How he beat it: Metamucil

Joe Drozd was hardly an unfit 44-year-old: He regularly lifted weights, played basketball, and actually enjoyed yard work. His diet was essentially healthy. But that wasn't enough; high cholesterol ran in his father's bloodlines, so it runs in Drozd's blood, too. After a November 1999 test, his total cholesterol came in at 232, and his LDL—the stuff that turns arteries into the equivalent of salami—simmered at 123.

Enter Metamucil. Drozd's wife, Shelley (a *Men's Health* senior researcher), had been taking it for more than 10 years as a fiber supplement, and her cholesterol readings always came in well below normal (128 total, last time it was checked), which Joe found strange. "We eat the same foods," he says. "My doctor told me that medication was the next step, so I decided to give Metamucil a try." The plan: 1 tablespoon dissolved in a glass of water daily. Six months later, Drozd returned to the doc. His new readings: 189 total and 96 LDL, a combined 25 percent drop.

Make it work for you: Metamucil is the brand name for psyllium husk, a natural plant fiber. While it's known as a laxative, psyllium also mops up cholesterol and carries it out with the rest of the refuse. "Psyllium binds with the bile acids that form cholesterol, a process that keeps them from reabsorbing into your blood," says Ruth Patrick, Ph.D., professor emeritus of nutrition at Louisiana State University in Baton Rouge. Research has shown that people who add psyllium to their diets reduce both their total and their harmful LDL cholesterol by up to 15 percent—while keeping protective HDL levels intact. The FDA recommends 7 grams of psyllium a day, which you can get in three doses per day.

SMOKING
How he beat it: Water

Alex Mutzak had smoked hard since he was 14 years old. He estimates that if he used nicotine patches to quit, he'd need "five or six an hour." So he never tried. Then, at age 23, he started having chest pains. After some x-rays,

Mutzak learned he had fluid in his left lung. His doctor gave him two options: Quit smoking, or drown internally.

Mutzak chose to drown—but in a far different sense. He went cold turkey, and anytime he craved a butt, he drank water. And cravings carpet bombed him. "You should see the backseat of my car," he says. "I have the biggest collection of empty bottles anywhere." Still, those 10 24-ounce bottles a day kept him from lighting up. And with time, his cravings evaporated. He cleaned his ashtray in January 2002 and hasn't used it since.

Make it work for you: Mutzak used a basic kick-the-addiction technique called substitution, according to Tom Horvath, Ph.D., a psychologist in La Jolla, California, who specializes in addiction and is the author of *Sex, Drugs, Gambling, and Chocolate*. In essence, Mutzak replaced his craving for cigarettes with a craving for water—not the water itself but the hand-to-mouth act of drinking it. "People can develop secondary addictions this way," says Horvath. "But a water addiction is definitely better than cigarettes." So if you're trying to kick the habit, find a sensible sub. Reach for water or lollipops every time you feel the urge—or exercise, which all of our experts recommend and which will keep you puffing in a better way than you are now.

BACK PAIN
How he beat it: Rock climbing

At age 63, George Knorr was the stereotypical old man shuffling down the street, holding his back. On the worst days, he'd go 50 feet before he'd have to stop to let the pain subside. His doctor diagnosed arthritis and recommended Tylenol. His chiropractor twisted him like origami for a full year. "And my back still didn't feel any better," he says.

Then his son opened a climbing gym in his hometown of Reading, Pennsylvania, and Knorr watched men of all ages pulling themselves up the walls. One day he reached up, grabbed a handhold, and hung from it. "My back didn't hurt any more than it already did. So I kept doing it," he says. After 2 weeks of hanging out, his back felt good enough to do easy climbs two or three times a week. After a few months, the pain was gone. Now a spry 69-year-old, Knorr still climbs. And walks. And runs. "I can do anything," he says.

Make it work for you: "Stretching is the bottom line for beating back pain," says Ronald Lawrence, M.D., founder of the American Medical Athletic Association in Bethesda, Maryland. "By climbing, George stretched muscles he would never have stretched otherwise." And he did it right—started slowly, saw results, and then upped his workouts. To get the same benefit (without wearing a harness), Dr. Lawrence recommends this wake-up stretch: Lie on your back and bring your right knee to your chest, clasping your ankle. Hold for a 10-count. Straighten your leg and repeat with the left leg, then do both legs at once.

BAD EYESIGHT
How he beat it: Optical calisthenics

Twenty-six-year-old Orlin Sorensen dreamed of flying combat missions like his grandfather, but his 20/80 eyesight kept him below standards for naval flight training (20/30, no glasses or surgeries allowed). Commercial airlines, however, aren't as strict—for several years, Sorensen flew for Horizon Air while wearing glasses. Then came September 11, leaving the airline industry decimated and Sorensen flying a lot less. "I was bummed, but I decided to try to turn my life around," he says.

He used the time to put a curiosity to the test: Can a man improve his vision by "exercising" his eyes? Inspired by World War II fighter pilots who used vision-training exercises, and by a 1920 book by Dr. William Bates (*The Bates Method for Better Eyesight without Glasses*), Sorensen stockpiled information until he had enough exercises to begin his own program. "I trained my eyes to do things they don't normally do," Sorensen says. "I treated the program like physical exercise." He "worked out" 25 minutes a day, 6 days a week, for 30 days, doing exercises like slowly rolling his eyes in a full circle. The results? The navy measured his vision at 20/30, he no longer needs glasses, and he's been accepted for pilot training.

Make it work for you: Improving your sight by retraining your eye muscles is "very doable," says William Moskowitz, F.C.O.V.D., an optometrist who has helped scores of patients with vision training at the Park Vision Therapy Center in Bridgewater, New Jersey. But different vision problems require different programs, so Dr. Moskowitz recommends you consult a behavioral optometrist. (Find one who's board-certified in vision therapy, at www.covd.org/membersearch.php.) After you're matched up with the right program, the follow-through is up to you—you have to do the exercises every day.

ALCOHOL ABUSE
How he beat it: Superstition

Alan Jamison was a young drunk. His poison of choice? "Anything. I was under 21," he says. By the time he graduated from high school, Jamison's GPA

PERCENTAGE OF VITAMIN AND SUPPLEMENT USERS WHO TAKE THEM TO TREAT COLDS: 53

PERCENTAGE WHO TAKE THEM TO TREAT HIGH CHOLESTEROL: 29

PERCENTAGE WHO TAKE THEM TO TREAT INSOMNIA: 20

had dwindled from 3.9 to 2.2; his all-state soccer career was stalled; and his shot at a national teen weight-lifting title (he benched 385 at age 15) gave way to "the party," as he calls it. The Phoenix resident didn't see this as a problem, however, until he started drinking alone. Then he knew it was time to stop, which he did, cold, at age 19. Starting out was difficult. He didn't have a lot of friends he could talk to, and anyone older chalked up his problems to teenage angst.

One morning Jamison attempted to climb Squaw Peak, a part of the Phoenix Mountain Preserve in Arizona. After a few successful ascents, he began alternating with nearby Camelback. Soon the climbs—both about a mile and a half up switchbacks—became mandatory for Jamison. "If I didn't climb, I knew I'd have a bad day," he says. "I'd feel like going back to drinking." But he never did. He just kept climbing. Now he's 30 years old, married, and the father of a 3-year-old son, and he's been stone-cold sober for 11 years.

Make it work for you: "It's all about taking your recovery into your own hands and using your own will to end your addiction," says G. Alan Marlatt, Ph.D., professor of psychology at the University of Washington in Seattle. Yes, that's contrary to the AA philosophy of powerlessness, but for some alcoholics it may be better to climb mountains than AA's 12 Steps. If you choose to go the DIY route, Marlatt recommends finding an activity that will give you the same benefits Jamison's climbing gave him: a good frame of mind first thing in the morning, a diversion from the booze, and a firm belief that it will help you stay on the wagon. (Exercise should be a top candidate since the endorphin rush Jamison experienced from climbing may have helped replace the physical pleasure of drinking.) Warning: If your activity doesn't keep you sober for 90 days, it's time to ask for help.

INSOMNIA
How he beat it: Acupuncture

John Martin suffered what he calls "seasonal" insomnia, which corresponded with allergy season and stressful periods at his Internet marketing job in Manhattan. He'd go to bed and just lie there. He tried Benadryl for the allergies, but that sped him up. He popped a prescription sleeping pill (Ambien), but it left him "fuzzed out." He stared at the ceiling for years. "It was exhausting," he says. "The sleeplessness built on itself and went on and on."

Finally, a doctor friend of Martin's suggested acupuncture. The first time, he says, was creepy: "Someone is actually leaning over you and sticking you

ONE OF THE MOST COMMON CAUSES OF CHRONIC INSOMNIA: DEPRESSION

with pins." For the first few minutes, Martin was skeptical, but soon—and involuntarily—he became more relaxed. The evening after the second session, he slept better than he had in weeks. As Martin continued his treatments—twice a week for 3 weeks—his sack time continued to improve and his allergies lessened. These days Martin goes for maintenance jabs once every few weeks, but his insomnia is gone.

Make it work for you: Don't like needles? Don't worry, says Christopher Trahan, O.M.D., a licensed acupuncturist and doctor of oriental medicine in New York City. "Acupuncture needles aren't hypodermic needles. They're superthin, almost like filament, and sterilized. It's not going to hurt, and there's generally no bleeding." For insomnia treatment, acupuncturists usually focus on two main points on your ears that induce relaxation. "Acupuncture enhances the release of calming endorphins and neurotransmitters in the brain," says Dr. Trahan. The time it takes to get results varies, but even severe insomnia sufferers usually see improvement within 10 treatments. (The need for maintenance sessions also varies.) Find a licensed acupuncturist at www.aaom.org, the Web site of the American Association of Oriental Medicine.

ANGER
How he beat it: Burning it out

On his 10th wedding anniversary, Thomas J. Harbin, Ph.D., a Fayetteville, North Carolina, clinical psychologist, gained a new patient: himself. "That day my wife said, 'If the next 10 years are going to be like the last 10, I'm leaving,'" he recalls. Harbin's chronic anger—a problem since he was a child—had finally reached the point where even he could no longer deny the problem. "I never got physical, and I never broke things," he says. "I just got into brutal arguments."

As a Ph.D., Harbin was savvy enough to know that his anger was not something he could resolve in an afternoon. So, short-term, he did the best thing he could: He walked away when he knew an argument was brewing. He also began exercising intensely. Long-term, he started writing what would become *Beyond Anger: A Guide for Men*. The book, in effect, became his therapist. "Writing helped me organize my thoughts and realize my own problems," he says. Now 48, Harbin specializes in anger therapy. He's treated more than a hundred chronically angry men, is much more happily married, and knows firsthand what boils inside tens of millions of men like him.

Make it work for you: "Anyone can get mad at being cut off in traffic," says Harbin. "But when you start taking it personally, as if the other driver has something against you, that's a problem." There's only one immediate solution when you feel the rage boiling: "Just walk away," says Harbin. "It's the best option until you learn how to control your anger more effectively." After that, flush the anger from your system with exercise and writing. You know how to do the former; for the latter, what are you afraid of? Making a list of what pisses you off can illuminate the real anger beneath—just shred what you write afterward. If you're still popping veins, Harbin suggests bringing in a pro.

Stop the Bleeding

Reddened eyes? Bloody nose? Aortic hemorrhage? Apply direct pressure and read on

By John Hyduk

Blood isn't destiny, but it is the original early-warning system—think red flag—of the body corporal. And it yearns to leak out at the most inopportune times. Should you panic? Never. But knowledge of the crimson tide, and what its unexpected appearance on your shirt, the bathroom porcelain, or some other inappropriate venue really signals, is critical. Anything less is just a Band-Aid.

WARNING: YOU'RE SEEING RED

Any number of things can cause bloodshot eyes, including bacterial and viral infections (commonly known as pinkeye), irritants such as pollen or smoke, and, of course, a hangover. If your red eyes are itchy and watery, the culprit is likely an allergen. Try an antihistamine. Skip any over-the-counter eye drops that promise "to get the red out." They can mask an infection during the contagious stage and cause rebound redness with prolonged use.

If you have any yellow discharge or still have redness and discomfort after 24 hours, hit your eye doctor up for antibiotics; you're probably battling a bacterial invader. And stop rubbing your eyes since that's the best way to reinfect your own tissues or spread the germs throughout your neighborhood.

WARNING: YOU'RE PEEING RED

During a bathroom break, all the other guys are dispensing a nice, golden lager, and you're (ulp!) serving up salsa. The presence of blood in the urine is called hematuria. Estimates are that 10 percent of the population pees red from time to time, and many of the causes are benign—a plumbing glitch caused by something hard (like a kidney pebble or bladder stone) rubbing against something soft (like bladder tissue). Interestingly, jogging can bounce your bladder, causing blood to leak into your urine in a condition dubbed "jogger's bladder."

We know you're a bright guy, but home diagnosis is not the smart call. "Since early detection is key," says Jon Pryor, M.D., chairman of urology at the

University of Minnesota in Minneapolis, "we think it's cancer until proved otherwise." Best way to clear your mind, and your stream, is a trip to your doctor.

One key to regaining mountain brook quality might be what you *don't* gulp. "Blood-thinning medications, even aspirin, can cause blood to show up in the urine," says Dr. Pryor.

WARNING: YOUR NOSE BLEEDS

"Most spontaneous nosebleeds are harmless," says Alexander Chester, M.D., a specialist in internal medicine at Georgetown University Hospital in Washington, D.C. "More often than not, they're caused by a crusting inside the tip of the nose, especially during dry, cold weather." Seems your proboscis is rich in tiny blood vessels that crowd the inner surface of the tip. Huffing frigid air causes a case of nasal freezer burn—the nose membranes split and crack, and even a sneeze can start the flow and cause permanent stains on your shirt. Another possible cause: high blood pressure, especially if you have nosebleeds frequently.

Dr. Chester suggests applying a preventive dab of petroleum jelly inside your nose during the winter and investing in a home humidifier. "Or you may want to change the nasal spray you've been using. Steroidal nose sprays (the kind your doctor prescribes) constrict the blood vessels, making a rupture more likely," he adds. Try saline, if your doctor agrees.

If the dam bursts, how do you stanch the flow? "Pressure," says Dr. Chester. Sit upright and lean forward slightly to avoid swallowing any blood. Apply firm, steady pressure to the tip of your nose for about 5 minutes. Bored silly? Pass the time by chanting, "Down goes Frazier!"

WARNING: YOU'VE GOT BLOODY NIPPLES

We really don't want to hear about your sex life and those mousetraps. Seriously, any sensitive skin area that comes into repeated contact with a rougher surface—like a T-shirt—can be subject to fabric irritation, redness, or even bleeding. The condition is called jogger's nipples because it's common among runners. Before lacing up, apply a thin coat of petroleum jelly to the affected area. Or run in a silk camisole.

WARNING: YOU RALPH IN GLORIOUS TECHNICOLOR

Vomiting blood is tricky to diagnose. "Circumstances are critical to an accurate diagnosis, but bleeding internally—and that's what you're doing—is always a big thing," says David Rothenberger, M.D., chief of surgery at the University of Minnesota in Minneapolis. "If you're vomiting blood, that might indicate severe gastritis, a duodenal ulcer, or even an esophageal tear." Your doctor will use a flexible camera (open wide), or he'll mix up a barium cocktail (step up to the x-ray and it's show time!) to seek the leak. Repair might

CHICKEN BLOOD AND OTHER DANGEROUS ENCOUNTERS

What are your chances of picking up something nasty . . .

In a tattoo parlor? About the same as when sharing a toothbrush or a barber's razor, getting a manicure, or using someone else's straw to snort cocaine. A recent study showed that even prison tattooers have a better safety record when it comes to spreading hep C than the body artistes at your local salon.

Risk factor: high

From the business end of a mosquito? Can a skeeter perform an unauthorized transfusion? Not likely. Even if you had the bad luck to be bitten by a West Nile–infected mosquito (fewer than 1 percent of the bugs), you have a less than 1 percent chance of developing the disease. Better you should immunize against Lyme disease.

Risk factor: low

On a steakhouse platter? Not to worry about that blood on the platter, says the nice lady at the USDA Meat and Poultry Hotline, as long as the center of your sirloin reaches 145°F. Your burger should reach 160°F.

Risk factor: low

In a poultry package? Campylobacter bacteria thrive in the soupy slop in your poultry package, so discard it immediately. Everything the raw yard bird comes in contact with gets a soap-and-hot-water scrubbing, and wash your cutting board in bleach after use.

Risk factor: medium

then go the medicinal route with antiulcer drugs, or the doctor may use a heat probe to cauterize the drip, plumber style.

WARNING: THERE'S BLOOD IN YOUR EJACULATE

"Here's one you probably haven't thought of," says Dr. Pryor. "Blood in your ejaculate." (Like we need this.) Funny thing, but blood in your ejaculate, or hematospermia, is more common than you'd guess. If you're under the age of 40, odds are you've traumatized yourself with too much bike riding or an STD. Antibiotics will be your get-out-of-Weirdsville-free card. If you're closer to 50, get checked to rule out prostate cancer.

WARNING: YOU SH— A BRICK (AT LEAST THAT'S WHAT COLOR IT IS)

As a diagnostic tool, stools rule. First question from your doctor: What color is your poop? "Bleeding in the gastrointestinal tract can cause blood in your stool," says Dr. Rothenberger. Dark stools mean dried blood from a stomach ulcer; a richer burgundy means you've sprung a leak farther down the pike (from an intestinal inflammation like colitis); bright red might signal something rectal—anything from a hemorrhoid to a tumor. Trouble is, a hemorrhoid alert and a cancer warning announce themselves, with precisely the same colors.

Consider any bloody out-of-booty experience a wake-up call. Best thing: Your physician will read your rainbow and save you a potentially embarrassing exchange with the color chart guy at the paint store.

WARNING: YOU SUFFER FROM JET LEG

As if air travel weren't already hell with pretzels, there's deep vein thrombosis (DVT). Researchers believe that this so-called economy-class syndrome results from the cramped conditions and enforced immobility that people endure in airline seats. As blood pools in the legs, clots may form. Should one of these swim to prime body real estate—like the lungs—the red-eye flight to Heathrow could become a short hop to the hospital.

Franklin Colon, M.D., a family practice physician in Cincinnati who did pioneering work on DVT, recommends being alert for tenderness, swelling, or redness in your legs on any long trip. He suggests taking an aspirin before boarding, staying hydrated by hitting the water bottle, and keeping in motion. "Stretch your legs as best you can, even if it's just walking the aisle or tensing and then relaxing your calf muscles," says Dr. Colon.

A Royal Pain in the Gut

Listen to the screams of a man with a kidney stone, and you'll do anything to avoid growing your own

By Michael Perry

In the end, what I remember most is how I would find myself *peeing hopefully*. I'd stand there over the bowl, with my little strainer in one hand and me in the other, and I'd be thinking, This time . . . maybe this time. And then I would finish, shake loose the last little drop, and *nothing*. Over and over again, five, six . . . 10 times a day for 11 days, from February into March, I'd peer into that strainer with the cheated pout of a little boy who finishes his Cracker Jack and finds no prize.

I had a kidney stone in me, and I wanted it out.

The stone struck on a Tuesday evening, somewhere along I-94 just east of Minneapolis. First came an upper-abdominal twinge, similar to gas pains at dawn (of the sort precipitated—I'm from Wisconsin—by excess bratwurst at bedtime), except that no amount of twisting or turning would break it loose. Then it seemed as if my right kidney had been run through with a super-heated knitting needle. I was veering in and out of my lane, gasping like a scuppered carp. Struck by this delusion that a hot bath would dissipate the pain, I careened to a motel. I'm certain the desk clerk pegged me for a meth fiend—I was pallid, shivering, and rolling in sweat as she ran my credit card—but she worked quickly. I staggered to the room, filled the tub full blast, and stripped out of my clothes.

By now, based on my experience as a nurse and an EMT, I had pretty much self-diagnosed. One in 10 Americans will experience the joy of kidney stones, and the pain I felt was my secret handshake into the club. I dropped into the steaming water and—drawing on my knowledge of anatomy, physics, and desperation—assumed a bizarre position calculated to roll the stone back into the kidney. (When Ben Franklin's kidney stone blocked his bladder, he used to stand on his head to pee.) After about 15 seconds of lying in scalding water with my butt hoisted above the Plimsoll mark, I ran up the white flag and dialed 911.

PAIN MANAGEMENT

On a pain scale of 1 to 10, kidney stones consistently ring the bell at 10. A mother of three who had a kidney stone once told me, "I'd rather give birth three times—in one day!" The pain is focused, relentless, and inescapable. I pride myself on a certain blue-collar hardiness and Scandinavian stoicism, but by the time a paramedic arrived, I was flailing around the motel room bed, spewing effenheimers. "Bet it's a kidney stone," said the paramedic. "Morphine?"

"Oh, yeah," I hissed.

While he slid the needle in, I puked into a bag. Puking is a classic kidney stone symptom, caused by overstimulation of stomach nerves. The morphine helped, but I was still twisting like a bug pinned to a board when they strapped me to the cot. In Woodbury, Minnesota, a nurse in the Woodwinds Health Campus ER gave me another bump of morphine, but during a CT scan, the pain came stabbing back. The nurse pushed a drug called Toradol. Sweet relief. I dozed until the ER doc woke me. "It's fairly large as stones go," he said. "It's borderline whether it will pass on its own." The next time I woke, my father and brother had arrived to retrieve me and my car. The nurse handed me a bottle of Percocet and a screened funnel. "Strain your urine," she said, "and save the stone." I tottered out the door, paused to puke in the parking lot, and set out for home.

I spent the week at my parents' farmhouse in Wisconsin. Now and then the pain would outdistance the Percocet, and I would try anything—hot baths, microwaved hot packs, incessant pacing—to distract myself until the drugs caught up. Once I was crawling out of the bathtub when I was swept with nausea. I scrambled for the toilet. Hearing the scuffle, my mom burst in to check on me, and so it was that at the age of 37 I found myself buck naked on all fours, head in the toilet, puking at the feet of dear old Mom.

She's been a nurse for 40 years and was unfazed, but a guy hopes for a little dignity.

The Percocet beat most of the pain and gave me freaky dreams. But it also made me more pukey, and since I couldn't keep anything down, I began to fall behind on my fluid intake. Not good when you're relying on hydraulic forces to flush a stone. On day 3, the knitting needle woke me with a vengeance. Back to the ER. "You got Toradol?" I asked. They did. By this time I was peeing thimblefuls of what appeared to be scorched corn syrup. They kept me overnight, pumped me full of fluids, and sent me home with Compazine to treat the nausea. Because long-term use of Toradol can affect kidney function, the doctor was reluctant to prescribe the pills, but I promised to use them only during peak pain moments. One kidney stone, 3 days, and I had become a craven junkie.

And so I pounded fluids and waited. I'd go an entire day without pain, then zing, it would be back. The stone was moving through the ureter toward the bladder. It was almost even with my hipbone. I took my little strainer everywhere. I carried it in my coat pocket, wrapped in a plastic bag. In public restrooms, I'd go into the stall (you really can't stand at a urinal in the Farm and Fleet peeing through a funnel and expect to escape arrest or injury), and I'm sure when people heard the crackle of the plastic they thought, Drugs! Perversion! Then there was the problem of rinsing the thing off. I resorted to feet checks and strategically timed dashes. Kidney stones are all about drugs and furtiveness.

ZEROING IN ON THE STONE

Researchers have identified 19 distinct types of kidney stones.

"Twenty, actually!" says Michael Rentzepis, M.D. He is a urologist in private practice in New York City. Nine days since the first attack and still no stone, so I was referred to him for a consultation. Dr. Rentzepis is young and trim. He has the large glasses and eager demeanor of your classic science geek, which I find to be a comfort, doctorwise. "A new variation has just been discovered!" he says. Excitement has drawn him right to the edge of his chair.

"Well, now," I say. "That'll be the talk of the annual urology convention."

"Oh, yes," says Dr. Rentzepis. He's lit up like a grade schooler describing the new teeter-totter. "It's just like adding another element to the periodic table!"

Bless his heart, my urologist is a geek for renal calculi.

"Let's look at your CT scan," says Dr. Rentzepis.

I was once arc-welding the underside of an equipment trailer when a molten pearl of slag dripped into my welding gauntlet, lodging against my fingernail. The pain was astounding. Flinging everything, I yipped and scooted from beneath the trailer like a poodle suffering a buttful of rock salt. On the

CT scan, the kidney stone is an incandescent dot amid all the half-tone grays. I think immediately of the molten slag droplet, sliding lazily through my ureter, burning white-hot until it finally plops into the watery bladder and the pain stops.

"The stone is right at the end of the ureter," says Dr. Rentzepis, pointing at the bright dot. "Almost out. Trouble is, a stone of this size, it's about 50-50 whether or not it'll pass on its own."

"What are my options?"

"Generally," says Dr. Rentzepis, "you want to let it pass. Although removal procedures are straightforward, you can have complications." He pulls

SKIPPING STONES

Any kidney is a potential quarry. This is because they all filter calcium and a food compound called oxalate out of the bloodstream. If enough of the stuff builds up, it'll bond together to form the world's tiniest torture device—a kidney stone. Most men just need to drink extra fluids to dilute the calcium and oxalate before it reaches critical mass. But if you have a family history of kidney stones, or have already had one, you'll need to do more. Here are four ways to prevent getting stoned.

Keep the calcium. It may seem counterintuitive, but a study published in 2002 in the *New England Journal of Medicine* found that male kidney stone sufferers who ate a calcium-rich diet—800 to 1,000 milligrams a day—were 50 percent less likely to get stoned again than those on a low-calcium plan. "Ingested calcium keeps oxalate in the intestine, preventing it from being absorbed into the blood and forming stones in the urine," says David S. Goldfarb, M.D., director of the kidney stone prevention program at St. Vincent's Hospital in New York City.

Hold the soy. You can eat extra calcium, but don't up your oxalate intake. In other words, eat soy sparingly. "Soy-based foods have some of the highest levels of oxalates and have been shown to increase urinary oxalate," says Linda Massey, R.D., Ph.D., professor of human nutrition at Washington State University in Spokane. Textured soy protein—used in veggie burgers—contains 638 milligrams of oxalate per serving, nearly 100 milligrams more than spinach, the previous record holder.

Roll over. Another reason to try new positions in the bedroom: A recent University of California at San Francisco study found that 76 percent of patients with recurring kidney stones developed them only on the side they consistently slept on. "Sleeping in the same position seems to alter the way bloodflow to the kidney is distributed, hurting its ability to stop stone formation," says Marshall Stoller, M.D., one of the study's authors. Every few nights, try to sack out on a different side to better distribute the flow of blood.

Watch what you chug. You lose fluids fast when you work out, but if you're stone-prone, skip sports drinks. "Unless you're training for something like a marathon that requires you to replace sodium, sports drinks aren't necessary, and the extra salt will increase calcium in your urine," says Dr. Goldfarb. Water too bland? Try Powerade; it has a lot less sodium than most sports drinks.

out a comic book: *Understanding Kidney Stones*. On the cover, a golfer clutches his back, his sweaty face gripped in a rictus of pain. On page 10, a man is reclining in a tub while shockwaves blast his stone to bits. Lithotripsy. Relatively painless, but the truck-mounted portable unit isn't due in town this week. On page 12, a doctor inserts a tube in the patient's back, blasts the stone with ultrasound, and plucks out the fragments, a treatment reserved for stones over 1 inch in diameter. My stone is big, but not that big. Another series of illustrations demonstrates how staghorn stones—huge things with spikes and projections—require surgical removal and a 4-day hospital stay. "I'll put a ureteroscope in your urethra, through your bladder, and up to the stone," says Dr. Rentzepis. "I'll pluck the stone with a little caliper-like device." No incisions. But right up the old main line. "Then we'll probably need to put a tube in the ureter for a few days, to keep it from swelling shut."

"Do you have to go back up there to get the tube out?"

"Oh, no," says Dr. Rentzepis. "We tie a string to it. After a few days, you come into the office and I'll pull it out."

"Um . . . let's give it another couple days."

THE BIG MOMENT

I was caught completely off guard when it finally happened. I was visiting friends. We were leaving to see a band, and I had run upstairs for a quick filtered pee. Urinating through a sifter was second nature by now, and my mind was somewhere else when—*boooiing!*—there was a sudden rubbery back pressure, my urine flow stopped dead, my bladder expanded, then—*clack!*—and I was peeing effortlessly again.

You know how sometimes if you turn the faucet off too quickly the pipes rattle? There's a term for that. It's called water hammer. When that kidney stone hit the homestretch, I had my own little water hammer moment. And now there it was: dark brown, rock hard, and the size of a chokecherry pit. I had a sudden urge to call friends and hand out cigars. Instead I rinsed the stone and looked at it closely. It was studded with tiny nubs and felt like sandpaper. I got a little creeped out and light-headed then.

I went to my follow-up appointment. No sooner had he closed the examining room door than Dr. Rentzepis turned to me eagerly. "Did you bring it?" It was like in third grade when Vinnie Boscoe wondered if you'd brought the fart cushion. I pulled the specimen bottle from my pocket and held it up to view. The stone rattled against the plastic.

Dr. Rentzepis's eyes widened.

"Oh, my God!"

Can I tell you what pride it gives a man to produce a thing in this way and have a board-certified urologist say, "Oh, my God!"? Fourteen years of medical training, stones of every type and dimension, and he says, "Oh, my God!"? I averted my eyes, flush with aw-shucks pride. Just as quickly, I drew back. "I bet you tell all your patients that."

"Oh, no," he said. "That really is a big one. Stones of that size, we usually have to go in after them."

I was glowing.

Dr. Rentzepis has known patients to mount their stones in resin. He made me turn mine in. He sent it to a lab to be crushed and analyzed. It was 80 percent calcium oxalate and 20 percent calcium phosphate. The most common sort. Based on that information, he says I have to drink 12 glasses of water a day for the rest of my life, basically to keep my system flushed, as recurrence rates run about 80 percent. ("Once a stone thrower, always a stone thrower," said my regular M.D. when he visited me in the ER.) I'll also drop in for an abdominal x-ray now and then, in the hope that we'll catch the next one earlier. Before we hit the "Oh, my God" stage.

The French essayist Montaigne wrote that kidney stones left him feeling great intellectual clarity. No sign of that so far. But I have noticed changes. I try to drink more water. Whereas I used to tolerate tales of childbirth with a sort of deferential politeness, I now find myself nodding in solidarity. And when I looked across the median of I-80 during a recent road trip and saw a westbound semi emblazoned with the words AMERICAN KIDNEY STONE MANAGEMENT, I got so misty I nearly left the roadway. Somewhere out there, someone else was gasping like a scuppered carp, and here, apparently piloted by angels, was a white Kenworth, its hood ornament aimed at kidney stones everywhere. Sweet, sweet relief, *hammer down.*

Show Your Back Who's Boss

Put your pain out of commission with these 7 strategies

By Bill Gottlieb

In the corporate hierarchy of the human body, your brain is the boss, your blood is the cash flow that keeps the company alive, and your bad back is the employee who's chronically late to work, often insubordinate, and occasionally under the influence of some pretty powerful narcotics. Unfortunately, you can't go ahead and fire its sorry ass because, in case you hadn't noticed, it's your ass, too. Besides, as much as it's hurting business, your back is still the best (and only) body part for the job.

What to do? One word: micromanage. Unlike employees in the typical brick-and-mortar outfit, flesh-and-blood workers respond surprisingly well to

WATCH YOUR BACK

Considering back surgery? The most common procedure is spinal fusion, in which bone from elsewhere in your body is fused to the compromised part of your spine. Some surgeons use screws to help stabilize the area during recovery; others use a back brace. Don't get screwed.

For starters, surgery with screws (called instrumentation) is a more difficult operation—it takes longer; you may lose more blood; hospitalization is sometimes longer; and there's greater risk of complications, such as a screw breaking. Then there's the study published in the journal *Spine*, in which doctors in Sweden evaluated 222 patients who had received different types of spine-stabilizing surgery for chronic lower back pain. They found that surgery with instrumenta-tion produced no additional reductions in pain or disability.

"Many surgeons claim that instrumentation produces immediate stability and allows patients to be more quickly mobilized and rehabilitated," says Peter Fritzell, M.D., the lead study author. "Our study found no clinical differences 2 years after surgery."

And yet, instrumented fusions are common. So don't be surprised if that's the way your surgeon wants to go, but do ask questions. "Discuss with your surgeon exactly why an instrumented procedure is the right choice in your case," says Dr. Fritzell. "Ask if the additional risks are really worth the possible gains."

this approach. See for yourself. Take one or more of the micromanagement strategies that follow, add them to your back's employee handbook, and then look over your shoulder to see how it's shaping up. In no time, you'll be logging fewer sick days and showing increased productivity. Heck, you'll feel so good, you may even want to merge with another company.

MICROMANAGER'S TIP #1: STAND UP TO THE ACHE

Every night, your back is booby-trapped by extra fluid that seeps into your disks, the spongy cushions that separate the 24 vertebrae in your spine. "When you bend over in the morning, that fluid creates more stress on your spine, making your back more vulnerable to pain," says Stover H. Snook, Ph.D., a lecturer on ergonomics at the Harvard University school of public health. In a recent study published in the *Journal of Occupational Rehabilitation*, Snook and his fellow researchers found that chronic-back-pain sufferers who followed a plan for staying upright in the A.M. had 23 percent fewer painful days than those who bent freely.

Here's the plan: Move to the edge of the bed, roll onto your side, and hang your feet off the mattress. With your back straight or slightly arched, use your arms to push yourself to a seated position and then to a standing position. Now stay standing. Stand to urinate (leave the seat up the night before). Don't bend over the sink when you brush your teeth or shave. Step into your pants without bending over. (Heed Micromanager's Tip #2 before you put your shirt on.) Even eat breakfast standing up. Save the must-bend activities, such as tying your shoes, for last.

MICROMANAGER'S TIP #2: PACK HEAT

Don't swallow your medicine; wear it. Researchers at UMDNJ–New Jersey Medical School found that people who wore disposable heat wraps every day had 25 percent less back pain than those taking either daily acetaminophen or ibuprofen. "Heat wraps increase bloodflow, getting rid of the by-products of tissue injury, and increase the elasticity of the tissues, improving mobility," says Scott Nadler, D.O., the lead study author. Simply place a wrap around your body, position its heating disks on your lower back, get dressed, and head out. Note: Only the ThermaCare brand has been studied for all-day use, says Dr. Nadler. (Other brands might get too hot and cause burns.)

MICROMANAGER'S TIP #3: TREAT YOUR ARTHRITIS

Known best as a knee saver, chondroitin sulfate may also help your back. In one 6-month study of people suffering from lower-back pain, Russian researchers found that 73 percent of those who took a daily chondroitin supplement had improved mobility and less pain. Why did it help? Because back pain is often caused by arthritis—the degeneration of the cartilage that cushions vertebrae, says Luke Bucci, Ph.D., C.C.N., an adjunct professor of nutrition at the University of Utah. "Chondroitin is a component of cartilage and works long term to slowly rebuild the tissue." Take 1,200 milligrams of chondroitin sulfate daily.

MICROMANAGER'S TIP #4: DON'T SHOW FEAR

University of Pittsburgh researchers evaluated people who were out of work due to lower-back pain, and found that those who feared their pain and avoided activities perceived as painful were the least likely to be able to return to work. "When you fear and avoid pain, you're more likely to fear and avoid strengthening and stretching exercises—the very exercises that can help you recover," says Steven George, Ph.D., P.T., an author of the study.

Understand that pain during recovery is normal and confront it, says George. "In terms of duration of exercise, go about 10 percent beyond your 'pain barrier,'" he says. If, for example, you're strengthening your back by walking on a treadmill and feel pain at 5 minutes, walk another 30 seconds. When is pain really a sign of something serious? When it "moves" to your thighs, changes to numbness, or is associated with weakness in your legs. In that case, you can be afraid—and see a doctor.

MICROMANAGER'S TIP #5: ACT DEPRESSED

Turns out the pain may be all in your head. In a study review published in the *Archives of Internal Medicine*, researchers found that back-pain sufferers who took antidepressants (such as Paxil) had 40 percent less pain than those who popped a placebo. Antidepressants reduce levels of serotonin and norepinephrine, brain chemicals that transmit pain signals between nerve cells, says Stephen M. Salerno, M.D., the lead study author. And their side effects—drowsiness, increased heart rate, and dry mouth, to name a few—may be preferable to those of nonsteroidal anti-inflammatory drugs. "If NSAIDs such as ibuprofen and naproxen are used for more than a few weeks, they can cause kidney problems and gastrointestinal bleeding, and can worsen high blood pressure," says Dr. Salerno. See if your doctor thinks an antidepressant is for you.

MICROMANAGER'S TIP #6: ENTERTAIN THE PAIN

Never mind the savage breast; music soothes the lower back. When Austrian researchers studied the effects of listening to relaxing music (and thinking equally relaxing thoughts) on back pain, they found that people who listened for 25 minutes daily for 3 weeks reported 40 percent less pain than those given the silent treatment. "Music diverts your attention from the ache. It also helps reduce stress hormones and muscular tension," says Franz Wendter, Ph.D., one of the researchers. The key here is *relaxing* music, meaning nothing by Monster Magnet. Instead, try *Silk Road Vol. 1* by Kitaro (all the yin of New Age music without the yang of Yanni) or *Aerial Boundaries* by Michael Hedges (another dead guitar god).

MICROMANAGER'S TIP #7: FIND A SUPPORT SYSTEM

Surgery is the last-resort remedy for a bad back. (See "Watch Your Back," on page 103.) The next-to-last resort? The partial-body-weight-support system. With the PBWS system, you walk on a treadmill while wearing a specially designed harness that supports some of your weight. (Relax—you do this at a physical-therapy clinic, not your gym.) In a clinical trial at the Lahey Clinic in Burlington, Massachusetts, researchers found that five out of six people who used the system for 6 weeks had significant reductions in back pain and improved functioning.

The PBWS system combines two back-pain busters, says David Joffe, P.T., the lead study author. One is endurance exercise, like walking. The other is "spine unloading," which can relieve the compression of the vertebrae that occurs whenever you sit or stand. Ask a physical therapist (or your doctor) if you should try the PBWS system, says Joffe. If he says yes, so will your insurance.

Meet Ralph

Introducing the only power in the universe that can bring a grown man to his knees and make him spill his guts

By Michael Perry

Apart from orgasm, no other natural human function overtakes our mental and physical faculties as thoroughly as a woofing good puke. Case in point: I recently barfed with such vigor that both my nasal passages became impenetrably jammed with chicken nuggets.

In part because I've always been a teetotaler, my personal puking experience is pretty unremarkable, limited mostly to run-of-the-mill spew sessions courtesy of the flu. I did once throw up as a direct result of eating a lukewarm, in-flight enchilada provided to me by a major airline. Then again, one suspects that the willful ingestion of an enchilada halfheartedly rewarmed at 35,000 feet is by definition a form of self-induced vomiting.

When not busy puking myself, I have studied the puking of others. For 15 years now, I have worked as an EMT (emergency medical technician), and while I'd love to project a more heroic image, I must say that in the field of medical rescue, puke is the great constant. Sick people puke, dying people puke, excited people puke; people puke while they're having heart attacks, they puke when their lacerated brains start to swell, they puke because they get carsick lying on the ambulance cot, looking up at the dome lights. Shoot, I have seen entire families puke purely out of solidarity. Ma blows potatoes across the bathroom, and Dad and the kids promptly lean over and hurl in unison. The sympathy puke, we call it.

And that's the complicated beauty of puking. It's so much more than a symptom of illness or a sign that one needs a new meat thermometer. Puking is a form of self-expression. It comes from the gut, yes, but also from the soul. And, sometimes, the heels.

Pursuant to my vomit contemplations, I resolved to consult experts on the subject. But because I so rarely attend birthing classes, fraternity hazings, or breakfast with waif supermodels, I settled for a Web search. No surprise, vomit is a subject tailor-made for the Web. In short order I turned up a slew of revolting jpegs, a handful of jaw-dropping mpegs, and reams of imaginative barfisms. Still, it was all so superficial, so thumbnail.

NUMBER OF PEOPLE WHO CONTRACT FOODBORNE ILLNESSES EACH YEAR: 76 MILLION

I needed depth. Science. I turned to the folks who wrote the book on vomiting. Or, more specifically, the "technical review" on vomiting, as approved by the American Gastroenterological Association (AGA) and published in the January 2001 issue of the journal *Gastroenterology*.

The AGA review defines vomiting as the "forceful oral expulsion of gastric contents associated with contraction of the abdominal and chest-wall musculature." Feeling, perhaps, that this initial description lacked the necessary punch, the authors revisit the subject a few sentences later, this time defining the central act as "a highly specific physical event that results in the rapid, forceful evacuation of gastric contents in retrograde fashion from the stomach up to and out of the mouth." Or, to put it another way, gastroenterologists can spank a thesaurus with the best of them. Though why they settled for "mouth" when "buccal cavity" was the obvious choice, I do not know.

The Merck Manual, bible of hypochondriacs everywhere, breaks down vomiting into two distinct types: physiologic and psychogenic. Physiologic vomiting occurs as the result of identifiable forces acting on the body, from tumors of the inner ear to bad shrimp to bad shrimp-boat rides. After you eat that piece of hinky shrimp, it produces toxins that enter the bloodstream and travel to the brain, where they trigger any of the five or so chemoreceptors capable of provoking vomiting. Then it's up and out with the offending crustacean.

Psychogenic vomiting, on the other hand, is precipitated by abstract elements such as intense fear or repulsion. Which is why your average IRS auditor is a little twitchy. *The Merck Manual* even goes so far as to indicate that psychogenic vomiting can be a sign of hostility. Not pent-up hostility, obviously. And again, bad news for the tax man.

PUKE PARTICULARS

Most of the time, vomiting is a good and necessary thing. On the other hand, it may indicate something more dire than a predilection for cheap Scotch. The AGA lists close to 100 vomit triggers, including bowel obstruction, strokes, Jamaican vomiting sickness, ear infections, closed head injuries, heart attacks, and, paradoxically, starvation. Vomiting, as it turns out, is the symptom for all seasons. Persistent vomiting, vomiting in the absence of nausea, or vomit containing blood or dark "coffee grounds"–type material (older blood) is worthy of a doctor's attention. In general, however, your main concern with vomiting is how to stay hydrated and avoid chipping your teeth on the toilet bowl.

Examples of vomiting-related injuries are rare in the scientific literature, but puke hard enough and you can blow a gasket, otherwise known as the esophageal artery. This is a nasty development doctors call Mallory-Weiss syndrome. The primary risk factors for incurring Boerhaave's syndrome, a potentially deadly puke-induced rupture of the esophagus itself, are alcoholism and overindulgence in food and drink, which makes me ask the question, Why not rename it the much-easier-to-pronounce NFL Stadium Parking Lot Pregame Tailgate Party syndrome?

And then there is the more recently recognized condition called prolapsed gastropathy. Midbarf, the upper end of the stomach collapses and is sucked up into the lower part of the esophagus. When you're not around to hear, board-certified gastroenterologists refer to this condition as Puking Your Guts Out.

THE ANIMAL KINGDOM

We do give it our all. We've all had that moment when we realized—right midhurl—that if we did crunches of this intensity on a regular basis, we would develop abs like marble speed bumps. By way of contrast, consider dogs, masters of the dispassionate puke. With a minimum of sound effects and hunching, they bring up supper and, just as quickly, put it back down. As if relief of the upset stomach were simply an issue of rearranging the gastric feng shui. Even cats hacking up hairballs don't slump to the floor in a spent heap when it's over.

Some animals—including mice and rats—don't puke at all. Others are veritable puking machines. Specifically, they're engineered to ruminate (defined by the AGA as "chewing and swallowing of regurgitated food that has come back into the mouth"). This last definition threatens to spoil a favorite memory, that of watching my father's cows chew their cud. Lacking television, I remember as a child watching for hours as the big Holsteins slowly worked over their previously stored meal. Reclining in the clover, they'd give out a nearly imperceptible heave, causing a bulge to emerge at the level of the brisket, work its way up the neck, and disappear between the jaws, at which point the cow would resume chewing at a contemplative pace.

Then there are the puking pioneers. The oldest recorded vomit—160 million years old—was discovered recently in an English clay pit, right where a dyspeptic ichthyosaur deposited it. I wonder if he gripped the sides of the pit with his flippers, got right down there, his scaly head hanging, his snoot dripping. *Praying Wisconsin-style*, as a friend once put it.

Ol' ichthy is extinct, but we're still bopping around the planet, in part because of our own urge to regurgitate. "Nausea and vomiting give us an evolutionary advantage," says David Fleisher, M.D., director of the division of pediatric gastroenterology at the University of Missouri School of Medicine in Columbia. "If we eat green meat, we vomit. The next time we see green meat, we don't eat it. This keeps us from repeating the same mistakes. It is very common in pediatrics, for example, where if a kid goes to McDonald's and for some reason throws up there, he will never go to another McDonald's again.

AVOID LOSING YOUR LUNCH

Here are four ways to keep from airing things out, so to speak.

Act allergic. Dramamine is the classic motion sickness medicine, but it's rarely handy when you feel the need to heave. The next-best thing? An antihistamine. The active ingredient in Dramamine is dimenhydrinate, an antihistamine that, like all antihistamines, blocks motion signals to the brain. "Other antihistamines, like Benadryl, can work," says Eric Muth, Ph.D., assistant professor of psychology at Clemson University in South Carolina. "The main problem is that they cause drowsiness, which I counteract with a beverage with caffeine."

Suck it up. Quick, find a 7-Eleven (or any other quick-mart) and hit the candy aisle. You're looking for nature's answer to nausea: peppermint. "It's an antispasmodic that works to decrease the stomach contractions causing your nausea," says Patti McCormick, Ph.D., R.N., president of the Ohio Academy of Holistic Health in Xenia. "Even sucking on a piece of peppermint candy can help." Or chew Wrigley's Extra Peppermint; it contains more natural peppermint oil than any other gum.

Give yourself the finger. Place the tip of your right index finger on the underside of your left wrist, an inch and a half from your hand. Now apply moderate pressure. Stop after 2 to 3 minutes. "This acupressure point is particularly calming and soothing to the gastrointestinal system," says Michael Reed Gach, Ph.D., founder of the Acupressure Institute in Berkeley, California. How calming? In a study published in the *Journal of Advanced Nursing*, this pressure principle reduced queasiness by 30 percent.

Strike a pose. Boat-rocking, stomach-emptying nausea arises from a sensory mismatch: Your eyes see one thing, your muscles feel another, and your inner ear registers yet another. The solution: "Reduce the input by pretending you have a neck brace on," says Muth. "Lock your head upright and look straight ahead. Then eliminate the visual input by closing your eyes, and you've minimized two-thirds of the problem." To eliminate the other third, get off the boat.

Or he gets nauseated every time he passes that particular restaurant." Which would explain why you so rarely see the elder George Bush at Benihana.

Evolutionary advantages aside, the human puking mode still seems grossly unfair.

If we must get "sick as a dog," then why can't we "vomit like a dog"? How, in contrast with our own, spasmodic chunk blasting, do dogs manage to toss their biscuits with such insouciance? "When I was in medical school, my pharmacology professor got a dog, put him in front of the lecture hall, and injected him with morphine, which is very emetogenic. The dog shivered and puked, and then it was over," says Dr. Fleisher. "My hunch is that if a dog sees something that is disgusting, it doesn't vomit. If I were a dog, I would be disgusted all day long, but dogs don't get disgusted."

Which helps in eating the puke, I suppose—the obvious drawback to doing things the dog way. Still, one man tried it. In the name of research, the

18th-century Italian naturalist Lazzaro Spallanzani studied human digestion by reportedly eating his own vomit, bringing it up again, noting any changes in consistency, eating it again, bringing it up, and so on, *ad nauseam*.

THE AFTER-PUKE

I was driving past a junkyard the day those chicken nuggets got the better of me. Overcome by a physiologic urge, I quickly pulled over, ducked between a pair of crumpled four-doors, and began to dispense chicken bits in a staccato, retrograde fashion. Oh, not out the nose, I remember thinking.

Kneeling weakly after the storm had passed, I tried to blow the nuggets clear. Nothing. Only one option: The dreaded retro-snork. I steeled myself, then snorked. The result was an immediate shift from physiologic to psychogenic vomiting triggered by disgust. I became locked in a horrific Spallanzanian loop: snork, hurl, snork, hurl, snork, hurl. Minutes passed. The nightmarish cycle was broken only upon the eventual depletion of nuggets. I knelt there, drooling and snot-ridden, eyes watering and bloodshot, rib and stomach muscles burning, teeth etched and bitter, nose stinging. . . .

What I'm trying to say is, I was feeling a lot better.

KNOW THIS

Drink to Your Health

Men who enjoy an occasional drink are less likely to call in sick to work than men who either abstain from alcohol or drink heavily. Researchers speculate that alcohol may kill viruses and bacteria, helping to protect you from illness.

Twice Burned

Cigarettes don't just singe your lungs; the smoke also worsens acid reflux—that burning, gagging feeling you get when stomach acid backs up into your throat. Researchers made the discovery after comparing the gag reflexes of a group of smokers with those of nonsmokers. Smoke appears to weaken muscles in the throat, making acid reflux more severe, says Kulwinder Dua, M.D., associate professor of medicine at the Medical College of Wisconsin in Milwaukee and the author of the study.

No Pain *and* No Gain

Most migraine medications cause users to pack on the pounds, but a new treatment appears to help people fight chronic headaches and lose weight at the same time. In trials, researchers found that men taking the drug topiramate (Topamax) experienced 50 percent fewer migraines than normal, in addition to losing nearly 4 percent of their body weight. Migraines can be caused by hypersensitive cells in the brain, and topiramate helps calm those cells, says one researcher.

Back Burner

A new heat treatment can repair many of the problems that cause chronic back pain. To perform the procedure, called intradiskal electrothermal therapy (IDET), doctors insert a small catheter into the damaged disk in your spine. The catheter is heated to a temperature high enough to toughen the outer layers of the disk while destroying any abnormal nerve endings inside that may be triggering pain. In a study of 58 men and women with back problems, IDET cut patients' pain levels by 50 percent or more. Results last 2 years or longer.

All Washed Up

There's absolutely no reason to buy antibacterial soaps, according to new recommendations from the American Medical Association. While close to 50 percent of soaps currently sold in the United States contain antimicrobial agents, the AMA claims that there's no solid scientific proof that these soaps are better at preventing infection than regular soap. In fact, the group argues that antibacterial soaps may be doing more harm than good—making bacteria stronger and more resistant to existing germ killers.

Ticked? Get Tested

If you're an outdoorsman, listen up: There's a new blood test for Lyme disease—a potentially debilitating condition you can develop if you're bitten by a tick that's carrying the disease. The C6 peptide test is 96 percent accurate in detecting Lyme disease during the earliest stages. "Older tests were highly inaccurate and produced a lot of false positive results for the disease," says Andrew Levin, Ph.D., CEO of Immunetics in Cambridge, Massachusetts, the company that developed the test. Although the C6 test is FDA-approved, Levin says many doctors aren't aware of it—so you may need to ask for it by name. Testing is covered by most insurance plans. Results take about 2 days.

DOWN THE PIKE

Hershey's Cough Syrup

A compound in chocolate may help fight sore throats. Researchers at London's National Heart and Lung Institute found that the cocoa-based chemical theobromine was more effective than codeine in the treatment of coughs.

Pollen Plugs

Researchers in Australia have developed nose plugs capable of trapping pollen from the air you breathe before it makes you sneeze or triggers your eyes to water. The plugs, made with sticky mesh filters, trap pollen without impeding your breathing. "Ideally, people with hay fever could put the plugs in before going outside on days when the pollen count was exceedingly high," says Tim O'Meara, Ph.D., of the Woolcock Institute of Medical Research in Sydney. In early trials, the plugs were significantly more effective at relieving hay fever symptoms than most current anti-allergy medications.

Stronger Suds

Researchers at the Colgate-Palmolive research center in New Jersey have developed a soap that makes it harder for bacteria to stick to your skin. In trials, the soap reduced the spread of bacteria by more than 50 percent. The cleanser is already available in Latin America under the brand name Protexa and should hit store shelves in the United States within several years.

A Tidier Bowl

A germ-free john may be right around the corner. Researchers at MIT and Tufts University in Boston have developed the first germ-free surfaces— pieces of glass and plastic that can kill bacteria on contact. To make the products, scientists attach disinfectant particles to an object's surface. "When germs touch the surface, tiny antibacterial particles pierce their cell walls, drilling holes through them as a knife would," says Joerg Tiller, Ph.D., a coauthor of the study. Once "popped," the bacteria become harmless and can safely be washed away. Within the next few years, researchers believe the technology will be used on everything from kitchen cutting boards to toilets and restroom sinks.

Something for the Pain

A new compound called ACV1 could be up to 10,000 times more powerful than morphine for fighting pain, without becoming addictive. The substance is harvested from a type of poisonous snail commonly found in marine reefs. A drug based on the discovery is still in development—but once ready, it could become the new standard for the treatment of back and knee pain, arthritis, and sports injuries.

GAME PLAN

Survive Your Visit to the Drill Sergeant

How to make sure you don't receive cruel and unusual punishment in the chair

Life is a series of ultimatums: work or starve, pay or leave, visit the dentist or end up gumming your steak. You might connive your way out of the first two choices, but not the third. These tips will reduce the screaming at your 6-month checkup.

Size him up. Choose a dentist who sees fewer than 15 patients a day, says Van B. Haywood, D.M.D., professor at the Georgia School of Dentistry in Augusta. If he gives you a 30-second glance after a hygienist works on you, he can overlook a serious problem. To find another dentist, check www.ada.org.

Feel no pain. As a preemptive strike against pain, swallow two ibuprofen tablets 1 hour before your visit, says Ray Dionne, D.D.S., Ph.D., of the National Institutes of Health in Bethesda, Maryland. Avoid aspirin; it can cause you to bleed more than usual.

Protect your heart. If you have a heart ailment of any kind (including a murmur), see your doctor before your dentist. Dental work could release oral bacteria into your blood and lead to a heart attack. Taking antibiotics can protect you.

Get the right anesthetic. For quick procedures such as fillings, ask for a short-acting drug like mepivacaine; lidocaine will numb you for hours. Speak up if you have hypertension or take Prozac, because epinephrine—a common anesthetic ingredient—can cause reactions. To ease the needle sting, ask the dentist to numb you with a "Denti-Patch."

Keep your head up. Reclining makes some people gag, says Mark Slovin, D.D.S., of SUNY Stony Brook. Ask the dentist to tilt the chair only about 135 degrees.

Take the silver. Any dentist who offers to remove your "toxic" silver fillings is trying to scam you, says John E. Dodes, D.D.S., a dentist in Woodhaven, New York. Silver fillings have never been proven dangerous, and at $150 for 10 to 15 years, they're inexpensive. Gold fillings can last 25 years, but they go for $500 each.

Don't glow there. You should have x-rays of your back teeth every 2 years. Get full-mouth panoramic x-rays once every 5 years; the dentist should send a copy of these to your doctor because they can reveal arterial blockages.

Open wider. Make sure that the dentist checks you thoroughly for oral cancer. He should scan your tongue, your gums, the roof of your mouth, and your neck for lumps and discoloration.

TAKE ACTION

We can think of a zillion things we'd rather do on our "sick days" than sniffle and sneeze: Hit the fairways, catch a ball game, reel in some lunkers. Heck, we'd even settle for crossing off a few items on the ol' "Honey Do" list. That's why we put the following feel-better-fast and don't-get-sick-in-the-first-place tips together. So practice up on your raspy "I'm-too-sick-to-work" voice and start dialing.

1. Fend off the flu. This winter, roll up your sleeve for a protective flu shot. Your local health department can direct you to a library, grocery store, or clinic on wheels that offers the shot. If the nurse or needle scares you, just look away. Four reasons to get jabbed:

To avoid getting lucky. One or two out of every 10 people will get influenza this winter. Look around the office. Why risk that lottery?

It won't make you sick. Forget the myth that you can catch the flu from a flu shot. Can't happen, says John Treanor, M.D., associate professor of medicine at the University of Rochester in New York. Your arm might be a little sore for a day, but only one person in 100 will feel some fever and aches.

It's practically free. Most insurance plans cover a flu shot. If yours doesn't, it'll be about 10 bucks. How does that cost compare with missing a week of work?

It could help the economy. If everyone got the flu shot, sick days would be reduced by 32 to 45 percent, says the Centers for Disease Control and Prevention. Do your part for the economy—the country would save $1.3 billion if all working adults were vaccinated, according to a federal study.

2. But get some shut-eye first. Before you roll up your sleeve for your flu shot, make sure you've had a good night's sleep. A study in the *Journal of the American Medical Association* found that flu shots are less likely to keep you from getting sick if you're sleep-deprived than if you're well-rested. In trials, researchers found that 10 days after getting the vaccine, sleep-deprived men had less than half as many flu-fighting antibodies as men who'd logged a full night's rest. The antibody levels eventually even out when you get more sleep, but until they do, sleep-deprived guys are much more likely to catch the flu, says Eve Van Cauter, Ph.D., professor of human nutrition and nutritional biology at the University of Chicago and the author of the study.

3. Kick a cold. Researchers at the University of Virginia may have found the quickest way yet to help you beat a cold: a three-part treatment consisting of anti-inflammatories, an antihistamine, and nose drops made from the hepatitis medication interferon. "The first two drugs temporarily relieve cold symptoms, while the interferon kills the cold virus," says Birgit Winther, M.D., in Charlottesville, Virginia, who helped devise the treatment. Interferon still needs FDA approval for the treatment of colds. Until that's given, Dr. Winther recommends fighting colds with a multisymptom cold medicine, an antihistamine, and an anti-inflammatory, taken once every 12 hours until your symptoms disappear.

4. Help the medicine go down. There's a possible cure for that terrifying face you make after swallowing liquid cold medicines: salt. Researchers at the Monell Chemical Senses Center in Philadelphia found that a bit of salt can help mask the bitter flavor of some liquid medications. There's no guarantee that a dash of salt will do the trick, but it's worth a shake.

5. Unstuff your nose. Blast a shot of saline nasal spray up your beak 2 minutes before blowing it. The solution will help clear out any crust and also help shrink swollen mucous membranes. "When they're swollen, you feel plugged up even if there's no buildup present," says Mark Gutowski, M.D., an otolaryngologist at Head and Neck Surgery Associates in Fort Thomas, Kentucky. And unlike sprays that contain oxymetazoline hydrochloride or phenylephrine hydrochloride, saline won't cause rebound congestion, no matter how often you snort it.

6. Sell the convertible. Breathing polluted air can worsen symptoms of a cold. Researchers at Johns Hopkins University found that air pollution and car exhaust can increase levels of inflammation in your body, worsening congestion and making cold symptoms more severe.

7. Make your bed. If allergies are making you miserable, toss the foam mattress that's on top of your bed. A study in Norway found that foam mattresses are magnets for dust mites, one of the leading indoor causes of allergy symptoms.

8. Halt a headache. Instead of hitting back with Tylenol or Advil, try pinching the webbed area between your thumb and index finger (either hand) for 30 seconds. It's called acupressure, and while Ivy League researchers haven't carried out a randomized, placebo-controlled study on the strategy, Marc Sharfman, M.D., director of the Headache Institute in Winter Park, Florida, swears by it. "The theory is that it stimulates nerve impulses to the brain and reverses blood vessel dilation," he explains. Expect your head to stop throbbing in about 10 to 15 minutes.

SINCE 1991, THE PERCENTAGE INCREASE IN THE NUMBER OF PEOPLE WHO RECEIVED THE FLU SHOT: 44

9. Relieve pain faster. When you have a headache or muscle aches, take the liquid gel capsule form of ibuprofen. The liquid gel form allows the drug to reach your bloodstream almost 60 percent faster than the solid form.

10. Heat things up. If you're suffering from back pain, heat is your best bet. Heat wraps are up to 50 percent more effective than over-the-counter pills at relieving lower-back pain, according to a study from the University of Medicine and Dentistry of New Jersey in Stratford. Researchers found that men who treat their sore backs with heat have less pain and muscle stiffness and are significantly more flexible than patients with similar back problems who take ibuprofen or acetaminophen. "Low-level heat increases bloodflow to the muscles, relieving pain and improving muscle elasticity," says Scott Nadler, D.O., a coauthor of the study.

11. Mend to music. Cranking your favorite music may help eliminate back pain as well. In a study of 65 people who'd been hospitalized for chronic lower-back pain, researchers found that men who relaxed and listened to music for 25 minutes a day slept better and had less pain than men who didn't listen to music. So while you're applying that heat, crank up the Beatles.

12. Watch your back. If you're not careful, your commute can kill your back. When you first get behind the wheel, your posture is nearly perfect. But gradually, whether due to fatigue or the climax of your air drum solo, you start to slouch, increasing the pressure on the disks in your spine. Fortunately, the rearview mirror is your silent alarm. Adjust it as soon as you slip into the driver's seat; when you can no longer see your reflection, it's time to sit back up. "There's a lot of pressure with sitting. Driving adds to it with the vibrations from the road. If you sit up, you at least put the disks in the proper position to handle that pressure," says Sue Bloom, a physical therapist in Needham, Massachusetts.

13. Save your own neck. There are 2 million rear-end crashes every year, which can be serious pains in the neck. But only 14 percent of drivers know how high the head restraint on the seat back should be. The Insurance Institute for Highway Safety says you can protect your neck by adjusting your head restraint as follows: The top of the head restraint should be as high as your head's center of gravity, or about 3 inches below the top of your head. Any lower is unsafe. The restraint also should be within 4 inches of the back of your head (less than 3 inches is best). If the restraint tilts, tilt it. If not, try adjusting the seat.

14. Speed up your recovery. If you spend more time on two wheels than four, try these tips from Jeffrey Neal, an avid mountain biker, who has left some blood and derm cells on the trail. He teamed up with dermatologist and adventure athlete Ezra Kest, M.D., who is in private practice in Los Angeles, to create Brave Soldier Antiseptic Healing Ointment ($12). Neal claims that using the ointment makes wounds heal faster than just leaving them alone. His road-rash rule: Never let it scab. "Keep the injury moist and covered with a bandage," he says. The company now has a whole line of athlete's skin care products, all field-tested by athletes. You can check them out by logging on to www.bravesoldier.com.

15. End the itch. Women powder their faces; you're going to powder your balls. Jock itch—tinea cruris, for the athletically disinclined—is caused by a fungus that thrives on the moisture trapped in your briefs. So, twice a day, wash the affected area, dry it thoroughly, and then douse it with powder to help absorb the day's dampness. But here's the key: Use a brand that contains one of the antifungal ingredients miconazole nitrate or tolnaftate, but no cornstarch; it actually feeds the fungus, making the condition worse, says Joan Spiegel, M.D., a dermatologist at Brigham and Women's Hospital in Boston.

16. Save your skin. Winter skin can be itchy, flaky, cracked, and red, and you don't want to have that much in common with Old Man Winter. For skin she'll want to snuggle against, do this:

Shorten your showers. Hot water removes natural oils that act as a protective barrier on the skin, which then loses moisture, according to Sheila Rose Boyle, M.D., a dermatologist in Boulder, Colorado.

Toss out your deodorant soap. It dries out skin. Substitute gentle cleansers like Dove or Cetaphil, says Dr. Boyle. And rinse completely—residue can further dry your skin.

Use moisturizing cream instead of lotion. Cream is made of oil emulsified in water and adds a thicker barrier than lotion, so it's better at preventing moisture loss from the skin, according to Dr. Boyle. And while you're at it, pick up one with alpha-hydroxy acids in it. It'll be less greasy and won't leave you feeling slimy, according to Stephen Webster, professor of dermatology at the University of Minnesota Medical School in Minneapolis. Try AmLactin 12 percent ($13, www.drugstore.com).

17. Lick chapped lips. You smear on the lip balm but still have a cracked kisser. Chuck the stuff you're using now; you could be allergic to one of the ingredients. Instead, pick up a balm that's pure petroleum jelly. No aloe. No vitamin E. No lanolin. "These ingredients can cause skin allergies, but no one is allergic to petroleum jelly," says Dr. Spiegel. But don't simply layer your lips with the goo; use your tongue to wet them first and then slather on some jelly to seal in the moisture.

18. Kiss that cold sore goodbye. Apply a milk compress, and soon the only thing on your upper lip will be a goofy mustache. According to Jerome Z. Litt, M.D., author of *Your Skin from A to Z*, a protein called lactoferrin in milk helps fight the herpes simplex virus and speed healing. "You need to use cold whole milk for the best results," says Dr. Litt. Hold the compress to your infected lip for 2 minutes four times a day.

ANY QUESTIONS?

Get in Position

What's the best sleeping position to avoid back pain?

—A.K., Austin, Texas

Facedown, with a firm grip on Paulina Rubio. Barring that, there really isn't one position that's best for everyone. However, you can do something to make your favorite position easier on your aching back. "Pillows are the answer," says Neil McKenna, a physical therapist at the Rehabilitation Institute of Chicago. Here's how: If you're a side sleeper, draw your legs up toward your chest and place a pillow between your knees. This will take stress off the hip joints and lower back, which may be causing your back pain. If you sleep on your back, place a pillow under your knees to save 8 hours of back stress. And if you like sleeping on your gut, stuff a small pillow under your abdomen to keep your lower back from sagging. You'll feel like a champ in the morning, when Paulina begins tugging at the drawstring of your PJ's.

Can't Take the Heat

How high can my temperature go before I need to see a doctor?

—R.G., Orlando

A fever below 103°F may be uncomfortable but usually isn't dangerous, but as soon as you hit the 103 mark, you have a high-grade fever. The fever most likely is caused by a virus or bacteria; in the latter case, you can get antibiotics to treat the infection. But see your doctor if any fever lasts for several days.

Healthy Appetite

Does the old wives' tale "Feed a cold, starve a fever" have any merit?

—B.C., Orefield, Pennsylvania

No. Starving anything is hazardous to your health, says Susan Moores, R.D., a spokeswoman for the American Dietetic Association. If you're fighting an infection or a cold virus, you need all the nutrients, fluids, and rest you can get. "You need to eat well in order to be well," she says. Her bedside bounty: fruits, vegetables, low-fat protein sources, and whole grains.

Don't Blow It

Is it better to barf and get it over with, or let nature take its course?

—S.M., Las Vegas

In painfully technical medical terms: It depends. If you've got chills and a low-grade fever along with nausea, chances are you've got a stomach virus. Praying at Elvis's Altar won't help. The bug must run its course, usually within 4 to 8 hours. "If it's a virus, you'll still feel sick afterward, even if you make yourself vomit," says Jorge Herrera, M.D., professor in the division of gastroenterology at the University of South Alabama College of Medicine in Mobile. "Just drink clear liquids and eat toast and try to ride it out." If you have nausea with no other symptoms, that Big Burrito breakfast is simply not being digested. "Food is not going down, so it will eventually have to come up," Dr. Herrera says. To help it along, swallow 2 tablespoons of ipecac syrup followed by 8 ounces of water. You'll vomit within 20 minutes. Second choice: Watch the Anna Nicole Smith show.

Stop the Bleeding

How long should I wear a Band-Aid?

—T.O., San Juan, Puerto Rico

Slap on a bandage within 2 hours of injury and keep it on for at least 48 hours, says Patricia Mertz, research professor of cutaneous surgery at the University of Miami. "Covering the cut will create a moist environment that allows epidermis to migrate faster and create new skin," she says.

Hate wearing bandages? Paint on Band-Aid Liquid Bandage. It forms a clear, breathable, flexible seal that helps prevent infection. Four drops and you're covered. But head for the ER if you apply direct pressure and the bleeding doesn't stop, or if the cut is jagged and can't be closed. You may need stitches.

Throw In the Towel

How many days can I use a towel before laundering it?

—P.L., Tampa Bay, Florida

Infectious bacteria and fungi (like the one that causes athlete's foot) can't survive on a towel once it's dry, says Syed Sattar, Ph.D., professor of microbiology at the University of Ottawa in Ontario. Each time you towel off, however, you rub bacteria from your skin onto the towel, slowing down the fabric's drying speed. After 7 days, your towel accumulates enough organic material to actually form a barrier that protects the bad bacteria. So after a week, do what Eddie Futch did in round 15 of the Rumble in the Jungle: Toss in the towel.

Hands Off

What's the worst thing to touch in a public restroom?

—K.P., Syracuse, New York

George Michael. Badum-bum! Seriously, it's not the toilet seat, which, given our hapless aim, was our first guess. Philip Tierno, Ph.D., director of clinical microbiology and diagnostic immunology at the New York University medical center, says the seat itself is not all that hazardous. It gets wiped down regularly. What's really bad is what lies beneath. The two top offenders: the toilet bowel rim and the curved outer surface of the bowl itself. "Once you flush the toilet, a spray of water and fecal matter can move up to 20 feet from the source and literally coat everything in its vicinity," says Tierno. "The rim and (outer bowl) aren't touched very often, and that's where layers and layers of this stuff accumulate." Your best defense against this slime that transmits salmonella and stomach flu? Fold a paper towel to create a barrier between your hands and the rim if you're going to lift the seat. Or simply leave it down. Tell your wife the doctor said so. We also recommend running like hell immediately after flushing.

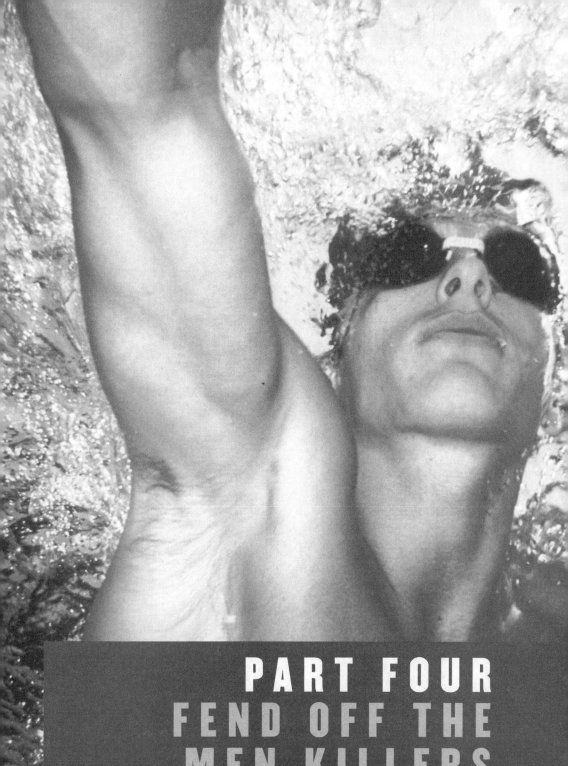

PART FOUR
FEND OFF THE MEN KILLERS

GAME SHOW

Who Will Get Colon Cancer?
All three of these men are at risk—are you?

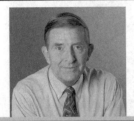

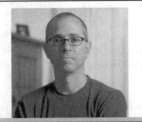

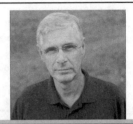

BOB QUICK
Age 61, 5'11", 165 lb
Sedentary smoker

STEVE PETERGAL
Age 44, 5'10", 165 lb
Has a family history

DON PEARSALL
Age 55, 6'6", 220 lb
Has had polyps removed

WHY HE MIGHT
Quick's age is a risk factor for colon and rectal cancers—simply called colorectal cancer (CRC). Incidence increases with age, beginning at age 40 and rising markedly after 50. He never exercises, and he's been a smoker for 34 years. Research shows that smoking increases risk of CRC, probably because some cancer-causing substances are swallowed and reach the digestive system.

WHY HE MIGHT NOT
About 5 years ago, Quick had a colonoscopy—a test in which doctors look into the colon—that showed no signs of polyps (potentially cancerous growths in the lining of the intestines or rectum). Quick eats a cancer-protective diet with plenty of fruits and vegetables, and he's not overweight. Excess fat in the waist area increases risk.

BOB'S PREDICTION
"I just don't see myself quitting smoking or starting to exercise after all these years. I've been okay so far."

WHY HE MIGHT
Petergal's sister was recently diagnosed with colon cancer at age 48. Having a first-degree relative—parent, sibling, child—with CRC roughly triples risk of developing the disease. Having a first-degree relative diagnosed under age 55 further increases risk. Also, Petergal has not yet had colon-cancer screening tests, which means he could have cancerous or precancerous polyps that are currently going untreated.

WHY HE MIGHT NOT
With an up-to-three-times-a-day apple habit, Petergal gets plenty of fiber. While inconclusive, some research suggests that a high-fiber diet may lower risk a bit. He eats plenty of other fruits and vegetables and avoids red meat. He also exercises for more than 10 hours weekly and maintains a healthful weight. All are believed to be habits that protect the colon.

STEVE'S PREDICTION
"I'm a healthy guy. My only risk is having a family history—but I think my sister is an anomaly. I won't be the winner."

WHY HE MIGHT
Last year, Pearsall had six polyps removed from his colon. Although they were not cancerous at the time, they were found to be adenomas. These types of polyps may become cancerous with time. A history like this increases Pearsall's risk of developing future adenomas and CRC in his lifetime. He is a meat eater who says, "Two hot dogs are better than one salad." Research suggests that a high-fat diet, especially from animal sources, may increase risk.

WHY HE MIGHT NOT
Chances are, Pearsall's colon is "clean" for the time being. It generally takes about 2 to 3 years for significant new polyps to form, and approximately 5 to 8 years for a polyp to develop into cancer, according to experts. Pearsall plans to have a colon screening again in a couple of years.

DON'S PREDICTION
"I'm changing my diet, and I'm getting more exercise. My polyps were removed, so I think I'm in good shape for now."

And the Winner Is . . .
Don Pearsall

Lester Rosen, M.D., a colorectal surgeon and professor of clinical surgery at Penn State Hershey Medical Center, helped us devise a test to determine our contestants' risk. The scorecard on the opposite page shows the major factors. Answer the questions and then add up your score. How clean are your pipes?

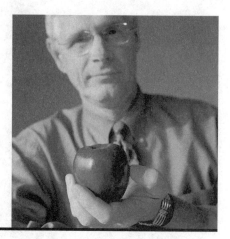

FINAL ANALYSIS

An argument could be made for both Pearsall and Petergal as "winners" since they both have higher-than-average risk of CRC. The major difference: Petergal has a family history of colorectal cancer, but no known personal history of polyps as does Pearsall. However, Petergal hasn't had a colon cancer screening yet, so he could be in trouble and not know it.

Researchers believe there is an adenoma-carcinoma sequence, meaning that about 95 percent of colorectal cancers begin as adenomas. So a person with adenomas is at greater risk than someone without them, regardless of family history. That means Pearsall has greater risk over time, according to Dr. Rosen. "The multiplicity of his polyps, that they were adenomas, and that they were distributed throughout make Pearsall's colon a target organ," Dr. Rosen says. "He has many years ahead of him, and his risk will increase as time goes on."

Petergal's risk is high because he has a family history of the disease, but also because his sister was under 55 when diagnosed, which increases his risk even further, according to research. A person should begin to get tested about 10 years before the age when an affected family member was diagnosed, says Dr. Rosen.

Quick has no symptoms or known predisposition to colorectal cancer. He has a risk of the disease, however, mostly because of age and smoking. Smokers who develop colorectal cancer are 30 to 40 percent more likely to die of it than nonsmokers, according to some research. Since his colonoscopy 5 years ago was clean, he should be fine for about another 3 to 5 years. "Quick's problem is the possible development of lung cancer," says Dr. Rosen.

To prevent colorectal cancer, the American Cancer Society recommends that all adults get colon cancer screenings starting at age 50, or earlier if they have a family history of the disease or a history of polyps. A diet low in animal fats and rich in fruits and vegetables may be helpful. Still, Dr. Rosen says, "even if you watch your diet, you need to have the screening done."

Tube Test

RISK FACTOR	POINT VALUE	BOB	STEVE	DON	YOU
AGE As you get older, your chances of developing colorectal cancer (CRC) increase.	40–50? —1 51–60? —2 61+? —3	—3	—1	—2	
PERSONAL HISTORY Previous CRC or adenomas increase risk.	Previous colorectal cancer? —9 Multiple adenomas? —4 Chronic bowel disease? —2			—4	
FAMILY HISTORY Having first-degree relatives with CRC increases risk. Also, a small percentage of families have inherited genetic conditions known as familial adenomatous polyposis (FAP) and hereditary nonpolyposis colorectal cancer (HNPCC), which greatly increase risk of developing CRC.	FAP? —10 HNPCC? —8 One first-degree relative with colorectal cancer? —3 The relative was diagnosed under age 55? —2 Two affected first-degree relatives? —5		—3 —2		
SCREENING Early detection may help prevent CRC.	Get colon screenings (as recommended by doctor)? +1 Should have had a screening but haven't? —1	+1	—1	+1	
DIET A healthful diet may reduce risk, according to some research.	Eat food mostly from high-fat animal sources? —1 Eat a balanced, high-fiber diet with lots of fruits and vegetables? +1	+1	+1	—1	
LIFESTYLE Smoking increases risk of developing CRC, as well as risk of dying of it.	Overweight? —1 Smoke? —2 Exercise 3 hours or more a week? +1	—2	+1		
TOTALS		—3	—5	—6	

▶ IF YOUR SCORE IS 1 OR MORE:
Colon power! You're a pipe dream.

▶ IF YOUR SCORE IS 0 TO —3:
Your pipes are only average, so keep a lookout.

▶ IF YOUR SCORE IS —4 OR LESS:
Pipe alert! Talk to your doctor about colon cancer screening.

MUST READS

Healthiest Homes for Men

Presenting our cross-country search for the places where guys can't help but be healthy—and those where they're likely to die trying

Edited by Matt Marion

If *Men's Health* had been on New World newsstands in 1607, we would have named Jamestown "The Healthiest Colony for Men." Okay, it was the *only* colony. But even though starvation, dysentery, and typhoid fever were rampant, Jamestown did protect its guys from the biggest health hazard of the day: eating an Algonquian arrow.

In 2004, a city needs more than a decent set of wooden palisades to support a healthy ZIP code—it has to be a statistical standout. Prostate cancer can deliver a low blow, but it can't score a knockout. Same goes for heart disease, stroke, and the other major man-killers. And, because a longer life span doesn't mean much if it's idled away in traffic, there can't be congested roadways. Or air that tastes like tailpipe.

The neighbors count, too. They have to be fit, not fat. Neither armed nor

PROSTATE CANCER

City Getting Hit below the Belt: New Orleans

Most Gland-Friendly: San Francisco

Men in San Fran rank 69 percent lower in prostate-cancer mortality than their cousins in the Crescent City.

"San Francisco has a robust health-care system—UCSF, Kaiser, Stanford—as well as an educated population that tends to be health-conscious," says Peter Carroll, M.D.,

chairman of urology at the University of California at San Francisco.

How men in New Orleans can catch up: Have your cPSA, or "complexed prostate-specific antigen" measured. Whereas PSA levels often go up because of an enlarged prostate or an infection, cPSA usually rises only when there's cancer. In a study presented at a meeting of the American Urological Association, cPSA testing was 67 percent more accurate than measuring PSA. Most urologists can administer the test.

IMPOTENCE

Mister Softee's Hometown: Atlanta
Most Uplifting City: Anchorage

Based on doctor visits for erectile dysfunction and number of Viagra prescriptions per man, the Atlanta man's love life has definitely gone south.

Southern diets tend to be high in fried foods. "That can lead to obesity, a risk factor for impotence," says Chad Ritenour, M.D., a professor of urology at the Emory University school of medicine in Atlanta.

How men in Atlanta can catch up: Make sure you don't have diabetes. In a study published in the *British Journal of Urology*, researchers tested 129 men complaining of erectile dysfunction and found that diabetes was causing the impotence in 22 of them, six of whom didn't even know they had the disease. If you're having difficulty achieving and maintaining an erection, ask your doctor to give you a fasting blood-sugar test.

dangerous. With a healthy smattering of white-coat professionals. Sound like too much to ask? It was for most of the 101 cities we looked at. Only a handful met our criteria for keeping a guy safe, sane, and scoring in the sack. You might be living in one of those cities right now, and even if you're not, that's okay, too; we'll give you the tools so you can build a healthy colony of one. Like disease, well-being is contagious—especially among our readers.

THE WORST: ATLANTA

Braves fans everywhere are glad that Greg Maddux didn't read this. For as his contract ran out, potential free-agent suitors no doubt could have rushed in and waved this story in his face. Yes, Atlantans can shout from Marietta to Buckhead about the glories of the Braves, the Falcons' "home-dome advantage," and the American institutions that are Southern rock and Coca-Cola. But the truth is that Atlanta is a 24/7 pressure cooker for men.

Is it all that deep-fried turkey at tailgating? A freeway system that looks less like the Old South and more like ol' L.A.? Or is it just that all those transplanted Yanks have erased the drawly, laid-back charm of the belles and their beaus and created all-day rush hours? Perhaps all of the above. Observe:

Atlanta hit the bottom 10 in homicide rate (or top 10, if you're an aspiring coroner) and had a higher overall mortality rate than 80 percent of the cities surveyed. Cancer and diabetes are the worst offenders (bottom 20 percent for both). But the biggest problem—a very treatable problem—is high blood pressure. If it weren't for Shreveport, Louisiana, and Akron, Ohio—not exactly booming population centers—Atlanta would be number one. "There could be several reasons," says L. Dana Wadsworth, a family practice M.D. in the Virginia Highlands section of town. "Atlanta has a large African-American

(continued on page 134)

THE CITY SCORECARD

Here they are, the final standings in the metro league.

City	Health Grade	Environ- ment Grade	Fitness Grade	Final Rank
Honolulu, HI	A	A	A	1
San Jose, CA*	A	B	C	2
Rochester, NY	C	A	B	3
Santa Ana, CA	A	C	B	4
Grand Rapids, MI	B	B	B	5
Denver, CO	B	B	B	6
Colorado Springs, CO	B	B	B	7
San Diego, CA	A	C	B	8
Boston, MA	B	B	B	9
Seattle, WA	A	C	C	10
San Francisco, CA	B	B	B	11
Albuquerque, NM	B	C	B	12
Raleigh, NC	A	C	C	13
Tucson, AZ	A	A	F	14
Des Moines, IA	D	B	A	15
Spokane, WA*	C	B	A	16
Lincoln, NE	B	B	D	17
Anchorage, AK	B	C	B	18
Minneapolis, MN	B	C	B	19
Sacramento, CA	B	C	B	20
St. Paul, MN	C	C	B	21
El Paso, TX	B	C	C	22
Yonkers, NY	B	C	C	23
Madison, WI	B	B	D	24
Wichita, KS	C	B	D	25
Omaha, NE	D	B	B	26
New York, NY	C	C	B	27
Corpus Christi, TX	F	A	C	28
Portland, OR	C	D	B	29
Anaheim, CA	B	D	C	30
Huntington Beach, CA	B	D	C	31
St. Petersburg, FL	B	D	C	32
Fremont, CA	B	D	C	33
Plano, TX	B	D	C	34
Austin, TX	B	D	C	35
Aurora, CO	A	D	D	36
Washington, DC	F	D	A	37
Tacoma, WA	C	D	C	38

City	Health Grade	Environ- ment Grade	Fitness Grade	Final Rank
Virginia Beach, VA	C	D	C	39
Pittsburgh, PA	F	B	B	40
Scottsdale, AZ	A	D	F	41
Glendale, CA	B	F	C	42
San Antonio, TX	D	B	C	43
Mesa, AZ	A	D	F	44
Phoenix, AZ	A	D	F	45
Jersey City, NJ	B	D	D	46
Long Beach, CA	B	F	C	47
Tampa, FL	F	C	B	48
Los Angeles, CA	B	F	C	49
Lexington, KY	D	A	F	50
Glendale, AZ	A	D	F	51
Oakland, CA	B	D	F	52
Toledo, OH	F	A	F	53
Hialeah, FL	B	D	D	54
Shreveport, LA	F	B	C	55
Miami, FL	B	D	D	56
Milwaukee, WI	F	D	B	57
Lubbock, TX	C	C	F	58
Mobile, AL	F	D	A	59
Las Vegas, NV	D	F	B	60
Fort Wayne, IN	D	C	D	61
Houston, TX	D	F	C	62
Fresno, CA	C	F	D	63
Akron, OH	D	C	F	64
Tulsa, OK	F	C	D	65
Bakersfield, CA	D	F	B	66
Richmond, VA	D	C	F	67
Newark, NJ	D	F	D	68
Buffalo, NY	D	B	F	69
Chicago, IL	F	F	C	70
Detroit, MI	F	F	A	71
Chesapeake, VA	F	D	C	72
Louisville, KY	F	D	D	73
Montgomery, AL	F	C	D	74
Cincinnati, OH	D	B	F	75
Greensboro, NC	F	D	D	76
Baltimore, MD	F	F	A	77
Baton Rouge, LA	D	D	F	78

City	Health Grade	Environment Grade	Fitness Grade	Final Rank	City	Health Grade	Environment Grade	Fitness Grade	Final Rank
Stockton, CA	F	F	C	79	Kansas City, MO	F	F	D	91
Fort Worth, TX	F	D	F	80	Jacksonville, FL	F	D	D	92
Cleveland, OH	F	B	F	81	Charlotte, NC	C	F	F	93
Norfolk, VA	F	D	D	82	Indianapolis, IN	F	F	D	94
Riverside, CA	C	F	D	83	Garland, TX	C	F	F	95
Arlington, TX	F	D	F	84	Oklahoma City, OK	F	B	F	96
Columbus, OH	F	C	F	85	Memphis, TN	F	F	D	97
Irving, TX	C	F	F	86	Philadelphia, PA	F	F	D	98
Augusta, GA	F	C	D	87	New Orleans, LA	F	C	F	99
Dallas, TX	C	F	F	88	Nashville, TN	F	D	F	100
Birmingham, AL	F	F	C	89	Atlanta, GA	F	F	F	101
St. Louis, MO	F	B	F	90					

*How does a city that got an "A," "B," and "C" (San Jose) place 14 spots higher than one with a "C," "B," and "A" (Spokane)? Just like in school, each letter grade represents a numerical range. So, while a test score of 91 is an A, it's not as high an A as a 98. Some cities' "A's," "B's," and, "C's" are worth more in the final ranking than others.

How It All Adds Up

Rather than drive around the country with a stethoscope in one hand and a thermometer in the other, we crunched numbers—a metropolitan phone book's worth—to diagnose the health of our nation's cities. This involved rating each according to 20 live-long parameters covering the general areas of health, fitness, and the environment. If we could adjust for age, we did. If women could be left out of the picture, they were.

Our sources? They included the Centers for Disease Control and Prevention WONDER database; CDC Behavioral Risk Factor Surveillance System data compiled and calculated by the Web site BestPlaces.net; the U.S. Census Bureau;

Health and Healthcare in the United States, County and Metro Area Data, Second Edition, 2000, put out by NationsHealth Corporation; and the American Lung Association's State of the Air: 2002.

After days of downloading data, we weighted, sorted, and sifted until we had our semifinalists. These were the cities that scored best or worst in each of the 20 parameters, be it blood pressure or body-mass index, weight training or the willingness to get off one's butt and run around the block a few times. Then we weighted the data again, but this time as it comprised the overarching health, fitness, and environment categories. Once everything was added up and averaged, we hit the Enter key.

population, which traditionally has more problems with hypertension. The traditional Southern diet is higher in fat. And this really is not a walking city."

If indeed you get sick, you might actually have a shorter wait flying to San Francisco to see a general practitioner, since the Bay Area has almost twice the number of doctors per person as Atlanta has.

Compounding all these health risks is an ozone problem so intense that for 45 days out of the year it's unhealthy even to be outside. Only southern California and Houston are worse. "The city has great parks," says Tanya Miszko, Ed.D., C.S.C.S., a personal trainer who has lived in the area for 4 years, "as long as you don't mind running in smog."

It makes little difference. No one's exercising indoors, either—Atlanta ranks near the bottom in overall fitness. "It's not a lack of availability," says Miszko. "There are plenty of health clubs to choose from."

The only men she sees in gyms these days are young college guys and middle-aged men trying to recapture that youthful sheen. But what about the catalysts of Atlanta's explosive growth in the past decade: the educated, bust-ass career guys? Maybe they're forsaking fitness for work, says Miszko—conquer the world, eat some takeout, start over tomorrow. "I see more blue-collar guys in the gym than high-powered executives."

So should all those Atlantans just chuck themselves onto the scrap heap? Give it up to bitter blood, constricted veins, and death from too much life? Hardly. There's one saving grace in all of this that most single Atlanta guys are forgetting about: single Atlanta women. They are legion, and they want you to get in shape. "Metro Atlanta has the largest concentration of college campuses in the state," says Miszko. "So single men are surrounded by educated, career-oriented women, as well as all the college women. There's lots of energy in this city."

Someone should start burning it off.

LUNG CANCER

There's Something in the Air: Baltimore

Breathe Easy: El Paso, Texas

Men in Baltimore die of lung cancer at a rate that's 64 percent higher than the national average and more than twice as high as in El Paso.

"At one time Maryland had one of the highest smoking rates in the nation," says Joseph A. Adams, M.D., F.A.C.P., a professor of medicine at the University of Maryland.

How men in Baltimore can catch up: Swap one stinky habit—smoking—for another—eating cabbage. According to a study published in the *Lancet Oncology*, a compound in cabbage slowed the lung cancer-causing activity of NNK, a substance in cigarettes. Eat more sauerkraut, stuffed cabbage, or cole slaw (with reduced-fat mayo).

OBESITY

Fat City: San Antonio
Trim Town: Boston

Bostonians are gutless; they have a body-mass index (BMI) of 25.4, two points lighter than the men in San Antonio (BMI: 27.7).

"Obesity is higher in Hispanic populations, and San Antonio is about 60 percent Hispanic," says Ken Goodrick, Ph.D., a professor of family medicine at Baylor college of medicine.

How men in San Antonio can catch up: Ask your doctor about the antidepressant bupropion. In a study published in *Obesity Research*, overweight people who took 400 mg of bupropion daily while dieting and exercising lost 8.6 percent of their weight after 48 weeks, versus 5 percent for the placebo group. Researchers believe the drug helps to control appetite by regulating neurotransmitters in the brain.

THE BEST: HONOLULU

What a shame that America's healthiest city for men is a place where so many of us live it up, but so few of us actually live. While you're getting lei'd, exploring black sand beaches, taking helicopter tours, and trying to score front row for Don Ho, the average Honolulan male is enjoying a daily bath of statistical immunity that makes your last blood panel look like a death warrant.

Only one city, San Jose, California, has a lower mortality rate. And why not? There's a lot to live for here. Twenty-footers on the North Shore. Dusk on Sunset Beach. Women in grass skirts, with hips that move faster than a paint-can mixer. And best of all, a climate that makes an unassailable argument for outdoor office space. Locals tap into all that positive energy to the tune of the lowest cancer death rate in the United States, and a heart-disease ranking in the top five. "People in general have good habits here," says Neal Palafox, M.D., a professor at the University of Hawaii's John A. Burns school of medicine. Along with fish, "they have access to very healthy foods that grow abundantly, like guavas, mangos, and papayas."

But that's just for starters. The men of Honolulu have run, swum, and lifted their way to a number-one ranking in overall fitness. Which makes a lot of sense, since anyone who's visited the city knows there aren't many reasons to stay inside. "It's the perfect training climate," says Barry Toyama, C.S.C.S., a trainer and lifelong resident. "Pristine natural environments lure all types of organized events."

Honolulu is also quick to confirm the old saw about friends in high places. And active men have some good ones here, says Toyama. "The partnership between the locals and the government is irreplaceable. Public land is easily

HEART DISEASE

Bum Tickers: St. Louis

Beat Goes On: Colorado Springs, Colorado

The Springs boasts 41 percent fewer male heart-disease deaths than the rest of the nation, and 62 percent less than St. Louis.

How men in St. Louis can catch up: Go for two cholesterol tests. UK researchers looked at how well a single measurement of systolic blood pressure and total and HDL cholesterol predicted heart-disease risk, and found it can be off by 25 percent. Get two tests, a week apart, and average the results.

accessible, and the governor has been influential in increasing and maintaining innovative park concepts."

The amount of that public land is staggering: 6,644 acres of parks, beaches, golf courses, tennis courts, and pools, and so much surfing, scuba diving, and snorkeling that when Aquaman visits, he requires an afternoon nap.

Beyond that, Dr. Palafox points to an even deeper cultural motivation for the men of Hawaii: "Being overweight is not something that goes over well here." Boys are exposed early to the community's widespread youth sports programs, awakening a competitive spirit that lingers for life. Toyama agrees. "Without a doubt, a sense of machismo proliferates in the islands."

So say aloha to Honolulu. Spend all your vacation days and all your money trying to untie the knots of your reckless mainland life. You might just be tempted to stay, which bodes well for your long-term survival. After all, once you're here, the deck is stacked against your escape, says Toyama. "The sun will always cast its perfect Hawaiian sunset, summer, winter, spring, or fall. And let's not forget, the most gorgeous women in the world live in Hawaii. That's motivation enough."

2. SAN JOSE, CALIFORNIA

It's the mecca of the microprocessor industry and the next-best thing to living in Honolulu. For one thing, guys don't die here—at least not very often. No other city has a lower overall mortality rate for men, in part because San Jose also has the lowest homicide rate. And if you do get shot or sick, there are more than enough doctors to patch you up and send you back out into . . .

The sunlight. It beams down for more than 300 unobscured days annually, which explains why San Joseans—anybody got a better nickname for these people?—report far fewer days of "poor mental health" (living near more than 50 world-class wineries probably helps) and why they get out and exercise more than men in 94 other cities. "The environment is a major factor," says Marty Fenstersheib, M.D., the San Jose-based health officer for Santa Clara County. "Whether it's the ocean or the mountains, active men have great opportunities here."

3. ROCHESTER, NEW YORK

Rochester? Put aside the 95-inch average annual snowfall and the 24-degree typical February temperature for a moment, and consider some of the evidence: The air makes for better breathing than in three-quarters of the cities surveyed, the commutes are half as long as in New York City, and the colon-cancer and stroke death rates are among the nation's lowest. "Overall, we receive a high level of medical attention, mainly because of the University of Rochester, which is the city's largest employer," says Eric Schaff, M.D., a professor of family medicine at the university's medical center.

Then there are the intangibles that help keep a man from killing himself, whether through disease or despair: fishing and golf. With Lake Ontario in its backyard and the Genesee River running through it, Rochester offers more chinook salmon, cohos, steelhead, and lake trout than you can shake a dry fly at. Omega-3 fatty acids (the heart-healthful nutrients in fish) are bustin' out all over. On higher ground, there are 65 golf courses in the surrounding area, including a Robert Trent Jones beauty that anyone can afford to play (just not necessarily well).

SKIN CANCER

Place Most in Need of Sunscreen: Oklahoma City
Toughest Hides: Chicago

Guys in Chi-Town succumb to skin cancer 61 percent less frequently than their Sooner brethren.

"The entire state has a very high incidence because it is a Southern state with a lot of outdoor activities and agriculture," says Mark Naylor, M.D., an associate professor of dermatology at the University of Oklahoma health-sciences center.

How men in Oklahoma City can catch up: Wear sunscreen and ask your dermatologist if he owns a "dermatoscope." A skin screening using one of these handheld microscopes is roughly 30 percent more accurate at identifying skin lesions than an exam with the naked eye. But according to one study only 22 percent of U.S. dermatologists use a dermatoscope. "In Europe, people demand their doctors use it," says Robert Johr, M.D., a dermatologist at the University of Miami.

4. SANTA ANA, CALIFORNIA

Disneyland is goofy; nearby Santa Ana is the *real* Magic Kingdom—for men. The price of admission entitles you to a prostate-cancer mortality rate that's 18 percent lower than the national average, a nearly nonexistent number of men stroking out, and a dearth of deaths-by-neighbor, i.e., homicides. "In the past 10 years, we've reduced our homicide rate by more than 50 percent," says Sgt. Baltazar De La Rive of the Santa Ana Police Department. "It's a combination of our strong law-enforcement programs and our close working relationship with our community."

Being a Santa Anian also means never having to hide your body inside a mouse or duck costume. Guys here boast a leaner body-mass index than their brothers in 83 other cities, no doubt due to the fact that they're bronze medalists in exercise rates. Their motivation: 39 parks, 11 bike trails, a daily average temperature of 65 degrees, and a duty to always be as fighting fit as the namesake of the city's airport: the Duke himself, John Wayne.

5. GRAND RAPIDS, MICHIGAN

In 2001, the Grand Rapids Rampage ran past 15 other teams to win the Arena Football Championship. The year after that, in another team effort, the city's men gang-tackled diabetes (seventh-lowest incidence), strokes (10th-lowest mortality), and colon cancer (12th-lowest death rate) to beat out 96 other cities for the number-five spot in our rankings. And they were in the shape to do it—guys in Grand Rapids spend more time on the running trails than almost anyone anywhere else.

Talk about covering ground; the average morning commute takes a blink-

EXERCISE

Least Likely to Break a Sweat: Oklahoma City
Staying in Shape: Madison, Wisconsin

Actually, the guys in Oklahoma City are no slouches, it's just that at any given moment, Madison men are more likely to be in the gym, on their bikes, or off on a run.

"The city caters to people being active by having a lot of bicycle paths and hiking trails," says John Porcari, Ph.D., a professor of exercise at the University of Wisconsin.

How men in Oklahoma City can catch up: Not into running your butt off? Lift more, but don't overtrain. "Muscle soreness generally peaks 2 days after your workout," says Darren Steeves, C.S.C.S., a trainer at Dalhousie University in Nova Scotia. "If you're exercising on a Monday-Wednesday-Friday schedule, overdoing it on Monday will make Wednesday's workout a pure pain-fest." Do eight repetitions with a weight that you can lift 12 to 15 times, and add an extra rep with each successive workout.

CAR ACCIDENTS

An Accident Waiting to Happen: Fresno, California
Designated Drivers: Sacramento

Perhaps Sacramento has such a low rate of fatal car accidents involving men (64 percent lower than the national average) because everyone's using public transportation, be it the light-rail service or the River Otter Water Taxi. But how do you explain Fresno's high roadkill rate—96 percent higher than the U.S. average?

"Most of our collisions are due to speed and alcohol," says Brian Hance, a fatal-accident detective with the Fresno P.D.

How men in Fresno can catch up: Don't trust your life to an airbag. University of Washington researchers found that a car's driver-side airbag reduces the risk of death by only 8 percent, compared with 65 percent for the seatbelt. Worse, airbags were also shown to be less effective for men than for women, perhaps because men are heavier and may overcome the bag's cushioning effect. "Unless you don't care about your risk of dying, buckle up," says Peter Cummings, Ph.D., the lead study author. And that means the back-seat too; a study published in *Lancet* found that unbuckled rear-seat passengers increase the driver's chance of dying because of the force with which they hit the front seat.

and-you-missed-it 19 minutes. It gets better on your lunch break: You can pop out of the office to angle for salmon as they make their way up the Grand River, which travels through the heart of downtown. Is it any wonder that the guys here rarely report feeling blue? "There are excellent resources for men and their families," says Thomas Spahn, Ed.D., a Grand Rapids psychologist. "A guy could go fishing all day and then come home and take his wife to a five-star dinner and the symphony. The economy has always been good. Men here have balanced lives."

Survive a Heart Attack

When chest pain struck, I made mistakes that nearly cost me my life. Read my story, and do as I say . . . not as I did

By Fred Abatemarco

It was not quite 8 A.M. To my mind, far too early to choose between life and death. But a red-faced doctor wouldn't let up. He was literally spitting as he shouted just a few inches from my face. "You need to tell me," he insisted. "Do you want the emergency angioplasty surgery or not?" I was having a heart attack. I had decisions to make.

Didn't I know it. I had been up all night making bad decisions. It was on an ordinary fall evening about 5 years ago when I felt the first twinge of chest pressure that ultimately landed me, strapped to a hospital gurney, in the emergency room of Mount Auburn Hospital in Cambridge, Massachusetts. I ignored the feeling at first, and then sipped some Scotch. Don't ask me why I thought that was a good antidote to indigestion—I just did.

I felt like one good heave of my stomach contents was all the relief necessary. The pain was nowhere near the "elephant sitting on my chest" description given by some heart attack victims. It felt more like heartburn. I thought I was coming down with the flu.

I went to bed early. But the uneasiness nagged on. The tightening in my chest kept waking me up. I ate some yogurt. I drank some water. Nothing changed. I was sweating and chilled. About 4 A.M. I began to worry seriously. This could be the Big One. But I stayed in denial.[1]

[1] My First Mistake

Drinking whiskey was a bad move. "The alcohol could have contributed to an arrhythmia" and caused cardiac arrest, says Nieca Goldberg, M.D., chief of cardiovascular rehabilitation at Lenox Hill Hospital in New York City.

It Didn't Feel like a Heart Attack

Men expect knife-in-the-chest pain. "It usually isn't that dramatic," says Robert Bonow, M.D., president of the American Heart Association. Never ignore a relentless fullness or tightness of the chest.

A life-threatening illness was unthinkable to me at the time. I was 48 years old, at the top of my career, having the time of my life away from home in a 10-week management program at Harvard. My life was a harmony of professional success, prosperity, and the love and security of a happy family. The balmy New England weather presaged a promising future. I had never had any serious health problems. At the time, I was bicycling 10 miles a day and feeling great. Only a month before, I had passed a life insurance physical, including the requisite electrocardiogram (EKG) test, with no reservations. I couldn't be having a . . . I wouldn't allow myself to consider the words.[2]

[2] I Was a Prime Candidate

Though I may have seemed like a healthy man, the warning signs were there—if I'd cared to notice. I was overweight. My cholesterol count, at 190, was coming precariously close to the recommended maximum of 200. I had smoked cigarettes since my teen years. Though I'd quit those more than a decade before, I remained a nicotine addict gratified by cigars, which I inhaled.

Two hours later, the sun came up and I gave in to what now seems obvious: I was in very serious trouble. I phoned the campus medical center, where a nurse had no problem thinking the worst when I explained my symptoms. "Chew an aspirin, call 911, and come to the hospital," she commanded. But 911 is for fires and domestic violence, I thought. "I'll just walk down to your office," I countered. "Do not walk anywhere!" the nurse shouted. So I took a cab.

Before I left my room, I did something that I still don't believe. Knowing the day ahead would be long, unpleasant, and not exactly according to my preferred routine, I made a pot of coffee and smoked a cigar. Oh yeah, I crunched down an aspirin, too, as the nurse suggested. Then I was ready to meet my fate.[3]

I was the medical center's first customer of the day—no waiting. They stuck electrodes to my bare chest and took an electrocardiogram. The EKG readout showed abnormal electrical pulses, quickly confirming that an MI (myocardial infarction, or "infarct") was in progress. Now I was genuinely terrified. The nurse called an ambulance, taped oxygen tubes to my nose, took a blood pressure reading, and slipped a nitroglycerin tablet under my tongue. It had a sour, nasty taste, but I wasn't about to complain or spit it out. Its purpose was to relax my constricted blood vessels, thus lowering my blood pressure. The ambulance paramedics started an intravenous feed of morphine to relieve the chest pain.

As I lay there, I thought about my wife and my teenage son and daughter beginning their day at our suburban New York home. I hadn't called. Didn't want to worry them. Now I wondered if that was a terrible, terrible mistake. I tried to force the thought from my head.[4]

[3]Big Mistake: I Waited All Night

Though most heart attack victims survive, the 5 percent who don't make it usually succumb to cardiac arrest in the early stages—and half of those die before they reach a hospital. "The worst thing you did was to wait," Dr. Bonow tells me. The second mistake I made was failing to call 911. "Trained personnel can monitor your condition, determine if you're having a large heart attack or a small one, call ahead to a hospital, and deal with arrhythmia or worse," Dr. Bonow says.

The One Smart Thing I Actually Did

Chewing an aspirin speeds the medicine to the bloodstream, where it thins the blood and can counteract some of the blood clots that cause a heart attack. "Aspirin is important because it prevents the blood platelets from sticking together," says Dr. Bonow.

[4]Get to a Hospital Fast!

The preferred hospital in Cambridge, at least as far as the staff of the Harvard Medical Center is concerned, is Brigham and Women's Hospital. But by policy, the paramedic crew was required to take me to the closest hospital—Mount Auburn—even though the difference was only 5 minutes by ambulance. "All our heart attack treatments are time dependent," says W. Douglas Weaver, M.D., chairman of the Heart and Vascular Institute at Henry Ford Hospital in Detroit. "Do anything you can do to reduce the time to treatment." There's good reason for this advice: Studies show that a clot-busting thrombolytic drug, such as TPA (Activase), can actually abort a heart attack if administered in the first hour. "But only 5 to 10 percent of heart attack victims reach the hospital in the first hour," says Dr. Weaver.

By the time I reached the emergency room, my pain, though never severe, started to dissipate. So I was back to my state of hopefulness. That lasted only a moment, as the spitting ER doctor grew impatient for my permission to do emergency angioplasty.

I wanted to know about the catheterization. "Are there any risks?"

"Of course there are risks." He was virtually screaming at me now. "You are having a heart attack!"

"Well, can I first call my wife?" I said sheepishly. He walked off in frustration.

Meanwhile, a host of ER technicians were having their way with me. One hooked up an echocardiogram to view my heart with sonar readings. Another redid the IV hookup and began feeding me clot-busting drugs. Someone brought me a phone. "Natalie," I said to my wife just before she left for a train ride to Manhattan, "I think you'd better catch the next shuttle to Boston."

A short while later, the hospital's chief of cardiology, Leonard Zir, M.D., strolled into the emergency room. Despite his casual and somewhat disheveled appearance, Dr. Zir is a gladiator of the cardiac catheter. His primary mission at Mount Auburn is cardiac intervention—emergency angioplasty. He lives for the opportunity to snake a thin wire up an artery—from your leg or groin right into your heart—and pump up a balloon to unclog a blocked artery while the heart attack is taking place. In my case, that opportunity had passed. In medical parlance, my heart attack had "evolved." Dr. Zir said angioplasty wouldn't help save heart muscle at this point. The good news was I was still alive. The extent of the bad news was still to be determined.[5]

I spent the next 5 days at Mount Auburn, first under close watch in the cardiac intensive care unit and later under more relaxed conditions. I was fed a steady stream of drugs, including heparin (a blood thinner) and oxazepam to ease my nicotine cravings. Mostly, I slept the first few days, with Natalie watching over me.

I had little appetite or energy. It was a combination of the medication and the fact that my heart had been severely "stunned." One medical student

[5] Agree to Angioplasty

At many hospitals, the standard procedure is to conduct an emergency, or "primary," angioplasty, though the patient must give consent. "For the patient, decision making can be totally irrational under these circumstances," says Dr. Bonow. "In a life-or-death situation, with trained professionals on hand, my attitude is 'Just do it.'"

Angioplasty is considered highly effective within the first few hours. But there is increasing evidence that it can make a difference even after as long as 9 to 12 hours, says Dr. Bonow, who adds that a so-called late opening of a constricted artery can sometimes save heart muscle from irreversible damage and make it easier for the laboring heart to recuperate. I simply had waited too long—through the night and by hesitating at the hospital.

PREVENT DEFENSE

The smartest plan for attacking a heart attack is preventing one from ever happening—and that means, of course, don't smoke yourself. But beyond quitting, choose three of the following preventive strategies that you're currently not doing. Make them a habit. The closer to the top of the list you get, the more you reduce your risk of heart disease.

1. Convince your wife to stop smoking. Nonsmoking husbands of smoking wives face a 92 percent increase in their risk of heart attack, according to a report in the *Journal of the American College of Cardiology*. Breathing secondhand smoke boosts LDL ("bad") cholesterol levels, decreases HDL ("good") cholesterol, and increases your blood's tendency to clot.

2. Walk, run, or lift weights for 30 minutes four times a week. Middle-aged men who exercised vigorously for 2 or more hours cumulatively per week had 60 percent less risk of heart attack than inactive men did, according to the *New England Journal of Medicine*.

3. Lose 10 to 20 pounds. If you're overweight, dropping 10 to 20 pounds could lower your risk of dying from a first heart attack by 16 percent. Being overweight drives up cholesterol and blood pressure, the precursors to coronary disease. A 10-year Mayo Clinic study found that overweight people had heart attacks 3.6 years earlier than normal-weight people did, and that obese heart attack patients tended to be 8.2 years younger than normal-weight victims.

4. Drink five glasses of water a day. In a study at Loma Linda University, men who drank that many 8-ounce glasses were 54 percent less likely to have a fatal heart attack than those who drank two or fewer. Researchers say the water dilutes the blood, making it less likely to clot.

5. Switch from coffee to tea. A Dutch study found that people who drank 3 cups of tea a day had half the risk of heart attack of those who didn't drink tea at all. Potent antioxidants, called flavonoids, in tea may provide a protective effect.

6. Grill salmon on Saturday, have a tuna sandwich on Tuesday. Researchers at the Harvard School of Public Health say that eating fish at least twice a week can lower your heart disease risk by more than 30 percent. The magic ingredient is the omega-3 fatty acids found in fish. In another study, men without heart disease were 10 percent less likely to die suddenly when their blood levels of omega-3s were high.

7. Ask your doctor about vitamin E and aspirin. Men who took the antioxidant and the blood thinner daily cut the plaque in their clogged arteries by more than 80 percent, according to a recent University of Pennsylvania study.

8. Eat a cup of Total cornflakes for breakfast. This cereal contains one of the highest concentrations of folic acid (675 micrograms) of any cold cereal. (Folic acid is the supplemental form of folate.) Taking in that much folic acid daily (the recommended amount is 400 mcg) cuts your risk of cardiovascular disease by 13 percent, according to researchers at Tulane University. Folate works by reducing blood levels of artery-damaging homocysteine.

9. Count to 10. Creating a 10-second buffer before reacting to a stressful situation may be enough to cool you down. Men who respond to stress with anger are three times likelier to be diagnosed with heart disease and five times likelier to have a heart attack before turning 55, say researchers at Johns Hopkins University.

10. Eat watermelon. It contains about 40 percent more lycopene than is found in raw tomatoes, and a new study by the Agricultural Research Service of the USDA shows that your body absorbs it at higher levels due to the melon's high water content. Half a wedge may boost heart disease prevention by 30 percent.

stopped by my room again and again, continually asking me to repeat my daily pre–heart attack regimen. She could not believe that I drank 10 cups of coffee a day. It was a revelation to me, too. But no one was even fazed that I smoked 20 cigarillos every day.[6]

After a few examinations and a thallium stress test, I was sent home with instructions to find a cardiologist and begin to exercise. For the first week, one trip up the stairs was about all I could manage. My overtaxed heart wasn't up to the task. Gradually, I was able to take 15-minute walks. But acclimating to the drugs was an ordeal. If I bent over to tie my shoelaces, I'd become faint. My family doctor, upon reviewing Mount Auburn's charts, shook his head gravely and suggested I make myself available as a heart transplant candidate. Transplant? My God, how bad was this heart attack?

While it didn't kill me, it was no trivial event. All those hours that night, while I was hoping my "gastric" problems would abate with one healthy belch, the lower half of my heart's left ventricle was being starved of blood by a clot in the left anterior descending artery. Doctors were amazed—and I must say I am quite pleased—that my heart did not simply stop or otherwise react cataclysmically to this suffocating blockage. The damage to my heart was so severe that a few months after my heart attack, my cardiologist got into a debate with a heart surgeon who insisted that bypass surgery wouldn't do me a bit of good. My cardiologist felt that bypassing the blocked artery would be worthwhile even though the area of the heart it served wasn't functional. Sometimes tissue can be revived when blood supply is returned to the area.

The two doctors agreed to a high-tech equivalent of a coin toss: They would let the results of a positron emission tomography (PET) scan decide my fate. If it revealed any signs of life in my heart's dead zone, the bypass surgery would proceed.[7]

The surgeon won the argument and lost the chance to slice and dice me. The PET scan showed convincingly that my heart's big gun in front was a mere memory, and that the area it served was long dead. As bad as that news

---

[6] Damned Smokes!

As a smoker, I had actually doubled my risk of having a heart attack. "Smoking is such a potent trigger that other factors are small bullets by comparison," says Dr. Weaver. Smoking increases heart rate and blood pressure, adding to heart stress that can cause long-term muscle damage. The ingredients of cigarette smoke can damage the lining of the coronary arteries, leading to the development of plaque.

[7] Get a PET Scan

This highly evolved, noninvasive imaging technology can help detect heart tissue's viability. If doctors see that the tissue is metabolizing glucose, they have good reason to believe that the tissue can be revived by restoring bloodflow to the area by means of bypass surgery.

THIS OLD HEART OF MINE

By Fred Abatemarco

There's a refrain in a favorite O'Jays song about mothers that can be applied equally to your heart: "You only get one, you only get one, yeah."

And after doing considerable damage to mine—my heart, not Mom—the challenge became how best to care for it going forward. Doctors decided I would commence with aggressive risk factor management. The keystone of this therapy is drugs, and more drugs.

Today, and likely every day for the rest of my life, I'll ingest a powerhouse of four pharmaceuticals: Lipitor, a cholesterol-lowering statin drug; Toprol XL, a beta-blocker that slows my heartbeat; Privinil, to lower my blood pressure; and aspirin, the over-the-counter blood thinner. "Each of these medicines can reduce risk of death by 25 percent or more, and together they may have some cumulative effect," notes Robert Bonow, M.D., president of the American Heart Association.

What has really changed is my lifestyle. I've switched to decaf. I take a multivitamin, plus vitamins E and C daily. My diet skews heavily in the direction of the Mediterranean: fish three or four times a week, chicken, vegetables, and salads. I work out with weights with a trainer or do aerobic exercise a minimum of 4 days a week. The exercise is beneficial to mind as well as body: It's a primary agent in raising the level of "good," HDL cholesterol. And I find it provides the best relief from the rigors of work and raising teenagers.

I've come to accept the slightly life-altering side effects of my medication: weight gain, diminished sex drive, slight fatigue, shortness of breath with heavy physical exertion. If not for these, I'm convinced I'd be feeling pretty close to normal and would probably be enjoying life to the extreme. But then, that's about the same attitude I had on October 1, 1998. Doing things to the extreme is how I got in trouble in the first place. So, better I should take a brisk walk.

was, I have to admit being somewhat relieved there would be no bypass. Having my chest cracked wide while my body is being run by machines is not my idea of a fun day.

The PET scan also revealed the first bit of really good news since this whole nightmare began. My circumflex coronary artery was functioning like a thing of beauty. Essentially, it was keeping me alive and accounting for the fact that my life was returning to normal. Or as normal as it could be for a man with a heart whose front and bottom parts are virtual wastelands of scar tissue.[8]

[8]I Had a Perfect EKG a Month Before

Heart attacks such as mine happen when some plaque—the nasty cholesterol and calcium buildup on a coronary artery wall—suddenly and mysteriously ruptures. The rupture sets off a chain reaction of events that causes a blood clot. Blood platelets are attracted to the arterial rupture as a natural defense mechanism. They sense an injury and instigate the blood proteins to coagulate. This is what triggers the blood clot that blocks off the flow of blood to a part of the heart.

As yet, no indicators can reliably predict if or when a heart attack will take place. "Even the smallest plaque can rupture," says Dr. Bonow. And standard annual physicals will never tell this tale. My perfect EKG exam was of absolutely no help in foretelling the events of a month later.

For the rest of my life, my doctors and I will have to be watchful that my heart doesn't become oversized. This commonly occurs when the good heart muscles overcompensate for the parts that don't work. If it enlarges, well, that's when arrhythmia danger comes in—and that could be it. So if you take only one thing from my experience, it should be that fast action is the key to not ending up like me—or worse, like the St. Louis Cardinals pitcher Darryl Kile. The sooner a doctor can remove a blockage, the less injury the heart will sustain. If I had sought help sooner, I might have saved part of my heart. But like many men, I thought I knew better. And I paid a high price for those many hours I tried to tough it out on my own.

Is Your Heart Sending Out an SOS?

Right now, a blood chemical called CRP is sounding a siren in the arteries of millions of men. Yet many doctors aren't listening

By Jonathan Wander

You might drop dead while reading this. Even if you're a model *Men's Health* reader—you eat right, your blood pressure is great over excellent, and your LDL cholesterol level is post-it-on-the-refrigerator low—you might feel any minute that gripping pain in your chest that tells you it's over.

It's the most confounding of all cardiac mysteries: Every year, heart attacks kill thousands of men who, frankly, have no business dying.

"Half of all heart attacks and strokes in the United States will happen among healthy, middle-aged men who have normal cholesterol levels," says Paul Ridker, M.D., director of the center for cardiovascular disease prevention at Harvard Medical School. "If you leave your doctor's office after being told that your cholesterol levels are low and that you're in good shape, it hardly means you're not at risk of a heart attack."

In fact, your risk could actually be quite high. For years we've been told to watch our cholesterol numbers to help us guess if we're headed for a coronary. But now many cardiologists are saying we should be looking beyond LDL and HDL. "CRP" may be the ticker symbol that saves your life.

CRP stands for C-reactive protein, a naturally occurring blood chemical. Your CRP level, which can be determined by a simple, inexpensive blood test, may be the single best predictor of future heart attack or stroke. According to the Physicians Health Study—a 19-year clinical trial of more than 20,000 doctors—elevated CRP can predict as much as a 300 percent increase in a person's heart attack risk, even if cholesterol levels are normal. Supporting CRP's diagnostic value is other landmark cardiac research, including the Framingham Heart Study, which has followed more than 5,100 participants since 1971.

"We got carried away with cholesterol," says Ishwarlal Jialal, M.D., director of the laboratory for atherosclerosis and metabolic research at the University of California at Davis School of Medicine. "Now we're catching glimpses of what's happening in the vessel wall, which is a quantum leap in this area."

In the history books, CRP may also stand for "Credit Ridker, Paul," the man who is recognized for doing the most extensive research on CRP. Dr. Ridker, of the Preventive Medicine Division at Brigham and Women's Hospital in Boston, is considered one of the top cardiologists in the world and is working to make CRP tests a standard part of the American diagnostic arsenal. In fact, he's already converted President Bush's doctors to the cause; they tested George W.'s CRP level at his last executive exam. (It turned out to be "very low.")

"The CRP test predicts risk even after you adjust for all other cardiovascular risk factors," Dr. Ridker says. "It's easy to use; it's widely available; and if patients ask their physicians for the test, they can get a better grasp of their true heart attack risks."

A RIGHT HOOK TO YOUR HEART

The science behind CRP begins with a fat lip. When you get popped in the mouth, C-reactive protein is released to sound the alarm that there's inflammation in the body. Something similar can happen inside your heart. Inflammation in an artery wall, which can be triggered by smoking or poor diet, causes blood levels of CRP to rise—often dramatically—in response.

By itself, an inflamed artery isn't a problem. But even those of us who have avoided eating a lot of saturated and trans fats have some degree of plaque spackling our artery walls. Inflammation can make that plaque more likely to break loose and form a clot that causes a heart attack or stroke. Enter CRP. If elevated levels are detected early enough, steps can be taken to reduce the inflammation before any plaque is dislodged.

In fact, CRP testing could identify an estimated 25 million Americans with normal cholesterol but above-average inflammation, says Dr. Ridker. (If you have elevated CRP—2 milligrams per liter or higher—and high LDL cholesterol, the risk of a heart attack is two times greater than if you had high cholesterol alone.) "A CRP test is an invaluable window into artery inflammation," says Eric Topol, M.D., chairman of the department of cardiovascular medicine at the Cleveland Clinic. "It's a vital part of cardiac evaluation."

Another advantage of testing CRP is that doctors can warn patients of a potential problem years in advance. "We've seen elevated levels 30 to 40 years before the onset of first-ever events," says Dr. Ridker. "We think that about half of the variation (in inflammation) is genetic and about half comes from environmental factors, such as smoking, poor diet, lack of exercise, and obesity." Especially obesity. The old adage "Being overweight puts a strain on your heart" is oversimplified. "The CRP phenomenon does a lot to explain why obese individuals have very high risks of heart disease," says Dr. Ridker.

So far, scientists are not exactly sure why environmental factors cause arterial inflammation. "We believe that they activate the cells that cause inflammation," says Dr. Jialal. "But there are no detailed studies on how."

AN ICE BAG FOR YOUR ARTERIES

You already know how to treat a fat lip: Apply ice and wait for the inflammation (and embarrassment) to subside. Fortunately, treating inflamed arteries is almost as easy.

"The things that we know reduce heart attack risk—a healthful diet, smoking cessation, exercise—all seem to lower C-reactive protein," says Dr. Ridker. Specifically, that means lowering your body mass index (BMI) to between 18.5 and 24.9, stubbing the cigs, eating less saturated and trans fats, and exercising 30 to 60 minutes three or four times a week. Popping low-strength aspirin may also sink your CRP.

For CRP levels that lifestyle changes can't budge, doctors can prescribe a cholesterol-lowering statin drug, such as Lipitor, Zocor, or Pravachol. "With statins you achieve a two-for-one effect," Dr. Ridker says, explaining that the drugs lower LDL cholesterol and work as anti-inflammatories. "Even people with great cholesterol levels will be prescribed statins to lower their CRP," adds Dr. Topol.

Other drugs that lower inflammation are also being prescribed or tested. According to Dr. Topol, his studies have shown that the clot-busting drug Plavix "lowers CRP substantially"; that drugs used for diabetes (such as Avandia and Actos) reduce inflammation, as do ACE inhibitors; and that high doses of niacin lower CRP while raising HDL cholesterol. For now, statins are the drugs of choice, but Dr. Jialal expects others to follow. "I think we'll see designer drugs that will directly lower CRP about 40 to 50 percent," he says.

AND IN THIS CORNER . . .

So why isn't your doctor telling you all this? Blame the medical bureaucracy.

In the near future, the Centers for Disease Control and Prevention and the American Heart Association are expected to issue their recommendations on CRP testing. Until then, "the American Heart Association does not recommend CRP testing for everyone," says Richard C. Becker, M.D., an AHA spokesman. "Accumulating data suggests that CRP is an important predictor. Further investigation is required, however, to determine the role of CRP in wide-scale risk assessment. We're close to that point, but not there yet."

Another argument is that CRP levels may be elevated for a reason other than arterial inflammation, which might result in a misdiagnosis. "While solid evidence is rapidly accumulating for CRP, there is controversy over whether the use of this test in clinical practice is ready for prime time," says Christopher J. O'Donnell, M.D., associate director of Framingham Heart Study of the National Heart, Lung and Blood Institute. "There are a number of conditions that raise CRP that have nothing to do with heart disease—most notably infections and arthritic syndromes."

But Dr. Ridker remains adamant that CRP can effectively be tested in all but the sickest patients. "It's not for someone who's hospitalized. But in an outpatient setting, it works fine," he says. "I think the data are extremely persuasive that the addition of a CRP level to the usual cholesterol assessment provides a better way to predict risk of heart attack."

Dr. Topol, who has routinely tested patients' CRP levels for 2 years, agrees that there's no need to wait. "CRP testing is a breakthrough in the field. Don't be on the trailing edge of optimal medicine."

Don't Blow Your Mind

Seven simple steps to clear your head and reduce your stroke risk

By Bill Gottlieb

A man's last years ought to be spent strapped to the fighting chair of a game fisher while battling a black marlin, not tethered to a nursing home bed, incontinent and unable to talk.

But the latter is a likely scenario if you're one of approximately 600,000 Americans who will have a stroke this year.

"Your chance of dying is 20 percent, but you have a 40 percent chance of being disabled and a 25 percent chance of being severely disabled," says David Spence, M.D., director of the stroke prevention center at the Robarts Research Institute in London, Ontario. An ischemic stroke—the kind that affects most men—occurs when an artery to the brain is blocked by arterial plaque that has broken loose and caused a blood clot. In fact, it's just like a heart attack, only instead of heart cells dying for lack of blood, brain cells are kicking off—thousands of brain cells. Perhaps paralyzing half of your body. Or slurring your speech. Or plunging you into senility.

PERCENTAGE LESS LIKELY YOU ARE
TO HAVE A STROKE IF YOU EAT
A SINGLE SERVING OF FISH JUST ONCE A MONTH: 43

But a "brain attack" is not inevitable.

"Fifty to 80 percent of strokes can be prevented," says David Wiebers, M.D., professor of neurology at the Mayo Clinic and author of *Stroke-Free for Life*. "Making the simple choices at 25, 35, or 45 years of age can make an enormous difference in preventing stroke when you're in your sixties, seventies, or eighties."

Strike back at stroke with these seven strategies.

SWALLOW NATURE'S BLOOD THINNER

Researchers at Loma Linda University in California found that men who drank five or more 8-ounce glasses of water daily cut their stroke risk by 53 percent, compared with guys who drank fewer than three glasses. Water helps to thin the blood, which in turn makes it less likely to form clots, explains Jackie Chan, Dr.P.H., the lead study author. But don't chug your extra H_2O all at

SURVIVE A STROKE

It's happening. One side of your body has suddenly gone numb, and your vision is blurry. Or perhaps you inexplicably feel confused and have trouble speaking. First, call 911. If you receive the emergency clot-busting drug tPA within 3 hours, your risk of brain damage may be reduced by as much as 50 percent.

Next, take these evasive maneuvers:

Get off your feet. If you're having a stroke, your balance is probably bad. So lie down before you fall down. This will also lighten the load on your cardiovascular system. "You don't want blood having to pump against gravity to get to your brain," says David Wiebers, M.D., professor of neurology at the Mayo Clinic and author of *Stroke-Free for Life.*

Shut up and breathe deeply. Every pause or hesitation in speech increases anxiety, which overloads the left side of your brain. This, in turn, activates the sympathetic nervous system, causing blood vessels to constrict. "This places a heavy demand on your cardiovascular system,"

says Ernest Friedman, M.D., professor of psychiatry at Case Western Reserve University in Cleveland. "Lessen the demand by staying quiet and taking slow, deep breaths to stay calm."

Do not take aspirin. In an ischemic stroke—the most common type—aspirin can break up the clot that's damming up a blood vessel in your brain. But if that vessel's ruptured and flooding your brain with blood—the case in a hemorrhagic stroke—aspirin can slow the clotting that stops the bleeding.

Take drugs. To the hospital, that is—or at least bring a complete list of the pills you're popping.

"Certain drugs can profoundly affect a stroke victim's treatment course," says Richard O'Brien, M.D., a spokesman for the American College of Emergency Physicians. Cases in point: The medications Plavix and Coumadin and the herbal supplements garlic and *Ginkgo biloba* are blood thinners. Like aspirin, they're bad news if you're hemorrhaging.

once. "You need to drink water throughout the day to keep your blood thin, starting with a glass or two in the morning," adds Dr. Chan.

SWIG LESS SODA

Unless it's the diet stuff. The Loma Linda University researchers also discovered that the men who drank large quantities of fluids other than water actually had a higher risk of stroke—46 percent higher. One theory is that sugary drinks like soda draw water out of the bloodstream, thickening the blood. Another explanation may be the boost in triglycerides caused by sipping liquid sugar. "Elevated levels of triglycerides—any level above 150—are a risk factor for arterial disease," says Daniel Fisher, M.D., assistant professor at the New York University School of Medicine.

COUNT TO THREE

You may have just lowered your stroke risk. In a study published in the journal *Stroke*, researchers noted that of 2,100 men, the anxious guys were three times likelier to have a fatal ischemic stroke than the more serene men.

"Anxiety causes chronic overproduction of dopamine, a neurotransmitter that regulates the brain's control of circulation," says Ernest Friedman, M.D., a professor of psychiatry at Case Western Reserve University in Cleveland. Counting to three—or reining in your racing mind in any other way—helps by stabilizing your levels of serotonin, the antidote to excess dopamine, says Dr. Friedman.

HOLD YOUR BREATH

At least when you're around a smoker. University of Auckland researchers found that people exposed to secondhand smoke were 82 percent likelier to suffer a stroke than those who never inhaled. It seems that carbon monoxide promotes clot formation by interfering with nitric oxide, a biochemical that relaxes blood vessels. "To get rid of every single bit of carbon monoxide after a night at the bar, you'd have to breathe fresh air for about 8 hours. But most of the carbon monoxide will be gone from your body in the first hour," says Laurence Fechter, Ph.D., professor of toxicology at the University of Oklahoma in Norman. So on your way home, make sure you roll down the car windows and start sucking in some clean air.

BEAT HOMOCYSTEINE

Research suggests that people with high blood levels of this amino acid are more likely to stroke out than those with low readings. Extra folate will help reduce the risk, but only for some people. "Fifty to 60 percent won't respond with lower homocysteine," says Seth J. Baum, M.D., medical director of the Mind/Body Medical Institute, a Harvard affiliate. Dr. Baum recommends 1,000 micrograms (mcg) of folic acid (the supplement form of folate), plus 25 milligrams (mg) of vitamin B_6, 1,000 mcg of B_{12}, and 1,800 mg of the amino acid N-acetyl-cysteine (NAC).

"With folic acid, B_6, B_{12}, and NAC supplements, almost everyone will have normal homocysteine levels," says Dr. Baum.

PICK UP AN IRON SUPPLEMENT

Aerobic exercise is antistroke medicine. Can't run or cycle to save your life? Then lift. "Regular resistance training decreases blood pressure, elevates HDL cholesterol, lowers LDL cholesterol, and decreases the stickiness of the blood," says Jerry Judd Pryde, M.D., a physiatrist at Cedars-Sinai Hospital in Los Angeles. If you don't already weight-train, try the American Heart Association program: Lift weights two or three times a week, targeting the major muscle groups. For each of the following, choose a weight you can lift eight to 12 times at most, and do one set to fatigue: bench press, shoulder press, lying triceps extension, biceps curl, seated row, lat pulldown, crunch, squat, Romanian deadlift, and calf raise.

NEVER MISS ANOTHER FLU SHOT

Think of it as a sort of stroke vaccine. French researchers found that people who received a flu shot every year for the 5 years prior to the study were 42 percent less stroke-prone than those who didn't. "Chronic infections and the resultant inflammation might cause damage to the arteries and increase the risk of blood clots," says Pierre Amarenco, M.D., the study author, who is at Denis Diderot University in Paris. And the best time to get stuck? The first week in November. That's because most flu epidemics start in December, and it takes about 2 weeks for the shot to kick in, says Robert Belshe, M.D., director of the vaccine center at St. Louis University.

This Is a Stick Up

You'd do anything to avoid it. Here's why you shouldn't

By Kevin Cook

Drop your pants," the doctor said. "Bend over." Next came the *thwupp* of a disposable glove. He casually lubed one finger. "Now relax."

Easy for him to say—he had his pants on.

As one of the nation's top urologists, Christopher Dixon, M.D., is an expert rectal spelunker. I was a rookie about to endure my first digital rectal exam (DRE), a test so dreaded and humbling that most men risk prostate cancer rather than endure it. Prostate cancer kills about 30,000 American men every year; the test embarrasses multitudes.

"Here we go," said Dr. DRE.

No problem, I thought. This is no worse than what women go through whenever they see an ob/gyn. It's routine, a common, simple ... *WHOA, POKEY!*

As his finger roved cavities I didn't know I had, I thought my butt was going to sneeze. And now Dr. Dixon's digit probed deeper, leaving me only two options—escape or cut to flashback.

HOME GLAND SECURITY

Like most men, I spent my first twoscore years thinking of my plumbing the way you think of a new car—sleek and trouble-free, with plenty of horse-power and no need for service, not for a long, long time. There was one scare, when I peed blood after doing too many situps, but my GP had a cure for that: "Don't do so many situps." But now I'm 45, getting into a prostate state of mind.

Most prostates can be safely ignored for half a century or so. The American Urological Association recommends regular DRE's and blood tests for men 50 and older, with testing at 40 for those in high-risk groups, including African-Americans and men with prostate cancer in their families. Not everyone agrees with the AUA, though. The National Cancer Institute opposes such widespread testing until further research can prove it saves lives. The stakes are high: Each day about 500 Americans learn that they have prostate cancer, the most common malignancy among men. The disease killed Frank Zappa and Steve Ross, chief of Time Warner. Its celebrity survivors include former New York mayor Rudy Giuliani, the Yankees manager Joe Torre, the NASCAR legend Richard Petty, and Gen. Norman Schwarzkopf, who boosted the DRE cause by declaring, "All it is, literally, is a temporary pain in the ass. . . . None of us enjoy the digital rectal examination—or I should say most of us don't enjoy it—but if you've got half a brain in your head, you'll make a point of asking for one."

But battling this killer isn't that simple. Unlike Stormin' Norman's rout of Iraq a decade ago, the war on prostate cancer is a rear guard action fraught with complexity. To test or not to test? The answer can be as slippery as Dr. DRE's digit.

Until 15 years ago, the DRE was medicine's lone sentry in the war on prostate cancer. Then came a blood test that measures a protein called prostate specific antigen (PSA). A high PSA score can signal cancer. It can also mean nothing more than a jumbo prostate.

"The prostate is a PSA factory," says Dr. Dixon, who is director of the benign prostate disease program at New York University medical center. "Some men have little prostates the size of a walnut. Another prostate might be healthy but two or three or even 10 times bigger. And size matters. A big prostate can give you a higher PSA, even without cancer." As a rule of thumb—or, should we say, forefinger—a 50-year-old man should have a PSA score under 4.0. Anything higher can send him to the hospital for a biopsy.

For a prostate biopsy, you start by lying bottomless on an exam table, your legs spread. A technician feeds a thumb-thick ultrasound probe several inches up your colon. Then a specialist threads a spring-loaded needle into the probe, and for the next 20 minutes that needle pistons up and down, taking samples of tissue. This will hurt like hell in a strange, insinuating way, unless your specialist has given you a local anesthetic. (If he hasn't, he's behind the curve. Next time, demand a local.) When it's over, you get a butt bandage to keep you from dripping blood on your way home. If your biopsy comes up negative, you can stop worrying until next year. If it's positive, you're given a new number to memorize—your Gleason score, which gauges the aggressiveness of your prostate cancer. A Gleason score around 6 may mean a moderately aggressive tumor.

THE PSA TEST: NOW? OR NEVER?

For me, the tough calls began the day I asked my family doctor for a prostate checkup. "I'm 45," I said. "I want to be safe, so I guess it's about time."

He surprised me by disagreeing. "Just because we can do a test doesn't mean we should," said Tom Kovachevich, D.O., who's in general practice at St. Vincent Catholic Medical Centers in New York City. "I'm almost 60, and my father had prostate cancer, but I haven't had a PSA." Dr. Kovachevich encourages all of his patients to weigh both sides of the story. Blindly screening a man can lead to a slippery slope—a diagnosis that can be accurate but harmful, and a cure that can be worse than the disease. "The disease is often indolent. It's slow," he says. "So slow that 80 percent of the men who have it would outlive it with no treatment. But once you undergo that test and it comes back positive, the patient thinks, I've got cancer."

At that point, treatment is often "watchful waiting," which can be excruciating. Some men are unsuited to it. Impatient, cancer phobic, unable to wait for years to clarify borderline results, they tell their doctors, Let's take it out. For them, as for those in more severe straits, radiotherapy and hormone treatment—chemical castration—can help, but surgery is often chosen. In the increasingly common radical retropubic prostatectomy, a surgeon cuts from the belly button to the pubic bone and removes the prostate, trying to spare nearby nerves, which the patient needs if he is ever to have another erection.

According to a study in the *Journal of the American Medical Association* (*JAMA*), 56 percent of patients were still impotent a year and a half after surgery. Every surgical patient endures several weeks, or even months, of impotence and incontinence—urinating through a catheter into a bag taped to his leg. The *JAMA* study also found that a small percentage never regain control of their bladders, and 40 percent have some leakage problems.

"That's devastating," says Dr. Kovachevich. "You're 50 years old and you're wetting your pants for the rest of your life."

Survivors will tell you that surgery saved their lives. Many of them are right. Others, however, might have been better off had they never known their PSA scores.

Still, something in me wanted to know. I left Dr. Kovachevich's office without dropping trou, but as the weeks passed, I played mental Ping-Pong with my prostate, bouncing from blissful ignorance to compulsive curiosity. There was information out there, and my male brain longed for that number, to compare it with other numbers and, by knowing it, to control the lurking thing it described.

GOING DOWN UNDER

The urologist's office was full of old men. The receptionist handed me a clipboard and a questionnaire. How often during the night do you wake up to urinate? How often is your stream weak or split into two streams? I checked all the right boxes. Hardly ever. Never. I had never stopped to think of it, but I am clearly a strong urinater. A pee-er of the realm. Handing over my clipboard, I felt urologically buff. Until I remembered what I was here to ask for.

"Dr. Dixon is ready to see you in the exam room," a nurse said.

But was I ready for him?

What a singular job this man has. He probes, pokes, squeezes, and laser-slices other men's nethers. He is 40-ish, casual, and as sharp as a spring-loaded needle.

"How you doing?" he said, shaking hands. I couldn't help thinking of all the places his hand had been. "What can I do for you?"

"I think I might want a DRE and a PSA."

"You might?"

I told him what Dr. Kovachevich had said. Dr. Dixon nodded, then rattled off paragraph after paragraph on prostate cancer policy that touched on every issue. Nobody had proved that screening saved lives, he said, though he thought it probably did. Until a research doctor sheds more light on this subject (and wins a Nobel prize in the process), there will be more nuances in his work than he'd like. More tough calls.

Dr. Kovachevich was right to urge caution, Dr. Dixon said. Still, he leaned more toward the activist approach. "Caution is fine," he said. "But if I can, I want to catch this cancer early, when I can still cure it. I've stuck my finger back there and felt prostates so diseased they were solid rock. I just saw a guy who had his prostate taken out. He's younger than you are."

Dr. Dixon sees his work as an art, one that calls for collaboration with patients. "The extremes are easy," he says. "For a 95-year-old man with low-grade prostate cancer, we probably won't do anything. If you're only 50 with a PSA over 10, we'll probably want a biopsy."

It's in the twilight zone—PSA scores between 4 and 10—that's when what he calls "the art of medicine" comes into play. A refined form of the test measures so-called free and complex PSA, adding yet another number to the mix. Still, even this more advanced test can lead to borderline calls. "So much of it comes down to the patient. Some will tell you, 'I don't want to know,' and they'll mean it. That's okay with me." Other patients want their prostates out ASAP, even if they have a four-in-five chance of outliving the disease. Dr. Dixon judges the data, never the patient.

He pointed at me. "So what do you think? Are you ready?"

"Let's do it."

My flashback ended. I had to face the finger.

"Drop your pants." *Thwupp.* "Now relax. Here we go."

Digitized for the very first time, I got that butt-sneeze feeling: a sudden fullness, as if I had to take a dump. (You should fight the urge to bear down. It'll be easier for both of you if you try to stay loose.) Dr. Dixon dug deeper, and deeper, until I swear his finger was about to come out the front.

"Fine, fine," he said, palpating my prostate. "Perfect."

"Big? Small?"

"Medium. About 20 cc's."

"I'm curious," I said through my teeth. "What shape is it?"

"Heart-shaped."

"How romantic."

In 20 seconds it was over. Dr. Dixon was washing his hands, saying he expected my PSA would be fine, too. "It's a quick blood test. We'll do it in the room across the hall. Then we can talk about the numbers."

But I had what I wanted. I was a DRE virgin no more. My golf-ball-size, heart-shaped prostate had received a big preliminary thumbs-up, and I was still 5 years short of my 50th birthday.

"I think I'll skip the PSA," I said.

"Really?" Dr. Dixon looked surprised.

"If I knew my PSA score, I'd probably just brood over it."

"It's your call," he said, and with a handshake and a wave, I was free.

The Wonder Drug

There's a miracle pill in your medicine cabinet right now. Here are 6 new ways to use it

By Brian Good

Last March, Mayo Clinic researchers unveiled a pill that helps prevent prostate cancer. Chemical name: acetylsalicylic acid. It has almost no side effects, is already FDA-approved, and costs just 3 cents a pop. Plus, studies show that the stuff can also help stop a heart attack, beat colon cancer, thwart Alzheimer's disease, and ward off strokes.

Want some? You already have a stash of acetylsalicylic acid. You just call it aspirin.

"There have been some amazing discoveries over the past 20 years in terms of what aspirin can do for your body," says Gerald Fletcher, M.D., professor of medicine at the Mayo Clinic in Florida and a spokesman for the American Heart Association. "There's simply not another medication out there that has as many varied uses, and that we're still finding out so much about."

Here are half a dozen benefits of dropping a little acid.

LOWER YOUR BLOOD PRESSURE

Nurse Vicky says your blood pressure is too high—even when you account for her tight white uniform. Ask her boss about aspirin. A recent Spanish study found that taking 100 milligrams (mg) of aspirin every day can lower systolic pressure (the top number) by an average of 7 points and diastolic pressure (the bottom number) by 6. One caveat: Pop yours before bed. The patients who took aspirin in the morning didn't lower their BP's at all.

WARD OFF PROSTATE CANCER

Research suggests that every man will get prostate cancer if he lives long enough. That must not be counting the aspirin addicts. When Mayo Clinic re-

BEFORE YOU TAKE TWO

Psyched to swallow an aspirin a day? Great. Now go tell your doctor. "There's a small chance daily aspirin could cause stomach bleeding and, in rare instances, cause a blood vessel in the brain to break, triggering a hemorrhagic stroke," says Richard Stein, M.D., a spokesman for the American Heart Association. That's why doctors check for a history of bleeding problems and calculate your risk of stroke before approving a daily aspirin regimen. All clear?

TIPS TO HELP YOU NAVIGATE THE ASPIRIN AISLE

Buy generic. Bayer. Anacin. Walgreens. "It doesn't matter," says Arthur Kibbe, Ph.D., chair of the department of pharmaceutical sciences at Wilkes University in Wilkes-Barre, Pennsylvania. "Aspirin is aspirin."

Go low. Unless your doctor recommends otherwise, low doses of aspirin seem to be more effective—and safer—than higher ones. "Scientists are still trying to determine the optimal dose of aspirin, but for many people, 81 milligrams a day

appears to be it," says Thomas Bryant, M.D., director of the Aspirin Foundation of America. Look for bottles labeled "low dose" or "low strength."

Save your stomach. Buy "enteric coated" aspirin; it's designed to pass through your stomach and into your intestines before dissolving. "Enteric coated aspirin takes longer to work, but it limits the amount of acid released into the stomach, which can help prevent damage to the lining," says Kibbe.

searchers studied 1,400 men for 5½ years, they found that the men who took nonsteroidal anti-inflammatory drugs, like aspirin, daily were half as likely to develop prostate cancer as those who didn't take them. The drugs appear to block production of and limit damage from COX-2 enzymes, which promote the growth of cancer cells, says Rosebud Roberts, M.D., the study author.

PREVENT A HEART ATTACK

Run down this checklist: High cholesterol. High blood pressure. Overweight. Smoker. Family history of heart disease. If you said "check" even once, the U.S. Preventive Health Task Force recommends you start popping aspirin. They found that taking at least 75 mg of aspirin daily can reduce a person's heart disease risk by nearly 30 percent, probably by thinning the blood and blocking blood vessel inflammation. And remember this: Chewing an aspirin at the first sign of chest pain may keep a heart attack from beginning or at least reduce the damage caused by one.

AVOID COLON CANCER

A family history of colon cancer entitles you to an annual colonoscopy beginning at age 50 and the right to ask your doctor about taking a daily aspirin now. Tell him that Dartmouth researchers found that men who took 81 mg of aspirin daily may have had up to a 50 percent lower risk of colon cancer than nonusers of aspirin. "Aspirin inhibits the growth of polyps, which are a known precursor to colon cancer," says John Baron, M.D., the study author.

SAVE YOUR BRAIN

Researchers at Erasmus Medical Center in the Netherlands found that people who used aspirin regularly for several years were nearly 80 percent less likely to develop Alzheimer's disease than those who used it infrequently. "One theory is that Alzheimer's is caused by inflammatory reactions within the brain, and drugs like aspirin may be able to block those reactions," says Peter Zandi, Ph.D., a researcher at the Johns Hopkins University medical center.

GUARD AGAINST STROKES

You can't have a stroke without a blood clot. Aspirin's specialty? Preventing blood clots. In a study review published in the *British Medical Journal*, researchers found that daily aspirin use can reduce stroke risk by more than 25 percent for men who've had a stroke or are likely to have one. Other studies suggest that the risk reduction may be even higher. "It's one of the best means we've found for preventing strokes—and for lessening their damage should one strike," says Dr. Baron.

KNOW THIS

Wake-Up Call

A 10-year, 70,000-patient Harvard study found that people who snored were twice as likely to develop diabetes as people who didn't—regardless of whether they were overweight or not. "Snoring impairs oxygen intake, which appears to trigger the production of compounds called catecholamines," says Wael K. Al-Delaimy, M.D., Ph.D., the study author. The more catecholamines you have in your system, the less effective the insulin produced by your body becomes.

Dead Weight

We've been saying it for years: Being overweight can increase your risk of a number of deadly diseases. Now Finnish researchers have calculated how much a man's risk of heart disease increases with every inch his spare tire expands. To see how you measure up, wrap a tape measure around the narrowest part of your waist, above your belly button but below the bottom of your rib cage. Then see where the number falls below.

Waist Size	Risk of Heart Disease
32 inches	Average
33 to 34 inches	38% increase
35 to 37 inches	89% increase
More than 38 inches	102% increase

Chemo Patients Beware

First came the news that the herb St. John's wort may not fight depression, and now a Dutch study says that it can make it harder for you to fight cancer as well. In trials, St. John's wort reduced the levels of a chemotherapy drug in the body by up to 42 percent.

Quit It

Here's even more incentive to quit smoking: Two new studies report that lighting up can increase your risk of developing kidney disease and colorectal polyps—a possible precursor to colon cancer. A third study suggests that secondhand smoke can harm your pet.

But quitting smoking is tough. Statistics show that between 60 and 90 percent of men who try to kick the habit start puffing again in less than a year. A new study from the University of Chicago found that if you can stay away from cigarettes for 24 months, you're nearly home free. After tracking the smoking habits of 483 men, researchers say that smokers who gave up cigarettes for at least 2 years had less than a 4 percent chance of relapsing. Even better: "After 10 years, that figure drops to less than 1 percent," says Elizabeth Krall, Ph.D., the study's lead author.

Another Shot against Hepatitis C

Tattoos, unprotected sex, and shared needles all increase your risk of contracting hepatitis C, a life-threatening disease with no known cure. Fortunately, dealing with the condition is getting easier. A new single-dose drug combination appears to be the best treatment yet for hepatitis C. In clinical trials, researchers at New York's North Shore University Hospital found that a mixture of PEG Interferon and Ribavirin eradicated the disease in nearly 60 percent of hepatitis C cases—a 20 percent increase over older treatments. What's more, the treatment requires only one shot a week, instead of the previous three.

PERCENTAGE OF AMERICAN ADULTS WHO SMOKE: 23

OF THOSE, THE PERCENTAGE WHO TRIED TO QUIT LAST YEAR: 41

DOWN THE PIKE

Cholesterol Vaccine

Researchers at Avant Immunotherapeutics in Needham, Massachusetts, are developing a new vaccine capable of boosting HDL (good) cholesterol levels while keeping LDL (bad) cholesterol levels low. The vaccine—called CETi-1—works by inhibiting production of a natural protein called CETP. "Without CETP, the body is no longer able to convert HDL cholesterol molecules into LDL molecules," says Una Ryan, M.D., the drug's developer and CEO of Avant. A single dose of the new vaccine could help keep your cholesterol levels in check for up to 6 months.

New Blood Sugar Tests

If you're a diabetic, checking your blood sugar level may soon be as easy as rolling up your sleeve or taking a look in the mirror. Researchers at Texas A&M and Penn State Universities are developing a new type of glucose monitor, a "smart tattoo" that changes color as blood sugar levels rise and fall. University of Pittsburgh scientists are developing a similar product: special contact lenses that change color according to the amount of sugar in your tears. Both forms of testing could be available within 5 years.

Quicker Diagnosis

If you had a heart attack today, it could take your doctor up to 30 minutes to accurately determine what had happened to you. But in the very near future, a test developed at Florida State University in Tallahassee may allow doctors to diagnose a heart attack in less than 3 minutes. The procedure works by detecting special proteins in your blood that form when you have a heart attack. "Speed is very important for heart attack patients," says Yousef Haik, Ph.D., the test's creator. "The sooner a doctor knows for sure that someone has had a heart attack, the sooner the patient will get the right medical treatment." Haik says that most ambulances in the country could be fitted with the testing equipment within 2 years.

Robo Doc

Robot bypasses are already being performed in Europe, and may soon be used in the United States as well. The California-built da Vinci Surgical System makes possible open heart surgery through a few pencil-size holes in the chest. Recovery is much faster than when you get your rib cage cracked open. The FDA requires more clinical studies showing that the device is safe and effective before it is approved for use in the United States.

Zero In on Arterial Plaque

A technology that helped NASA scientists spot rocks on Mars may soon help doctors save your life. Using a procedure called near infrared spectroscopy, doctors are now able to scan your arteries to detect clusters of plaque that have the greatest likelihood of bursting or breaking free and triggering a heart attack or stroke.

Skin Savers

Researchers at Stanford University may have discovered a new drug that can slow or stop the growth of skin cancer cells. "In trials, we found that the drug Apomine inhibits the growth of melanoma cells, as well as their ability to spread," says Marianne Powell, Ph.D., the study author. Besides helping to treat existing melanoma cases, Powell says that Apomine could be added to sunscreens to prevent skin cancer for those at high risk of the disease. The drug is still in the testing phase, but could be available within a couple of years.

In related news, scientists are determining whether a common acne medication may be another new weapon in the fight against skin cancer. Researchers at the University of California found that mice given a prescription vitamin A cream called tazarotene were up to 85 percent less likely to develop skin cancer tumors than mice that weren't treated with the cream. "If tazarotene has the same effect on humans, the possibilities for cancer prevention would be huge," says study author Ervin Epstein Jr., M.D., of the dermatology department at the University of California School of Medicine in San Francisco.

NUMBER OF NEW CASES OF SKIN CANCER DIAGNOSED EACH YEAR: **1 MILLION**

NUMBER OF AMERICANS WHO DIE OF MELANOMA—THE DEADLIEST FORM OF SKIN CANCER: **NEARLY ONE PER HOUR**

GAME PLAN

When You're a Guest Star on ER

How to navigate a trip to the emergency room

You got a little chop happy with your new Ginsu. Now you're in the ER, and unless you heed these suggestions, you'll be sitting in that plastic chair until Saddam Hussein surrenders. Take these tips along to minimize the agony.

Find the best hospital. Rate the nearby hospitals before you need one, says Stephen Epstein, M.D., an emergency physician at Beth Israel Deaconess Medical Center in Boston. Find out which are known for trauma care, cardiac treatment, and parking lot muggings. If you're clueless, head to the biggest university hospital in the area.

Phone first (with your good hand). "If your life isn't in danger, call your insurance provider before checking in at the ER," says David Meyers, M.D., of Sinai Hospital in Baltimore. They might send you to a doctor to save cash. "If you don't call, you might be responsible for the whole ER bill."

Use 911 wisely. For head wounds, chest pain, stomach pain with vomiting, loss of consciousness, or other potentially serious afflictions, call an ambulance. For broken bones and other non-life-threatening conditions, find a cheaper ride.

Bring your dossier. They'll ask for your Social Security number, insurance card, name and telephone number of your family doctor, current medications, allergies, and a medical history going back to your first-grade tonsillectomy. Put all this info in your wallet before you head to the hospital.

Don't try to snow the woman in white. A triage nurse will greet you first, and she knows all the "rush me in" tricks. Dramatic chest clutching will only anger her, the doctors, and the guy ahead of you with the protruding crowbar. A crowd won't help, either. "No more than two people should accompany the patient," says Dr. Meyers.

After 30 minutes, bitch. "If you feel like you're being ignored, ask to see the charge nurse or attending physician," says Dr. Meyers. As long as you keep your cool, talking to the head honcho might speed you onto the exam table before the next shift change.

Know the hierarchy. Remember, you decide who treats you. Typically an intern is a fresh grad; a resident has at least 1 year of experience; a fellow has at least 3; and attending physicians are the top dogs. All are fine for stitches. Tap the latter two for life-and-death matters.

TAKE ACTION

We're all trying to get ahead—in our careers, our bank accounts, our stock portfolios. Another place it pays to get ahead: your health. As you reach middle age and beyond, Mr. Grim Reaper starts gaining ground on you. To stay several steps ahead of the hooded hound, here are 15 simple actions you can begin taking *right now*. Go ahead, read on.

1. Brush up. Your toothbrush may be one of the best tools for protecting your brain. A new Harvard study suggests that regularly flossing and brushing your teeth could cut your risk of stroke in half. In a 12-year study of 14,000 men, researchers found that individuals with the healthiest teeth and gums were also the least likely to have a stroke. "It's not the loss of a tooth you should worry about, though; it's the disease that causes the tooth to fall out," explains Kaumudi Joshipura, Sc.D., the study author. The bacteria that cause periodontal disease may slip into the bloodstream, damaging blood vessels and increasing stroke risk, she says.

And next time you need a new tube of toothpaste, check the label for the ingredient silica. A separate study found that after 6 months of twice-daily use, patients brushing with silica toothpaste had 44 percent less plaque and tartar than patients using pastes without the ingredient.

2. Mark your calendar. You may be able to reduce your heart attack risk significantly in as little as 3 weeks. We've known for years that diet and exercise help fight heart disease, but a new study from UCLA shows that intense exercise and rigorous changes to your diet can shrink your heart disease risk fast. In the study, researchers put 11 men on a low-fat, high-fiber diet combined with up to an hour a day of aerobic exercise. After just 3 weeks, the men's blood pressures dropped by as much as 14 percent, while their total-cholesterol and triglyceride levels plummeted by 20 and 41 percent respectively, says R. James Barnard, Ph.D., the study author.

3. Steam things up. Japanese researchers report that spending 15 minutes a day in a sauna can improve blood circulation. The finding is especially encouraging for men with heart problems who would benefit significantly from better bloodflow. If you have any health problems, be sure to check with your doctor before getting steamed.

4. Go for garlic. Garlic keeps away more than just vampires. It's been shown to fight infections, lower cholesterol, and possibly slow the spread of cancer. And now research from India suggests that eating garlic may help limit damage to your heart after a heart attack or heart surgery. In the study, researchers found that animals that were fed garlic regularly had more heart-protecting antioxidants in their blood than animals that weren't. The only catch? Garlic in pill form isn't as effective. For maximum protection, you need to eat the real thing.

5. Talk to your doctor, stat! If you're recovering from a heart attack, don't let your doctor take you off cholesterol-lowering statin medications until you've discussed this new research: In a study of 1,616 patients recovering from heart problems, German researchers found that patients who stopped using statins after being hospitalized for chest pain had up to three times the risk of death or a second heart attack, compared with patients who stayed on the drugs. The benefit comes from statins' ability to reduce arterial inflammation and clotting.

6. Consider taking Tylenol. You've already read about the health benefits of aspirin. Well, a new study from Rutgers University suggests that over-the-counter medications containing acetaminophen—such as Tylenol—may also help treat angina, a painful tightening in the chest that occurs when your heart doesn't get enough oxygen. A separate animal study from New York Medical University found that a daily dose of acetaminophen may help prevent colon cancer as well. Acetaminophen offers an additional benefit to aspirin's blood-thinning and circulation-improving effects; it acts as an antioxidant, preventing cellular changes that lead to disease.

7. Make an appointment. If you're an African-American age 45 or older, pick up the phone and start dialing your doctor. Not only are Black men twice as likely to develop prostate cancer; they're also twice as likely to die from it. But when the disease is caught and treated early, cure rates for Blacks are identical to those for Whites, according to a study from the Radiological Society of North America. Experts recommend African-American men get their first prostate cancer checkup at age 45.

8. Eat more fruit and flaxseed. Here's why.

Flaxseed. Toss a few tablespoons of finely ground flaxseed on your morning cereal. Flaxseed, available at health food stores and most supermarkets, is the richest source of plant-based omega-3 fatty acids, the heart-healthy fats also found in fish. And flaxseed may also be good for your prostate. A new study at Duke University medical center found that men with prostate cancer who ate 3 tablespoons of flaxseed daily saw a reduction in the growth of prostate cancer cells.

Pectin. This fiber, found in apples, oranges, and grapefruit, reduces cholesterol and may prevent prostate cancer by improving the transmission of signals between cells, researchers say.

9. Step outside. Getting just 15 minutes of sunlight on your hands and face every day could reduce your risk of developing certain cancers. "A series of recent studies shows that the vitamin D your body produces when you're in the sun may be helpful in slowing or preventing the growth of a number of different types of cancer cells," says Gary Schwartz, Ph.D., an epidemiologist at the Comprehensive Cancer Center of Wake Forest University in Winston-Salem, North Carolina. And if you can't get enough sun or you live in perpetual darkness, Schwartz recommends taking a vitamin D supplement. "Even if you don't need the extra D, the worst that will happen is you'll end up with a strong, healthy skeleton," he says. Just keep in mind that Boston University researchers found that the vitamin D your body produces while in the sun is not only better for you than the D you get from food or vitamins, but lasts longer within the body, too.

10. But first, lube up. Before you head outside, you should slather on some sunscreen to protect against damaging UVA and UVB light. For outings longer than a few minutes, rub on vitamin C or E lotion before you apply sunblock. You'll eliminate up to 96 percent of cancer-causing free radicals brought on by sun exposure.

11. Buckle up. Seat belts save more lives than air bags do, according to a study published in the *British Medical Journal*. Air bags reduce your risk of dying in a crash by just 8 percent, while seat belts can slash your chances of dying by up to 65 percent, researchers say.

12. Pull over. Talking on your cell phone? Do yourself a favor and get off the road. Motorists talking on cell phones have reaction times an average of 30 percent slower than those of people who've been drinking alcohol. Cell phone users also have a harder time maintaining a constant speed and keeping a safe distance from the car in front of them than regular drivers, say UK researchers.

AMONG DEVELOPED COUNTRIES, THE ONE WITH NEARLY THE LOWEST SEAT BELT USE RATE: **THE UNITED STATES**

PERCENTAGE OF MALE DRIVERS WHO HAVE BEEN INVOLVED IN (OR NEARLY INVOLVED IN) AN ACCIDENT BECAUSE THEY WERE DISTRACTED WHILE DRIVING: **34**

THE TOP SECONDARY ACTIVITY DRIVERS ARE MOST COMMONLY ENGAGED IN: **EATING OR DRINKING**

THE SECOND MOST COMMON ACTIVITY: **TALKING ON A CELL PHONE**

13. Let her lean on you. Researchers at Yale studied 300 couples over the age of 65 and found that men who believed they were a source of strength to their wives were more likely to be alive 6 years later than men who felt that their wives did not depend on them.

14. Look on the bright side. Researchers at the Mayo Clinic had 450 people complete two personality tests, one in the 1960s and a follow-up one more recently. After analyzing the data, they found that individuals who were optimistic lived longer and remained more physically and mentally fit in old age than their more pessimistic counterparts.

15. Save someone else's life. You've likely seen them hanging on walls everywhere lately—in airports, malls, even casinos. Automated external defibrillators (AEDs) are portable, idiot-proof versions of the cardiac crash carts that TV docs grab before yelling, "Clear!"

Because of growing awareness and dropping prices, about 225,000 AED's are now standing by. Seventy AED's are deployed at Chicago's three airports and, in a 2-year period, were used to save 11 of 18 people who went into ventricular fibrillation. All but two rescuers were Good Samaritans.

Some AED's literally talk the rescuer through the process. So be a hero: Start with CPR, find an AED, and do what it says. ASAP.

PERCENTAGE OF MEN TRAINED IN CPR WHO HAVE
NOT BEEN RECERTIFIED SINCE THEIR CARDS EXPIRED: **68**

HOW LONG YOU RETAIN YOUR CPR SKILLS
BEFORE THEY BEGIN TO FADE: **6 TO 12 MONTHS**

ANY QUESTIONS?

Heartburn or Heart Attack?

How can I tell the difference between routine chest pain and heart attack symptoms?

—P.M., Boston

It's a matter of pressure, duration, and location. "If you're having a heart attack, you'll feel as if someone's sitting on your chest," says Donald LaVan, M.D., clinical associate professor of medicine at the University of Pennsylvania and spokesman for the American Heart Association. "It's pressure, as opposed to sharp pain, and it may radiate to the jaw, the left shoulder, the left arm, or the area between your shoulders." If you think you're having a heart attack, call 911 within 5 minutes. *Under no circumstances should you drive yourself, especially if you also are feeling queasy, sweaty, or fatigued and are short of breath!*

Okay, we'll calm down now. Not all chest pain is 911 material. Michael Crawford, M.D., a cardiologist at the Mayo Clinic, offers this menu of chest pain that won't kill you:

Heartburn. Sloshing stomach acid can cause a painful burning sensation behind your breastbone. "You'll also get a bitter taste in your mouth, usually a couple of hours after eating," Dr. Crawford says.

Panic attack. This one leads off with escalating fear, and general physical symptoms follow—including, for some men, rapid heartbeat and chest pain. But if the terror comes first, you probably need the help of a shrink, not a bypass.

Pleurisy. "This is sharp, localized chest pain that increases when you breathe in or cough," Dr. Crawford says. You'll feel this when an infection inflames the sac around one of your lungs, causing a big pain on one side. Call a doctor.

Sore muscles. "If it hurts when you twist from side to side or when you raise your arms, you probably have muscle-related chest pain," he says. So lay off the one-rep maxes for a few days.

Injured ribs or pinched nerves. A bruised or broken rib or a pinched nerve can cause chest pain that tends to be localized and sharp. Next time, charge the mound when Clemens brings the heat. When the fight is over, see your doctor.

Don't Dig Yourself an Early Grave

I've heard horror stories about guys croaking while shoveling snow. What are the health risks, and how can I best prepare to tackle my driveway?

—S.M., Shoreview, Minnesota

A study conducted at North Dakota State University in Fargo (a city that got hammered with a record-breaking 117-inch snowfall in 1996) should make us all sit down and take notice. Fifteen healthy, college-age students shoveled snow for 14 minutes. Within 1 to 4 minutes, their heart rates of about 72 beats per minute (resting) ramped up to a roaring plateau of 175 to 180 bpm.

"It's pretty stressful," says Brad Strand, Ph.D., one of the researchers. "Especially when you consider that most people shovel snow for more than 30 minutes." At that rate and duration, people who have a history of heart disease, angina, or high blood pressure are at risk. So go ahead and worry about your dad, too. "As one gets older, blood circulation is not as efficient," Strand says. "In cold weather, our blood vessels constrict, and circulation becomes even more difficult. When the heart tries to pump harder, it can't be healthy." Four good tips: (1) Warm up for 15 minutes prior to shoveling. Do anything to break a light sweat. (2) Do some flexibility exercises to stretch your lower back and hamstrings. That's where most injuries occur. (3) Start slowly and speed up. (4) Use large-faced shovels for removing fluffy, light snow, and small-faced shovels for wet, heavy snow. It might take longer to clear the driveway, but your last words won't be "One, two, three, heave!"

Supplemental Advice

I'm 39 years old. My dad had a heart attack at age 46. Which vitamins and minerals should I be taking?

—L.S., Chicago

Start with a good multivitamin that meets 100 percent of the Daily Value recommendations, except for iron. "As you get older, your need for iron de-

PERCENTAGE INCREASE IN THE AVERAGE GUY'S RISK OF DYING OF HEART DISEASE OR STROKE IF HE DOESN'T ATTEND WEEKLY RELIGIOUS SERVICES: 44

NUMBER OF YEARS HE COULD ADD TO HIS LIFE IF HE DID ATTEND WEEKLY: 3

creases, and excess iron can increase your risk of heart disease," says Jeffrey Blumberg, Ph.D., professor of nutrition at Tufts University in Boston. Look for a multi that contains no iron, like Mega-One Iron Free, or Centrum Silver. Multivitamins like these ensure that you'll get the vitamins and minerals you need even when you're on the road eating chimichangas. But there are two other supplements you should swallow daily: You need 1,000 to 1,200 milligrams of calcium per day (with vitamin D) to combat age-related bone loss and colon cancer and 400 International Units (IU) of vitamin E, which helps prevent heart disease. Most men don't get enough of these nutrients from food or even from a multivitamin.

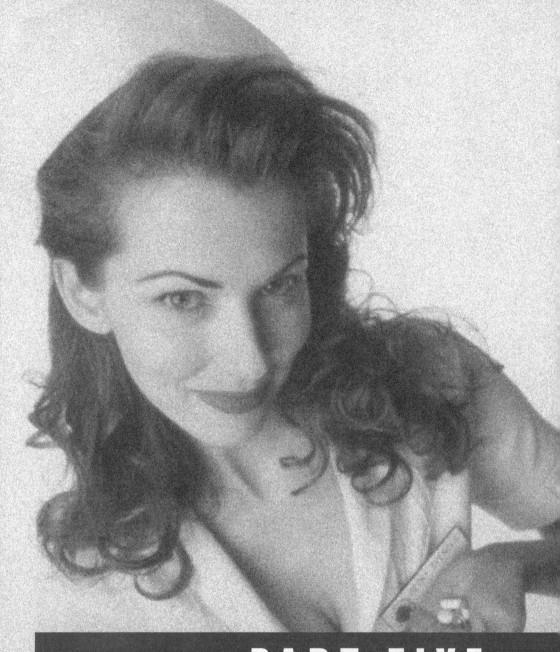

PART FIVE
BEAT THE HEALTH CARE SYSTEM

GAME SHOW

Who Will Lower His Cholesterol for Good?

One of these get-healthy guys? Or you?

Campbell is berry confident.

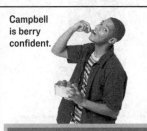

COREY CAMPBELL
Age: 26 Weight: 160
Health assessment specialist

Vaillancourt swears by soy.

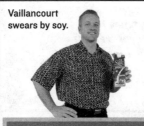

BRIAN VAILLANCOURT
Age: 39 Weight: 195
Associate publisher

Cusick is on the pills.

MIKE CUSICK
Age: 45 Weight: 163
Sales representative

HIS NUMBERS
• A year ago, Campbell's total cholesterol was 211, his HDL 47 (LDL and triglycerides weren't measured). Today the numbers are 133, 53, 49, and 157, respectively.

HIS PLAN
• Lifestyle changes. Campbell cut saturated fat and simple carbohydrates from his diet. He upped the intensity of his weight-lifting workouts and joined a Spinning class.

ADVANTAGES
• Campbell dropped 20 pounds. Losing weight helps reduce total cholesterol, triglycerides, and LDL (bad) cholesterol.

• He works in an office full of nurses. "They keep me in check," he says.

DISADVANTAGES
• To have had borderline-high cholesterol this early in life is a bad sign since cholesterol rises naturally with age.

• Because he's young, with a negligible heart attack risk, he may be less motivated than older men to stick with this program.

• Both of his parents have high cholesterol.

HIS NUMBERS
• About 3 years ago, Vaillancourt's total cholesterol was 236, HDL 36, LDL 173, and triglycerides 134. When last checked, his numbers were 188, 37, 129, and 105.

HIS PLAN
• Vaillancourt was already running and lifting weights, so he focused on his diet—ditching butter for Benecol, eating less saturated fat and more whole foods. He added ¼ cup of soy milk to his oatmeal and takes soy lecithin and saw palmetto.

ADVANTAGES
• The American Heart Association recommends 25 grams (g) of soy protein daily.

• Moderate alcohol consumption raises HDL, as does vigorous exercise.

• Benecol contains plant stanol esters, which help reduce total and LDL cholesterol.

DISADVANTAGES
• There's little support for saw palmetto and soy lecithin as cholesterol busters.

• He has a family history of high cholesterol.

• He prefers not to take medication.

HIS NUMBERS
• Three months ago, Cusick's total cholesterol was 243, HDL 20, LDL 165, and triglycerides 290. Now his numbers are 224, 37, 162, and 126.

HIS PLAN
• Medication and more exercise. He takes Zocor (a statin drug) and niacin (a B vitamin).

ADVANTAGES
• Statins are effective drugs.

• Niacin reduces LDL and triglycerides while raising HDL.

• Cusick does 4 to 6 hours of aerobics and several hours of weight lifting weekly.

• Diet changes helped him lose 22 pounds.

DISADVANTAGES
• At 45, Cusick is getting a late start. Bad habits are hard to break.

• His HDL is very low. (HDL of 60 or more protects against heart disease.)

• Most men in his family have high cholesterol.

• Taking medication can make you less dedicated to lifestyle changes.

And the Winner Is . . .
Corey Campbell

J. Michael Gaziano, M.D., associate professor of medicine at Brigham and Women's Hospital in Boston, helped us devise this quiz to estimate which contestant has the best chance of controlling his cholesterol for life. Take it yourself and see which direction your numbers will go.

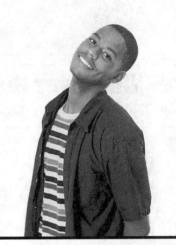

FINAL ANALYSIS

First, keep in mind that total cholesterol, HDL, LDL, and triglyceride levels are not the only indicators of heart disease. You can evaluate your 10-year risk of heart attack using the Framingham Risk Assessment tool at www.americanheart.org. (Click on Diseases, then Risk Assessment.) Your score will take into account other important risk factors, such as blood pressure and body mass index.

Campbell proves you can significantly cut your cholesterol—without taking prescription drugs. It was a good move for him to have his cholesterol checked at such a young age. "If he had waited until his forties or fifties, as many men do, his cholesterol could have been 280, and he might have been on the verge of a heart attack," says Dr. Gaziano. "My guess is that, long-term, Campbell is going to maintain his numbers the best. What's interesting is that his total cholesterol dropped as much as that of someone on lipid-lowering medication. This is the time of life to make lasting lifestyle changes."

Vaillancourt's secret weapons may be helping, but he really needs 3 cups of soy milk daily to meet the 25-gram requirement. (Roasted, salt-free soy nuts are another good source.) Dr. Gaziano is also skeptical about the soy lecithin, but he says the red wine, Benecol, and soy milk are good steps that may bring modest improvements. "Having a positive attitude about lifestyle changes is also a really good thing, and Vaillancourt has shown that he can stick with his effort long-term," says Dr. Gaziano.

And Cusick? "I like the treatment his doctor has chosen—the statin plus the niacin," says Dr. Gaziano. "It's too early to say whether he'll stick with the medicine and the lifestyle changes, both of which are important. It's possible that he'll come off the medication, so he has to be very aggressive about the lifestyle changes."

Drop Box

FACTOR	POINT VALUE	COREY	BRIAN	MIKE	YOU
AGE Cholesterol levels rise naturally with age.	Age 21–29? 0 30–35? −1 36–44? −2 45+? −3	0		 −2 −3	
TOTAL CHOLESTEROL Alone, it's a poor predictor of heart disease.	Total cholesterol lower than 200? 0 200–239? −2 240 or higher? −4	0	0	 −2	
LDL CHOLESTEROL This is the bad stuff that fouls arteries.	LDL lower than 100? 0 100–129? −1 130–159? −2 160–189? −4 190 or higher? −5	0	−1	 −4	
HDL CHOLESTEROL This is the good stuff that moves LDL to the liver for disposal.	HDL 60 or higher? +3 41–59? +1 31–40? −2 30 or lower? −4	 +1	 −2	 −2	
TRIGLYCERIDES Another dangerous blood component that increases heart attack risk.	Triglycerides lower than 150? 0 150–199? −1 200 or higher? −2	 −1	0	0	
WEIGHT Losing weight lowers LDL, triglycerides, and total cholesterol, and raises HDL.	Healthful weight? 0 Overweight? −2	0	0	0	
DIET Ideally, it should be low in saturated fat, simple carbohydrates, and dietary cholesterol. Soy (in food) reduces total and LDL cholesterol.	Good diet? +1 Bad diet? −1 Get 25 grams of low-fat soy protein from whole foods daily? +2 Eat some soy? +1	+1	+1 +1	+1	
EXERCISE Physical activity lowers LDL and raises HDL.	Get 30 minutes of physical activity daily? +2 Don't exercise regularly? −1	+2	+2	+2	
MEDICATION Statins lower LDL and triglycerides while raising HDL. Other cholesterol-lowering drugs, such as bile acid sequestrants, niacin, and fibrates, also work.	Taking a statin drug, such as Zocor, Mevacor, or Lipitor? +3 Taking one of the other drugs? +2			+3 +2	
HEREDITY High cholesterol can run in families.	Uncle, aunt, or grandparent with high cholesterol? −1 Mother, father, or sibling with high cholesterol? −2	 −2	 −2	−1	
TOTALS		+1	−3	−4	

▶ **IF YOUR SCORE IS +2 OR MORE:** You've mastered your lipids.

▶ **IF YOUR SCORE IS +1 TO −2:** You're doing a pretty good job.

▶ **IF YOUR SCORE IS −3 OR LESS:** What's that shooting pain in your chest?

MUST READS

Critical Condition

Overworked doctors. Bankrupt hospitals. Thousands of unnecessary deaths. Exactly what you'd expect in a country whose health care ranks below that of Colombia, Morocco, and Costa Rica. That country? You're living in it

By Christopher McDougall

Todd Taylor, M.D., doesn't waste any time when he comes banging through the emergency room doors at the start of each shift. If he did, he'd be distributing body bags instead of bandages.

"There can be 30 to 50 patients waiting, so I have to find the worst cases and dive right in," says Dr. Taylor, an ER physician at Good Samaritan Hospital in Phoenix. "I'll examine them in the hallway, in the waiting room, in the bathroom—just making sure everyone will stay alive."

This kind of Hail Mary health care is common for a MASH unit in a combat zone—except Dr. Taylor works far from firefights, in a relatively high-brow hospital. But to hear him tell it, he and the rest of the nation's ER docs are on the front lines of another kind of war: the battle to practice quality medicine as America's health care system falls apart.

"Most Americans still have no idea how dangerous it has become to be ill or injured and end up in an emergency room at the wrong time," says Dr. Taylor, who doubles as vice president for public affairs at the Arizona College of Emergency Physicians, also in Phoenix. "The chance of surviving a heart attack now depends more on the time of day, the day of the week, and your type of insurance than any other factor."

During a recent medical conference, Dr. Taylor asked an audience of doctors if they'd had firsthand experience of patients dying as a result of crowded ERs. One by one, about half the hands in the room went up. This isn't just stressed-out griping from overworked ER docs. According to the World Health

THE AVERAGE WAITING TIME FOR NONURGENT VISITS TO THE EMERGENCY ROOM: 67.7 MINUTES

TAKE MATTERS INTO YOUR OWN HANDS

Our health care system is listing—badly. So what are you going to do? Swim to Morocco? No, you're going to start bailing. Here are four ways you can help right the ship.

I. Choose a primary care physician: This is the family doctor you stopped seeing when you grew up and decided you knew better. "Men use the health care system only when they're banged up, but if they come in for regular checkups, I can catch minor problems before they manifest in larger ways," says Richard Roberts, M.D., chair of the American Academy of Family Physicians. "Regular checkups" means every 5 years in your twenties and thirties, every other year in your forties and fifties, and yearly from age 60 on. Log on to the AMA's Physician Select Web site at www.ama-assn.org/aps/amahg.htm to check the credentials of physicians in your area.

2. Quiz your HMO: Call your HMO and pose these two questions: "Do you provide any financial incentives to any of your physicians to limit diagnostic tests and referrals to specialists?" and "If a particular medical treatment is turned down, is there an appeal process?"

The correct answers are "No" and "Yes."

3. Or skip the HMOs entirely: One alternative is a "defined contribution," which provides $1,000 a year ($2,000 for families) to use in whatever way you want for your health care. What you don't spend stays in an account. Another grand is added annually. And since $1,000 won't go far for a serious illness, most plans have catastrophic coverage, which takes effect $500 after your account runs out. "Forty-three percent of company benefit managers have interest in consumer-driven programs, and they'll soon be available nationwide," says Clelland Green, founder of America's Choice Healthplans, a defined-contribution provider.

4. Know three numbers: Your ratio of LDL (bad) cholesterol to HDL (good) cholesterol. Your blood pressure. And your body mass index (BMI). Keep them within the ideal ranges—less than 100 for LDL and over 45 for HDL cholesterol, 120 over 80 for BP, 19 to 24 for BMI—and you may never need this number: 911. "The key is making this part of your routine," says Bill Williams, M.D., president of the National Association of Managed Care Physicians. Hit the blood pressure station in your local drugstore, calculate your BMI at www.nhlbisupport.com/bmi, and check your LDL-to-HDL ratio with the Biosafe home test (www.drugstore.com).

Organization (WHO), it's a dead-on assessment of the state of American medicine. When it comes to keeping ourselves healthy, the United States doesn't even make the WHO's top 10 list of countries. In fact, we're barely in the top 40.

Based on our health system's responsiveness to the needs of the population, the cost of health care to the individual, the allocation of public and private funds, overall population health, and the ratio between the current state of our health and the state that could be achieved, the United States limps in at 37th, far behind first-place France and second-place Italy. By those standards, you'd get better cradle-to-grave care in Podunk-y pit stops like Luxembourg (16th) and Morocco (29th).

Morocco? What the hell is going on? Aren't we the richest, most advanced nation on the planet? Aren't our doctors the miracle workers, the inventors of an artificial heart, the perennial Nobel laureates? Then why are we only slightly better off than Cuba (39th)? We're actually worse, in one sense: At least every Cuban citizen has state-provided medical care, but nearly 40 million Americans don't have health insurance, meaning they receive virtually no health care—or have to crowd ERs and hope for the best.

"They don't have health insurance, or it won't cover the procedures," Dr. Taylor explains. "They hope by some miracle we can help them in the emergency room." There's sometimes nothing he can do, but by law he has to at least make sure they have no immediate life-threatening problems. All the while, other patients can be stuck for up to 2 hours in an ambulance, waiting for an open ER gurney.

Whatever the cause, the overcrowding of emergency rooms has placed hospitals across the country in a bind between compassion and compensation: ERs have to treat everyone who's seeking care, but they're reimbursed only a fixed fee by Medicare and managed-care plans.

"Emergency medicine is an essential public service with no funding source," says Gary Tamkin, M.D., an emergency room physician in Vacaville, California, and president-elect of the California chapter of the American College of Emergency Physicians. Last year, emergency room doctors in California delivered $110 million in unpaid care.

That's a major reason that hospitals are laying off staff, going into bankruptcy, and closing. Two-thirds of the hospitals in Massachusetts are running a deficit, while nationwide, 128 general acute-care hospitals closed in 1999 and 2000. The direct result? Dangerously overworked ER physicians. Doctors, especially residents, are often forced to extend their work hours from an already grueling 80 per week to 90, 100, even 110. The effect, say medical researchers, is a level of sleep deprivation comparable to chugging five beers: Staying awake for 24 hours impairs psychomotor performance to a point comparable to a 0.1 percent blood alcohol level, according to a study published in the journal *Occupational and Environmental Medicine*. Put it this way: How'd you like your doctor to cannonball a six-pack before opening you up and operating?

"That's why we all make errors," says one first-year medical student. "You can't work 36 straight hours without making a mistake. But we cover them up. There's no push to change."

Dr. Taylor doesn't pull day-and-a-half shifts. He made a deal with his colleagues at Good Samaritan Hospital that he would work every Friday and Saturday night—the busiest time for ERs—in exchange for weekdays off. By the time Dr. Taylor's shift ends, at 7 A.M., there are often patients still waiting to be seen. "I look at them and wonder how desperate they must be," he says.

"Sitting all night, suffering. I can't believe it when they thank me—until I find out they already waited at another ER for several hours or called their primary care doctors and were told they couldn't be seen for a week."

DEATH OF THE FAMILY DOCTOR

The search for a culprit in the American health care crisis leads from the emergency room back to the family medical practice. ERs are dangerously overcrowded not only because of the masses of sick and uninsured but also because of a dearth of do-it-all generalists once known as "family doctors." According to a recent American Medical Association report, 20 percent fewer graduating med students entered family practice residencies in 2000 than in 1996. As a result, people are turning more and more to the emergency room for all their primary care needs.

That's why if one thing can put a smile on the face of every ER doctor in the country, and possibly even boost the United States toward the top of the WHO rankings, it's the promise that a few thousand medical students are about to become primary care physicians.

David Grande, M.D., is just the kind of guy they have in mind. He's a youthful-looking 28-year-old who often bustles around in a skateboarder's green sweater and cargo pants, a stethoscope slung around his neck. He's insanely hardworking and would probably be the star of any medical practice—except he's decided not to work in one.

"It's a very hard decision to make, especially after borrowing so much money for medical school," Dr. Grande says. "But I can't participate in a health care system that doesn't work without trying to make a change."

The way he sees it, American medicine has become a money pit that will keep falling apart no matter how many millions are dumped into it. The time has come, he's convinced, to tear the structure down and rebuild from the bottom up. To back up his conviction, he's forgone a big-bucks medical specialty to become something more valuable: a primary care physician who only makes house calls.

Today he's in north Philadelphia's infamous "Badlands." Here, amid the neighborhood gangstas, crack addicts, and heroin dealers, Dr. Grande and his fellow volunteers are setting up shop inside a secondhand mobile home that's been converted into a crude mobile medical truck. Soon they'll begin treating any wounded, diseased, or delirious person who stumbles in off the street.

It's not long before a line forms. A pregnant young woman comes in with a fever; an older woman has an infection deep inside her ear; a gray-haired geriatric pries off his tattered construction boot and reveals toes that have swollen into fat, pus-filled grapes. Last week, a diabetic who couldn't afford insulin turned up with blood sugar readings that were off the chart; Dr.

Grande sped over to a nearby drugstore and bought him a prescription out of his own pocket.

"Our supplies here are really limited," Dr. Grande says with a shrug. "We depend on donations, so sometimes we need to supplement on our own." More than 60 percent of the people treated here have no insurance, and many others are senior citizens whose ailments have progressed past the point of an easy fix because their health plans don't subsidize their medications.

The problem isn't that our country lacks the cash. Already, the United States' annual tab for health care is over $1.3 trillion—not only way more than any other country's, but also more than that of some of the higher-ranked countries combined. "The American health care system is at once the most expensive and the most inadequate system in the developed world," the *New England Journal of Medicine* noted in 1999. Sure, our nation has some of the most respected and innovative medical specialists in the world and more state-of-the-art gizmos than almost any other nation on the planet. In fact, when it comes to the availability of such high-tech gadgetry as MRI's and CAT scans, the United States is second only to Japan.

But whereas we pour a huge amount of that $1.3 trillion into developing superadvanced technology, Japan focuses as much on primary care as it does on miracle cures. The results are unmistakable: According to the WHO, Japanese men have the longest life expectancy on the planet—74.5 years— while American men can expect to die nearly a half decade sooner. That may not mean much to you right now, but ask your 69-year-old father what he thinks.

"What the World Health Organization ranking points out is that it's not important *how much* you spend," explains Dr. Grande, "as opposed to where you spend it." While we have some of the greatest hospitals in the world, their budgets are balanced on revenues from radical procedures, instead of the early diagnosis and preventive care that would make them unnecessary. Even Fidel Castro puts more into primary care than we do: *Los cubanos* have one generalist per 255 people, while we *americanos* have only one for every 430. We're becoming the world's best firefighters, in other words, while the rest of the world just keeps its oily rags away from the stove.

Med school students learn the lesson early on in their education: Specialists get rich. "That's a very powerful draw when you've taken out a fortune in loans and have to figure out a way to pay them back," says Amy MacKenzie, a first-year medical student at the Drexel University College of Medicine in Philadelphia, who now has to decide her future. The difference in pay is dramatic: According to a 2001 compensation survey by the journal *Modern Healthcare*, pediatricians and primary care doctors make $156,000 a year on average, while cardiologists and urologists, for instance, earn about $277,000.

The solution to America's health care woes, therefore, might seem simple. All we have to do is pay generalists more, and in no time we'll have empty ERs, well-rested residents, and longer life spans than any other country. But of course it isn't that simple, and you can spell the reason with just three letters: H . . . M . . .

Care to buy a vowel?

BADLY MANAGED CARE

HMOs have a nickname for primary care physicians: They call them "gatekeepers." The way managed care works, general practitioners are a critical first obstacle to a patient's request for specialized—read: "expensive"—medical care. Without that magic referral slip, there's no chance an HMO will cover a consultation with a high-priced specialist. The result is a huge disincentive for a med student to become a primary care physician: Succumb to HMO pressure and your patient will want to sue you, but appease the patient and you're relegated to HMO hell—no insurance payments.

"Given a choice between saving money and saving your life, which way would your HMO go?"

Linda Peeno, M.D., lobs the question up there, inviting you to think the worst of the health care industry. But before giving way to cynicism, you have to ask the question: Are managed care executives *really* that cutthroat?

"Absolutely," replies Dr. Peeno. "Without a doubt."

As a former medical reviewer for Humana, one of the nation's largest publicly traded managed health care companies, she should know. Dr. Peeno scrutinized doctors' medical requests and either accepted them for reimbursement or denied them as unnecessary or not covered by the patient's plan. Her duties went further, however; whenever possible, Dr. Peeno says, she was supposed to cajole or bully doctors into avoiding pricey procedures. "Intimidation, hassling, humiliation—I did it all," Dr. Peeno says. It's hard to believe, coming from a petite Kentuckian whose bluegrass drawl makes her sound like a schoolmarm, but that's what made her perfect for the job: She could deny Grandma's procedure and make the decision stick.

PERCENTAGE OF DOCTORS WHO SAY THAT MANAGED CARE HAS HAD A NEGATIVE IMPACT ON THE WAY THEY PRACTICE MEDICINE: **76**

PERCENTAGE WHO SAY IT HAS HAD A NEGATIVE IMPACT ON THE MEDICAL SERVICES AVAILABLE TO THEIR PATIENTS: **75**

Another part of Dr. Peeno's job was to consult with marketing executives to find ways to "monkey with the language," as she puts it, so the plan would appear to promise one thing while preserving loopholes for denial of care. She got so caught up in the challenge of cost cutting, she says, that it became "like a game" in which she tried to find any possible reason to deny payment.

But even when the necessary treatments are approved, doctors say, they're being pushed too hard to speed patients along. More than 2,000 Massachusetts physicians published a call to action in the *Journal of the American Medical Association*, complaining that they were being forced to treat patients like parts on an assembly line. "The time we are allowed to spend with the sick shrinks under the pressure to increase throughput," they charged. "Doctors and nurses are being prodded by threats and bribes to abdicate allegiance to patients, and to shun the sickest, who may be unprofitable."

According to the Massachusetts doctors, the HMOs are ruthless when it comes to wielding incentives and punishments. If the doctors demand too many expensive procedures, they say, they risk being dropped by the insurer. If they minimize care, however, they receive bonuses. State medical societies in California, Georgia, and Texas have gone so far as to accuse the insurance industry of Mafia-style practices. Backed by more than 75,000 physicians, they recently filed a federal lawsuit that says that denying necessary medical care is tantamount to racketeering and that paying doctors to limit tests and treatments is unfair business.

Dr. Peeno saw it all, and played along. But in 1987, one case jolted her so badly, it haunts her to this day. A patient in California, she says, had been scheduled for a heart transplant. While Dr. Peeno was reviewing the case, one of her colleagues dropped by. "Someone came in my office and said, 'Have you called yet about this case? We can't pay for this. This is going to occur at a hospital where we don't have a contract, and we've got to figure out a way not to pay for it.'" Dr. Peeno wavered, and rationalized, and finally stamped the request "Not medically necessary."

Because the decision saved Humana about $500,000, Dr. Peeno says, she was given a raise and promoted. She was also stricken with self-loathing. She quit Humana and went to work for another HMO, and then another, thinking each one might be different. Nothing changed. "I always had the same task," Dr. Peeno says. "Using my medical expertise for the financial benefit of the organization, often leading to great harm, and potentially death, for some patients."

While Humana has stated that Dr. Peeno was never in a position to be the final arbiter of any medical, health care, or insurance matter, copies of her work contract with Humana indicate otherwise. The company also said it could find no record of the foiled transplant patient she describes. But Dr.

Peeno passionately insists that it happened. At first she chose not to find out the patient's fate, preferring to hide the truth from herself as long as possible. But 12 years later, spurred by Humana's steadfast denial of the case, she tracked down the patient's death certificate. He had died 28 months after the benefit denial without having received the transplant. Dr. Peeno's medical expertise tells her he lived out his days in end-stage heart failure. "I live with that act, and many others, eating into my heart and soul," Dr. Peeno says. "A physician's basic rule is Do no harm. I did worse. I caused death."

ARE YOU PART OF THE PROBLEM?

But HMOs are victims, too, one doctor contends: victims of bad timing. Just look at their customers.

"Let's face it, this is a terrible time in history to be responsible for American health," says Frederick deBeer, M.D., chief of medicine at Veterans Affairs Medical Center in Lexington, Kentucky. "We see patients every day who neglect their health until they start coughing up blood from lung cancer. Then they expect a miracle cure to drag them back from the portals of death. And then they want it regardless of the cost!" Dr. deBeer concludes indignantly, his South African accent punctuating his point that this is an American phenomenon.

Dr. deBeer was raised and trained in the United Kingdom and South Africa and, since coming to the United States, has been consistently amazed at how little attention Americans pay to their health. Poor access to primary care may contribute to men's neglect of their health, or it may be the other way around—perhaps the fact that men don't bother getting checkups has made primary care less lucrative for doctors. Dr. deBeer can't say which is cause and which is effect, but in his budget-monitoring capacity as the chief of medicine at a major veterans' hospital, he's certain of this: The failure of Americans to take responsibility for their health has contributed significantly to the country's health care problems.

"Everyone complains about how expensive health care is, but the costs are largely patient-driven," Dr. deBeer explains. "Many Americans live their lives with little regard for the consequences, then go to specialists for what are essentially very expensive end-of-life procedures." As examples, he points to the ever-increasing obesity rate and never-increasing blood pressure exams. "It's so well-established that men in their thirties need annual blood pressure exams, but we've failed miserably in convincing them to get them," he says.

PERCENTAGE OF DOCTORS WHO REPORT THEIR ENTHUSIASM FOR PRACTICING HAS DECREASED: 58

"Then they have a stroke, and the cost to keep them alive is far more than it would have been for 10 lifetimes' worth of early care."

In this regard, Dr. deBeer says, HMOs aren't completely at fault for hiring screeners to dissuade patients from relying on specialists. Where they are to blame, however, is in allowing these decision makers to become both intimidators and a money-sucking entity of their own. By trying to save money, HMOs have created massive administrative machinery that costs as much to run as the hospitals. On average, administrative costs in the United States swallow about 24 percent of health care costs. That's more than double the administrative costs in Canada, which manages to provide universal health care while holding the bureaucratic overhead at 11 percent.

"As managed care enrollment has soared, so have administrative expenses," says Steffie Woolhandler, M.D., associate professor of medicine at Harvard University and cofounder of Physicians for a National Health Program. "The percentage of workers in the health system dealing with paperwork has increased from 18 percent to nearly 30 percent, belying the myth of HMO efficiency."

NO SIMPLE SOLUTION

America's health care system is bloated and bleeding, and it's just been wheeled into the trauma unit. You're the doctor. What do you do? Pump more money into the nation's emergency rooms? Odds are, patient loads will continue to outpace funding due to the paucity of primary care physicians. Bring the salaries of family doctors more in line with those of specialists? It'll still be a thankless job as long as HMOs continue to pit primary care physician against patient. So overhaul the HMOs? Won't make a difference if, because of laziness or lack of insurance, most Americans don't receive the early preventive care they need.

The only way to effectively stabilize the patient may be a phrase we don't want to hear: national health insurance, better known as "socialized medicine." There are dozens of reform plans, but most share the same core philosophy: High profits and healing cannot coexist. Nearly all propose using tax dollars to finance health care for every citizen, taking medicine out of the hands of for-profit companies.

AMONG CITIZENS OF THE UNITED STATES, AUSTRALIA, CANADA, NEW ZEALAND, AND THE UNITED KINGDOM, THOSE WHO ARE THE LEAST SATISFIED WITH THEIR HEALTH CARE SYSTEM: AMERICANS

Although governments control health care in nearly every other first-world nation (including most of those ranked higher than the United States in health care performance), Americans are unrelenting in their opposition to so-called socialized medicine. The HMOs are against it, naturally, and so are the overwhelming majority of physicians, particularly the specialists, who fear that their salaries will be capped at bus driver levels. But more important, the American public has never accepted the idea. This is partly because of its "commie menace" ring, but even more from the belief that state-run health care will be as incompetent and crushingly bureaucratic as, say, the Department of Motor Vehicles.

"But there's no reason it has to be that way," says Dr. Grande, the crusading young doctor who's hoping to champion just such a radical health care overhaul. "There are all kinds of national systems, and if the right one is created, it can be far more beneficial—and cost-effective—than most for-profit businesses." After all, we do it with the military, public education, and trash collection—why not medicine?

Perhaps because, in practice, socialized medicine improves the health of the overall population but shortchanges the individual who truly needs that expensive specialist. Just look across the border. In one national poll, eight in 10 Canadians said they believe that their country's much-extolled cover-everyone health system is in crisis. That's why (among other reasons) any such program considered for the United States would need to give every citizen the option of paying for care at a private clinic, possibly through a voucher system of the sort used for charter school programs. Even then, proponents of socialized medicine will have an extraordinarily difficult time selling it as a cure-all for our ailing health care system.

Dr. Woolhandler, for one, makes a more pragmatic argument: "How much worse could it get?"

Pushed to the Limit

Across the country, tens of thousands of pushers battle one another in a fierce turf war to get their drugs into the hands of users. But it's not your kids they want to sell them to. It's your doctor

By Tom Zoellner

Jerry Rice is working hard tonight. The former 49ers wide receiver is now 50 handshakes into the evening and still greeting strangers as if they were his new best friends. The San Francisco Hilton conference room has been mocked up to look like a football stadium—Astroturf on the floor, fake goalposts, piles of ballpark food; there's even a chain-link fence that separates Rice from a line of orthopedic surgeons waiting to have a picture taken with him. The party's sponsor is the drug company Pharmacia, whose representatives are here to tout the benefits of their new anticlotting drug, Fragmin. At the nearby convention of the American Academy of Orthopaedic Surgeons, the Pharmacia guys are giving away a free 35-millimeter camera to anybody who looks like a doctor.

I don't look much like a doctor, but I manage to slip into the drug company's party anyway. Here, Thomas W. Jackson, M.D., a surgeon from Riverside, California, is munching on a free hot dog. As we watch Rice doing his grip-and-grins, I ask Dr. Jackson if going to an event like this makes him more inclined to prescribe Fragmin to his patients.

"To tell you the truth, yes," says Dr. Jackson, a tall, mustachioed fellow in his forties. "If there are five drugs that are equal in quality, and if the pharmaceutical rep does a favor for me, then I'll be inclined to use his drug. You scratch my back, I'll scratch yours. It's the American way. I'm not offended by it."

Dr. Jackson goes on. "Now, you have to keep in mind that I'm more scrupulous than most. I know a doctor in my town who explicitly asks for stuff before he prescribes a drug. He'll actually say to the rep, 'Now, I sure would like to start giving my patients your drug, but it sure would be nice to go fishing in Cabo San Lucas first.' And you know what? He'll go." And his patients will get the drug—whether or not there's a safer or more cost-efficient alternative out there.

Free NBA tickets, lavish dinners, golf outings, ski trips to Aspen under the guise of "medical education," even free tanks of gas—drug company representatives dole out all these and more to get doctors to listen to their pitches. In 2000 these companies, including the likes of Merck, Schering, Pfizer, and Hoffman-LaRoche, spent a total of $11 billion to court doctors. That comes out to about $11,000 a year for every physician in America. In fact, these firms spend more on marketing and administration than on research and development. And the number of salesmen to spread the bounty has doubled in 5 years—from 41,800 in 1996 to 83,000 in 2000, according to Scott-Levin, a firm that tracks the industry.

New York City physician Barrie Raik, M.D., was well-accustomed to the sales-heavy culture of the medical field, but never thought much about it until

"This is not a small thing. This is a major problem.
And it goes very deep. It affects both the costs and quality
of medicine."   **—James Norris, M.D., Portland, Oregon**

"The prescribing decision is very much based on how much the doctor was wined and dined. And sometimes, the decision is inappropriate." **—Ashley Wazana, M.D., Montreal**

1993, when an antiheartburn prescription drug called Propulsid hit the market and salesmen hit doctors' offices with a vengeance. Dr. Raik says she was stunned to see sales reps—bearing basketball and Broadway musical tickets—urging doctors to assign Propulsid immediately to any new patient who complained of acid reflux. Her main concern: Prescription drugs were usually the last course of action for treating heartburn.

"This was a treatment that bypassed any incremental steps, such as lifestyle changes and over-the-counter antacids," she says. Her worries, it turns out, were justified: Propulsid is now suspected of causing irregular heartbeats in some patients and has been linked to 80 deaths. It was withdrawn from the market by the FDA in 2000.

This is the major reason Dr. Raik has joined a small but highly vocal group of doctors called No Free Lunch. The group is run by an internist named Bob Goodman, M.D., whom I met for coffee in a diner down the street from Co-lumbia-Presbyterian Hospital in New York City. Since 2001, Dr. Goodman has succeeded in convincing about 100 other doctors to "take the pledge" and refuse all gifts from drug companies. The entire culture of American medicine is addicted to the handout, he believes.

"Doctors learn from their medical school teachers and their role models that gifts are acceptable," says Dr. Goodman. "They even feel they're entitled to them."

Dr. Goodman, a father of a 3-year-old son, says his own feelings on the subject were solidified in 1996 when his 9-year-old nephew came down with strep throat and was taken to see a pediatrician in Brookline, Massachusetts. To Dr. Goodman's disbelief, the child was prescribed Keflex, an expensive an-tibiotic that had the potential to cause resistance to future antibiotics. A shot of penicillin—not a drug that anybody cares to market aggressively these days—was all that was necessary, says Dr. Goodman.

"You see this all the time," he says. "Drugs that cost $60 for a 5-day course are favored over older drugs that cost pennies."

UNDER THE INFLUENCE

At the Kaiser Permanente Hospital in Portland, Oregon, James Norris, M.D., is chairman of the formulary committee, which oversees the dispensing of drugs in the hospital. He says the perk problem used to be so bad that re-

"I had begun to feel like a prostitute, selling myself for dinner." —**Mark McConnell., M.D., La Crosse, Wisconsin**

quest forms for new drugs—the forms are internal hospital documents—often came to the dispensary filled out in handwriting that did not match the requesting doctors' signatures. Apparently some salesmen were filling out the doctors' own paperwork. Dr. Norris's committee instituted a new rule—each future request had to be in a physician's own hand.

If Dr. Norris were a basketball fan, he'd probably spot a few of his colleagues at Portland's Rose Garden Arena. "I know doctors who accept Trailblazers tickets," he says. "They may have a short conversation with the drug rep before tip-off, and then go in, sit back, and enjoy the game. These people don't realize how blatantly they're being manipulated. They are in denial about it."

The average physician meets with a drug company representative approximately once a week, according to a study review published in 2000 in the *Journal of the American Medical Association (JAMA)*. The study's author, Ashley Wazana, M.D., of McGill University in Montreal, says he was offered an all-expenses-paid trip to a resort in the Canadian Rockies last spring. He turned it down. "Doctors are influenced, even if they think they're not," he says.

And it appears that they've been under this influence for some time. Consider the pediatricians at the Cleveland Clinic who in the early 1990s studied the usage rate of two drugs at their hospital before and after doctors there were flown to two all-expenses-paid "symposiums," including one in the Caribbean. The study, published in the medical journal *Chest,* showed that usage of the drugs increased out of proportion to the rate at other hospitals of similar size.

Mark McConnell, M.D., an internist in La Crosse, Wisconsin, says he is becoming wearily accustomed to seeing patients with high blood pressure who've been prescribed expensive calcium channel blockers like Norvasc as a first step. The conventional first treatment for high blood pressure is a diuretic and a beta-blocker—a program that costs a tenth of what a calcium channel blocker costs.

"There is no explanation for this kind of treatment except that the doctor has been influenced by a pharmaceutical representative," says Dr. McConnell.

He himself used to accept dinners and other gifts from drug salesmen. But Dr. McConnell's conscience was stirred when he saw a pharmaceutical company paying doctors in his hospital $250 cash for each prescription they wrote for a certain drug. The company was supposedly conducting a "study," but Dr. McConnell says it was a transparent attempt to get patients hooked. He now turns down all perks. "This winter, I could have gone skiing every weekend if I'd wanted. Not just me, but my family and all the nurses in my office, too."

THE NEED FOR SPEED

The surge in marketing money being thrown at physicians is in part due to the best intentions of the Food and Drug Administration. The spread of AIDS gave rise to an enormous population of people who needed help right away, but the ponderousness of the drug approval process kept them waiting. The resulting pressure convinced the FDA to give "priority approval" to certain critical medications. Instead of facing years of clinical trials, a new drug could be on pharmacy shelves in just months.

One unintended side effect of the amped-up approval process is that it's now much easier for rival companies to move competing drugs quickly onto the market, even if it's not a matter of life and death. This creates fiercer competition for the attention of a physician with no strong feelings on the matter.

Under this kind of pressure, drug company representatives are striving to stick their feet in the door, so to speak, earlier and earlier. The calls—and the perks—from drug reps start coming almost as soon as a student enters medical school. "They're trying to reach us early so we'll be loyal to them later," says one first-year resident at a New England hospital. This resident is years away from writing his first prescription, but he never has to bring his lunch to work. It's always there in the hospital, buffet-style and hot, and paid for by the pharmaceutical companies. Dr. Goodman, of No Free Lunch, told me about a doctor who did his residency at a Bronx hospital where catered food was not just frequent, but an expected part of each lunch hour. "Every day, he had different companies coming in, bringing lunch to the staff," he says. "It got to the point that the hospital would send out a special bulletin if there wasn't a catered lunch that day."

But the really intensive selling to doctors takes place once they have begun their careers and are actually writing prescriptions. Then they're treated to small, one-on-one meetings at five-star restaurants and exclusive golf courses. Some companies have perfected the art of what they call the "dine-and-dash," in which a doctor will agree to meet a representative at a

"A few of the doctors on my rounds just hand me a menu and tell me what they want before they'll see me."   —"Willie," pharmaceutical sales representative, California

fancy restaurant. The doctor listens to a sales pitch for 5 minutes and then leaves with his meal. Drug reps can individually pitch dozens of doctors in one night with this method.

WHAT'S THE DEAL?

"Willie," as we'll call him, covers northern California for a large pharmaceutical company and cheerfully calls himself a "drug dealer" when asked about his line of work. He has managed to perfect his golf game through all the free rounds he's given to doctors. Tall, friendly, and fond of his work, he consents to an interview only if I agree to keep his real name out of the story—so he won't get in trouble with his company.

"The key is repetition, repetition, repetition," he says. "You always want to be the last guy who visits the doctor because more than likely, that's whose drug he's going to go with." Willie admits he's envious of a rival company that runs a variation of the dine-and-dash known as the "gas-and-go." The rep makes arrangements to meet the doctor at a local gas station and, while standing on the fuel island, discusses the drug of the moment while the doctor fills his tank with gas—which the drug company then pays for.

Besides the meals, the free gas, and the knickknacks, pharmaceutical reps also carpet-bomb doctors with professionally boxed "free samples" of their new drugs. Detail men—drug industry jargon for reps who pitch physicians—handed out a staggering $8 billion worth of samples in 2000, more than the gross national product of Brunei. Physicians like the practice because giving away free 2-week supplies of expensive medicines helps them build goodwill among their patients. Drug companies like it because they know full well that a single free sample stands an excellent chance of turning into a longtime—and profitable—prescription. "Getting those samples in the doctor's cabinet is like putting money in the bank," says Dr. Goodman.

Mary Anne Rhyne, a spokeswoman for the drug giant GlaxoSmithKline, says that her company has a policy that permits the representative to buy only "modest meals" for the doctors. And, she points out, free samples and get-togethers with physicians are critical in educating the medical community about the latest breakthroughs.

"The goal is to have a conversation with the physician and to provide information to the physician and have an education exchange," she says. "The

"I may be a whore, but I'm not as big a whore as some of these other guys."   **—Anonymous M.D., Illinois**

FAST-ACTING DRUGS

Faster FDA approval means more drug money for anyone holding a prescription pad.

Average Time It Took the FDA to Review and Approve a Drug (in months)

1993	20.8
1994	15.8
1995	15.3
1996	14.8
1997	12.2
1998	12
1999	11.8
2000	10.9

SOURCE: Food and Drug Administration

Total Amount the Drug Companies Spent on Marketing to Doctors and Consumers (in $billions)

1997	11
1998	12.5
1999	13.9
2000	15.7

SOURCE: IMS Health and PhRMA

best drug in the world is of no use unless the doctors and the patients know about it."

GlaxoSmithKline takes this concept seriously. In 2000, it spent 37 percent of its revenues on marketing and administration. Only 14 percent went to research and development.

Across town from the Jerry Rice meet-and-greet, an even better party has attracted more doctors. Pfizer has rented out San Francisco's new baseball stadium, Pacific Bell Park, for the night. I manage to slip in with equal ease. Waiters wander about the glassy mezzanine level with trays of canapés and wine, and sports legends Ozzie Smith and Dick Butkus are on hand to pose for buddy-buddy photographs with doctors they'll never see again. The party is technically an educational event. A doctor brought in by Pfizer stands in a recessed alcove and gives a 15-minute lecture on some of the glowing clinical trials of Celebrex, a new anti-arthritis drug. Almost nobody is listening. Butkus is the big attraction (how could he be anything else?), followed closely by the open bar.

Out in the empty ballpark seats, I find orthopedist Wayne Johnson, M.D., of Colorado Springs, looking out at the darkened field. He says he will sometimes prescribe a drug based on the personality of the salesman pitching it. "If there's no difference in the quality of the drugs, I'll go with the one whose rep I get along with best," he says. "It'll be in the back of my mind when I'm writing the prescription."

A NOT-SO-RANDOM DRUG TEST

You wouldn't trust a politician who took gifts and payola from a contractor bidding on a new baseball stadium, right? Well, we're talking about a more important structure here—your body. Philadelphia-based psychiatrist (and pharmaceutical perk opponent) Amy Brodkey, M.D., suggests six discreet questions to ask when your doctor is writing you a prescription.

1. "How long has this drug been on the market?" Anything brand-new might imply that the doctor has been a target of a whirlwind launch.

2. "What advantages does this have over similar drugs?" See if he knows anything about the competition.

3. "What potential side effects does it have?" This might not have been included in the representative's pitch, or the doctor might not have been paying attention.

4. "Are there nondrug options for my condition?" There often are, but drug reps would prefer there weren't.

5. "Can I get free samples?" If the answer is yes, that's a sure sign that a drug company representative has paid the doctor a visit and wants to get you hooked.

6. "Where did you get that pen?" If it's branded with a drug company label, that's like a whiff of perfume from the femme fatale.

But how do doctors know if drugs really are equal in quality? Celebrex is an excellent case study. It was introduced in February 1999 after FDA approval. But no substantial information about the drug was available to doctors or the public for 9 months—except the information provided by pharmaceutical sales teams. It wasn't until November 1999 that *JAMA* published the results of the first clinical trial comparing Celebrex with another drug. By that time, Pfizer had already cleared roughly $1 billion in sales of Celebrex. According to Larry Sasich, Pharm.D., of the Washington, D.C., watchdog group Public Citizen, there is still no solid evidence that Celebrex is any more effective as an anti-inflammatory than the old workhorses Motrin and Advil— a.k.a. ibuprofen, which was introduced more than a quarter-century ago.

"Why would someone purchase an untested drug that wholesales for $2.43 a dose versus a drug that wholesales for about 7 cents a dose?" asks Sasich. "Celebrex is just not as good a pain reliever as and is no safer than Motrin."

A COSTLY DRUG HABIT

Huge marketing campaigns, including budgets for salesmen's salaries and doctors' perks, are usually mapped out long before new drugs win formal approval by the FDA. The detail men themselves are prohibited by federal law from touting unapproved drugs before they hit the marketplace, but one common way around that ban is to pay a cooperative physician a cash honorarium to give a "scientific presentation" about the drug at a medical conference. According to the industry tracking firm Scott-Levin, there were 314,000 such events in 2000, ranging from catered lunches in hospitals to getaways at top-tier resorts.

Pharmaceutical marketing is "a fractured system" that is unique within the world of capitalism because the end user—the patient—has almost no say in the buying process, says Mick Kolassa, Ph.D., professor of pharmacy administration at the University of Mississippi School of Pharmacy in University. "It can get problematic. Often a doctor doesn't have the foggiest idea how much a drug is costing the patient."

The ultimate costs to a patient can be more than financial. A 54-year-old deaf man named Jerry Keen is one example. Keen, from Holmes County, Mississippi, has only a fourth-grade education and, because of his hearing disability, has never held a job. A recent diagnosis of diabetes drove him to a doctor, who gave him a new oral drug called Rezulin, a drug that was given priority approval by the FDA. The 215-pound Keen was delighted not to have to endure twice-daily insulin shots. But what he didn't know—and what his doctor, who had been offered golf outings and speaking fees by the drug's manufacturer, might not have known either—was that clinical studies had shown evidence of potential problems with the drug. At least 18 patients had been diagnosed with damaged livers.

Yet, despite the fact that other established diabetes drugs were safer and less expensive, the manufacturer continued to convince doctors to prescribe Rezulin. According to *Washington Monthly* magazine, in the spring of 1999, selected doctors in the New York City area received a fax from the drug's manufacturer, Parke-Davis, inviting them to a dinner and a short lecture on the benefits of Rezulin, to be held at the Club Bar and Grill in Madison Square Garden. After the talk, the doctors got to watch the New York Knicks play the Toronto Raptors. This was nearly 2 years after the drug had been removed from the market in Great Britain because of concerns about liver damage, and about the same time the FDA revealed that the drug had injured more than 400 patients. Rezulin allegedly went on to kill 63 people before it was finally pulled off the market in March 2000. As for Keen, today he suffers from chronic abdominal pain because of early cirrhosis of the liver; he's suing for

PERCENTAGE INCREASE IN THE NUMBER
OF BIOTECH DRUGS THAT WERE APPROVED
IN THE UNITED STATES FROM 1995 TO 2000, COMPARED WITH
THE PREVIOUS 13 YEARS: NEARLY 200 PERCENT

$50 million. Parke-Davis has since been purchased by Pfizer, whose corporate spokesman Bob Fauteux declined to comment on the litigation.

Fauteux did, however, defend the practice of pushing perks at physicians, including the occasional free lunch, in an effort to educate them about the latest pharmaceuticals.

"Physicians are very busy individuals, and it's well-recognized that it's tough to schedule a spot on their calendars," says Fauteux. "If a doctor can't see us in the office, then sometimes we'll say, 'Well, can you make it for lunch or dinner?' These meetings are an important way for doctors to hear about the latest advances in pharmacology."

But Dr. Goodman points out that truly important breakthroughs get more than adequate attention in the medical press and that a doctor who relies solely on what the salesperson says is like any other consumer ripe for a swindle. "A doctor's choice of drugs should be based solely on the legitimate scientific literature and nothing else," he says. "So you can blame doctors for this as much as you can blame the drug companies."

And maybe you can blame the American Medical Association, too. Sure, the AMA has a policy on how much doctors can accept from drug manufacturers; its 1990 guidelines limit the gifts a doctor may receive to "textbooks, modest meals, and other gifts" that are not of "substantial value." But those guidelines are nonbinding. "We don't police it, and we're not going to suspend anybody's membership," says Bob Musacchio, Ph.D., an AMA senior vice president. "But it is universally understood what the guidelines mean." Perhaps, but why, then, did the AMA launch a 19-month campaign to "raise awareness of the guidelines" just a few months after being contacted for this story? And how is it that Dr. Wazana's review found that as many as half of all medical school residents are unaware that the AMA guidelines (as well as those of other organizations) even exist?

It's fair to ask just how serious the AMA is about its own guidelines, when it assists drug companies in their marketing efforts. The organization supplies pharmaceutical manufacturers with the "physicians' master file," a database that contains detailed biographies of member doctors, as well as their individual DEA (Drug Enforcement Agency) numbers. By itself, a doctor's DEA number isn't that valuable, but combine it with the prescription records that

NUMBER OF PRESCRIPTIONS FILLED BY AMERICANS IN 1992: 2 BILLION

NUMBER FILLED IN 2000: 3.15 BILLION

ALTERNATIVE MEDICINES

If not that expensive and possibly dangerous new medication, then what? Something less expensive and safer. Here are some options, courtesy of Larry Sasich, Pharm.D., of the Washington, D.C., watchdog group Public Citizen.

Drug: Relenza, an antiflu inhalant
Effective alternative: Tylenol and water

Drug: Xopenex, an asthma drug
Effective alternative: Albuterol, a generic drug with a virtually identical chemical formula

Drug: Geodon, an antipsychotic
Effective alternative: Haldol, an antipsychotic

Drug: Avelox, an antibiotic
Effective alternative: Cipro

Drug: Cardura, an alpha-blocker for high blood pressure
Effective alternative: Hydrodiuril (a thiazide diuretic commonly used to treat high blood pressure)

drug companies purchase from pharmacies, and suddenly you're looking at every medication a doctor is prescribing. Of course, the drug manufacturers have to pay for the information.

Sales of the file to drug companies made the AMA an estimated $20 million in the year 2000 alone.

Just Say "No" to Drugs

Four life-threatening conditions. Four lifetime prescriptions for costly, risky drugs. The way to avoid all four: Act fast and act naturally

By Christian Millman

A friend of mine, Adam, has high blood pressure—probably a genetic gift from his mom. Sometimes he clocks in as high as 150/100 mm Hg, well above the optimal score of 120/80 mm Hg. And like any father of three who just turned 40, he doesn't want to have an early heart attack, so he follows his doctor's advice. He doesn't smoke. He takes vacations. He stays extremely fit: He runs about 35 miles a week and competes in two marathons a year, so his heart is in near perfect shape.

It's a lot of work, but Adam has motivation: He doesn't want to take hypertension drugs for the rest of his life.

"The pills my doctor prescribed made me dizzy, and I just feel better without them," he says. "What's more, I resented dropping $40 a month on medication that didn't seem to be doing me any good."

Adam's doctor warns him that he's taking a risk by forgoing drugs, but a lot of men make the same decision. And doctors support it. In fact, some believe that taking lifelong prescription drugs is an unnecessary drill for thousands of men. We asked physicians to weigh the pros and cons of the typical drug therapy for four common health problems and to outline the drug-free strategies that might put your pharmacist out of business.

If you're in the early stages of one of the following conditions, ask your doctor to let you try the drug-free option first, and make sure he monitors your progress. If he refuses, he'd better have a pretty good reason. If he doesn't, you have a good reason to find another doctor.

YOU'RE SEEING THE DOCTOR BECAUSE . . .
. . . Your blood pressure is in the 150/90 range.
Your risk: *Heart disease or stroke*

The drug fix: There are six classes of hypertension drugs available by prescription, all capable of lowering blood pressure by an average of 10 points within 2 months, says Nicholas P. Tsapatsaris, M.D., of Tufts University School of Medicine in Boston and the Lahey Clinic in Burlington, Massachusetts. Some work by reducing your heart rate and cardiac bloodflow; others dilate your blood vessels, reducing pressure. The downside: They can be expensive and occasionally cause dizziness, persistent coughing, or even that most unpleasant of side effects, sexual dysfunction.

The natural fix: It's simple, but that doesn't mean it's easy. You need to exercise aerobically for at least 30 minutes three or four times a week, cut your fat intake to less than 30 percent of your diet, and eat more fiber and less salt. For example, researchers placed 412 people with high blood pressure on the DASH diet—it stands for "dietary approaches to stop hypertension"—and lowered their sodium intake. Their systolic BP (the top number, which measures pressure as your heart beats) dropped as much as 11.5 points within 30 days. The DASH diet is rich in fruits and vegetables, light in red meat and cholesterol, and low in both saturated and total fats. It also contains 31 grams of fiber daily, or almost twice the amount the average American man eats. (Check out the DASH diet online at www.nhlbi.nih.gov/health/public/heart/hbp/dash. They provide the meal plan; you just have to eat it.)

Why natural might work for you: If you're diagnosed with stage 1 high blood pressure (your BP is between 140/90 and 159/99) but are otherwise fit and healthy, lowering your blood pressure with drugs may not give you much added protection against cardiovascular disease.

"The slight protection you gain may not be worth the risks or side effects of taking blood pressure medicines," says Dr. Tsapatsaris. Hypertension (defined as BP higher than 140/90 mm Hg) significantly raises your risk of heart attack and stroke only when it's coupled with another risk factor, such as obesity, diabetes, high cholesterol, kidney disease, smoking, or a family history of heart disease. Eliminate the factors you can control, and you can probably lose the drugs, too.

But if you have any of these additional risk factors or moderate to severe high blood pressure (160/99 mm Hg or higher), taking antihypertension drugs can help you avoid a heart attack or stroke. And death is worse than any side effect.

. . . You're peeing a lot more, especially at night.

Your risk: *Benign prostatic hyperplasia, or BPH.* No, it's not prostate cancer, but that weak dribble is a lousy thing to wake up for.

The drug fix: If your prostate is enlarged, it will put pressure on your ure-

GO AHEAD, TAKE THE DRUGS TO . . .

Quit Smoking

Studies have proved that using a smoking cessation drug doubles your chances of quitting successfully, says Lowell Dale, M.D., of the nicotine research center at the Mayo Clinic in Rochester, Minnesota. In a University of Wisconsin study, 181 people who used a nicotine patch and bupropion (Zyban) were half as likely to resume smoking within a year as the 82 subjects using placebo patches and pills. Talk to your doctor about a prescription.

Ease Back Pain

This is one case in which taking drugs is the medicinal means to the natural end.

"The right kind of exercise can remedy most back problems," says Lewis G. Maharam, M.D., a sports medicine doctor in New York City and author of *A Healthy Back.* "But first we need to treat the pain." Ice may help initially, but anti-inflammatory medication will speed your healing—and the sooner, the better.

"Lying in bed for a week only makes your pain worse and your rehabilitation longer," says Dr. Maharam. Ibuprofen works well, but if your stomach's sensitive, ask the doctor for a COX-2 inhibitor such as Celebrex or Vioxx—and have him design a customized daily regimen of stretching and exercise to treat your condition.

Avoid Gum Disease

Really, really, hate to floss? Those deep pockets in your gums will come in handy. Your dentist can stuff them with a PerioChip (chlorhexidine, a topical antibacterial agent) and the oral gel Atridox (doxycycline, an antibiotic). Both can treat severe gum disease—or periodontitis—better than planing and scaling alone, says Raul G. Caffesse, D.D.S., of the University of Texas at Houston health science center. Periodontitis can not only make you toothless but even invite a heart attack, so spend the money if your dentist recommends the procedure.

thra. Your doctor will likely prescribe the prescription drug finasteride (Proscar) or the newer tamsulosin (Flomax). Studies show that Flomax effectively treats 50 percent of men, but it can cause dizziness and low blood pressure.

The natural fix: Take a daily 320-milligram pill of standardized saw palmetto extract that contains 85 percent fatty acids. (ProstActive fits that bill.) The herb saw palmetto seems to help block the conversion of testosterone to dihydrotestosterone, the form that causes prostate growth. (Dihydrotestosterone is also implicated in hair loss—another reason to consider taking the supplement.) Look in the supplement aisle at any well-stocked pharmacy, or go to www.naturesway.com.

Why natural might work for you: Saw palmetto works just about as well as the prescription drugs and offers minimal side effects. A study review by the Department of Veterans Affairs involving 2,939 men found that saw palmetto improved urinary flow nearly as well as the drug Proscar. And saw palmetto will cost you a lot less—a good thing since you should give the herb a 6-month trial. If it hasn't alleviated your symptoms by then, consider stronger BPH drugs.

. . . You occasionally have trouble breathing.

Your risk: *Asthma*

The drug fix: If it turns out you're one of the millions of men with adult-onset asthma, you probably suffer at least one severe attack per month, and mild attacks a few times a week. So you carry an inhaler filled with albuterol (Ventolin) or ipratropium (Atrovent). Two good shots will stop the attack within 5 minutes. But the drugs often cause dizziness, headaches, and tremors.

The natural fix: Many cases of asthma can be helped by strength training and breathing exercises, says Wayne M. Samuelson, M.D., of the University of Utah in Salt Lake City. In his preliminary study, he found that a "pulmonary rehabilitation" program of strength training and aerobic workouts sharply reduced the subjects' dependence on their inhalers. For more information, call (801) 585-1015 or see www.med.utah.edu/pulm/index.htm.

PERCENTAGE OF AMERICANS WHO USE PRESCRIPTION DRUGS: 66

PERCENTAGE OF AMERICANS WHO HAVE FAILED TO HAVE A PRESCRIPTION FILLED DUE TO COST: 26

Why natural might work for you: "Pulmonary rehabilitation can reduce the number of attacks you have and, consequently, your dependence on inhalers," says Dr. Samuelson. "You may need to use drugs only to stop acute attacks." Do yourself another favor: Stay thin. A study of 86,000 nurses found that those who were overweight were twice as likely to develop adult-onset asthma—and this finding is applicable to men, says Dr. Samuelson. Researchers think extra fat may stop the tiny airways in your lungs from expanding.

. . . You're sluggish after eating, you can't see straight, and you fear that soon you might become a blind, obese, impotent guy with an insulin habit.

Your risk: *Diabetes mellitus*

The drug fix: Develop type 2 (adult-onset) diabetes and you'll be on a first-name basis with your pharmacist in no time. Oral medications such as Dia-Beta, Micronase, and Prandin may help keep you from injecting insulin for a couple of years, but their effectiveness tends to wear off. Then it's on to insulin injections plus, possibly, more drugs—more often—to keep your fasting plasma glucose levels normal (between 70 and 110 mg/dl). This routine can cause side effects like weight gain, hypoglycemia, and needle tracks. Besides, it's one hell of an expensive hobby.

The natural fix: You know the drill: Exercise frequently and eat a high-fiber, low-fat diet. Work out aerobically 20 to 60 minutes at least three times weekly and you'll torch body fat. Lift weights to build muscle mass and boost your metabolic rate so you're a better blubber burner. An active guy needs up to 3,000 calories daily to sustain that level of activity—no more than 30 percent of those calories should come from fat (and only 10 percent of those from saturated fat), 60 percent from carbohydrates, and the rest from protein. Get fiber from whole fruits, vegetables, and grains. Lean dairy products, poultry, and meats will supply the protein and spare you the fat. Beans, beans, they're good for your . . . average diabetic since they deliver plenty of protein and fiber with zero fat.

Why natural might work for you: There's plenty of research that shows you can fight off diabetes with exercise, according to Sheri Colberg, Ph.D., assistant professor of exercise science at Old Dominion University in Norfolk, Virginia, and author of *The Diabetic Athlete*. Physical activity enhances insulin's effectiveness, which helps your body use glucose more efficiently. Fiber slows your body's absorption of sugar, which helps stabilize blood glucose levels.

That said, this condition is nothing to mess with. You'll need your doctor to watch your progress carefully in case your condition worsens. Potential blindness and loss of limbs are two of the best reasons we know to go ahead and take your drugs.

Scan Artists

Full-body scans could be one of the most important preventive medical breakthroughs ever. But not everyone thinks so

By Stephen Rae

If you'd had the misfortune to watch *The Oprah Winfrey Show* on October 10, 2000, you would have seen Oprah reveal an ugly part of herself that she had theretofore kept buried deep, deep inside: her pancreas. Unable to contain herself, she also laid bare her liver, lungs, heart, and kidneys. On that day, the full-body scan had arrived.

Two years later, in 2002, more than 100 full-body-scan centers were operating across the country, with that number estimated to reach 4,000 by 2007. Utilizing breakthroughs in computed tomography (CT) imaging that yield dazzlingly sharp 3-D pictures of the organs and the plumbing connecting them, the clinics sell early disease detection to the worried well-heeled. (Full-body scans, usually not covered by insurance, can run more than $1,000.) To the scan centers' boosters—their owners, but also impartial doctors such as Ronald R. Blanck, M.D., former surgeon general of the army—CT scanning is the future of medicine and a vehicle for consumer self-empowerment.

To the centers' critics—several professional medical associations and the Food and Drug Administration—they're a waste of time and money and a possible health hazard. Who's right? We did an organ-by-organ appraisal to figure it out.

THE HEART

What isn't up for debate is the speed and simplicity of full-body scanning. A technician attaches three electrodes, and then a motorized examination table slides you faceup and feetfirst through the CT scanner—a huge, doughnut-shaped portal containing a rotating x-ray tube. Twenty seconds and a few "hold your breath"s later, your entire torso has been mapped with 3-D digital images.

In the case of your heart, those images are of your arteries and any calcified plaque lining the walls. Scan center doctors analyze these midbeat snapshots and grade the degree of plaque with "coronary scoring"—a zero-to-over-400 scale, with higher scores indicating more buildup. In an oft-cited study of nearly 1,200 patients at St. Francis Hospital in Roslyn, New York, people with coronary scores above 160 were 35 times more likely to have a heart attack within the next 19 months than those who pulled in a zero.

Scan or scam? If you suspect the plaque may be piling up (due to lifestyle or a family history of heart disease), a scan could be the shock therapy you need. "Actually seeing the calcium can be very helpful in motivating people to make difficult lifestyle changes," says Rose Marie Robertson, M.D., a past president of the American Heart Association. Simply looking for a clean bill of arterial health? Don't rely on a scan. "A low score can create a false sense of security," says Dr. Robertson. That's because CT scanning doesn't measure other markers for heart disease, such as cardiac arrhythmias and "soft" plaque, which is just as lethal as the calcified kind.

THE LUNGS

CT scanning also checks your air bags. In a Cornell Medical Center study of 1,000 current and ex-smokers, chest x-rays detected only seven lung tumors, compared with the CT scan's 27, most of the latter in the treatable, stage I phase. "For a lung tumor to show up on an x-ray, it has to be about the size of a penny," says Stephen Koch, M.D., medical director of Imaging for Life, a whole-body imaging center in White Plains, New York. "With CT, we can pick up a 1-millimeter nodule—one-tenth the size." Others in the radiology community—those without a financial stake in scanning—agree that such early detection can save lives. "Common sense–wise, it's a no-brainer," says Elliot Fishman, M.D., head of radiology at Johns Hopkins Medical Institute.

Scan or scam? It's the best thing for smokers since the patch. But if you've never lit up, there's a danger: false positives. In this case, CT scans are actually *too* sensitive, detecting not just small tumors but also benign nodes, harmless cysts, and scars from childhood infections. In one Mayo Clinic study, 66 percent of CT lung scans found abnormalities, but only 1 percent turned out to be cancer. That's a lot of people getting false positives—or false maybes—and needlessly entering the health care system. "We're very good at picking which suspicious nodules to follow up on," says Dr. Fishman. "It's just that following up costs money." And peace of mind.

THE KIDNEYS

What could go wrong in a maintenance-free filtration system? Two things: cancer and kidney stones. CT scans are the standard for detecting kidney cancer, but not for spotting rock formations. "You can see a stone in the bladder with a CT scan, but if it's in the kidney itself, a sonogram is better," says Donald E. Wesson, M.D., chief of nephrology at Texas Tech University Health Sciences Center in Lubbock. And by the time a jagged little pebble hits your supersensitive bladder, you won't need a CT scan to tell you there's a problem.

Scan or scam? Your chances of developing kidney cancer are too slim (1.4 percent) to justify a scan—unless you were a smoker, in which case the risk shoots up by 40 percent (the carcinogens in cigarettes build up in the kidneys over time). And while stones are more common than cancer, their mineral makeup may make them invisible to a CT scan. "Some stones do not contain 'radiopaque' substances such as calcium and so cannot be seen by CT," says Dr. Wesson.

THE COLON

In the past, there were basically two ways for a doctor to conduct rectal reconnaissance: sigmoidoscopy and colonoscopy, both of which involve inserting a lighted scope into the colon. But today consumers have the à la carte option of adding a "virtual colonoscopy" to the basic full-body scan. In a head-to-head comparison published in the *New England Journal of Medicine* (*NEJM*), virtual colonoscopy was shown to be just as effective as traditional colonoscopy at finding tumors, and nearly as good at detecting large precancerous polyps.

Scan or scam? How about "better than nothing"? In the same *NEJM* study, virtual colonoscopy detected only 55 percent of the tiny precancerous polyps that were spotted by the traditional procedure. Plus, "virtual colonoscopy can miss a sessile, or flat, lesion," acknowledges Dr. Koch. "They're not that common, but they're out there." And while it's true that with a virtual colonoscopy there's no risk of a scope's accidentally perforating your colon— a one-in-1,600 chance with a colonoscopy—that advantage doesn't overcome the procedure's deficiency in polyp detection, especially considering that colon cancer is 90 percent curable if caught early.

EVERYTHING ELSE . . .

Scan centers also tout gee-whiz images of your liver, pancreas, stomach, and prostate as part of the virtual dissection. But unless you have hepatitis or have been a boozer (both cause cirrhosis), there's no need to see your liver in 3-D. And stomach and pancreatic cancer are very rare (a 1.29 percent and 1.25 percent lifetime chance respectively). In fact, the condition that men could use an instant test for—prostate cancer—is also the one that CT scanning is lousy at detecting.

Scan or scam? You feel fine but want to see your pancreas anyway. Consider this: One full-body scan bombards your body with up to 500 times more radiation than a conventional chest x-ray, says Thomas B. Shope, Ph.D., a radiation physicist with the FDA. "The risk of having a fatal cancer later in life from the radiation associated with a CT scan is probably between one in 2,000 and one in 10,000," says Shope. "A lot of people getting a lot of CT scans for no reason probably does add to the overall cancer burden."

Whether elective scanning ultimately saves more lives than it costs has yet to be determined in the United States. But in Australia the practice is being tightly regulated. The Environment Protection Authority in New South Wales now requires that consumers have an independent doctor's referral before getting a full-body scan and that they be told of the possible dangers of radiation exposure. "These machines have a place in the medical world," says Craig Knowles, the New South Wales health minister. But, he adds, "they are not moneymaking wonder toys. Consumers have a right to know they can be dangerous."

Time to Play Doctor

A step-by-step game plan for choosing the most qualified and convenient physician for you

By Jonathan Wander

Your new 11-amp reciprocating saw slipped. Oops. And now your severed middle finger is flipping you the bloody bird. It's times like these when being selective about your medical care isn't all that important.

But, power-tool mishaps aside, choosing a primary physician—a hall monitor for your general health, if you will—is one of the most important decisions you'll ever make. Unfortunately, you'll probably make it with the yellow pages.

Now, how smart is that?

But it makes sense because (a) few people know how to go about choosing a doctor, and (b) most of us figure that those stoic men and women in white coats are all cut from the same Hippocratic cloth.

Hardly. As in anything, some doctors are A players, and others are B's and C's. You deserve the A's. Here's how to find them—in a little game we call the Physician Playoffs.

ROUND I: REVIEW THE ROSTER

Call the number on the back of your health-insurance ID card and ask your HMO or PPO (or whatever acronym your plan uses) to fax or e-mail you a list of approved physicians in your county or region. (Of course, if you have an indemnity plan, every doctor is "approved.") When we're finished, you'll have crossed out every name on this list but one—that of your new doctor.

Let's start crossing. While almost anyone with "M.D." after his or her name is qualified to cure you, doctors of internal medicine (a.k.a. internists) have a slight edge. These are the do-it-all doctors that pick up where your pediatrician left off; they handle the whole adult package, from, well, your package to your postnasal drip. "They're known as 'medical detectives' for their diagnostic savvy," says Sara Walker, M.D., president of the American College of Physicians. Married with children? Find yourself an internist and pick a pediatrician for the kiddies. Or, if that sounds like too much trouble, go with a doctor of family medicine.

IS A D.O. OKAY?

The short answer: Yes. Doctors of Osteopathy are as qualified to treat your sick self as their M.D. brothers. In addition to their standard medical training, D.O.'s learn spinal manipulation (yep, like a chiropractor) as well as other nondrug treatments. They also tend to emphasize preventive medicine, but so should any good M.D.

ROUND 2: BREAK OUT A MAP

Going to the doctor is like going to the gym: Convenience will keep you coming back. So pick one who's close to home *and* work. "We all spend so much time at work that it makes sense to have a physician who's close by," says Michael O. Fleming, M.D., president-elect of the American Academy of Family Physicians.

Visit the American Association of Health Plans at www.aahp.org and click on "Health Plan Site Links." Find your health plan's Web site, click on its doctor finder (almost all have one), and type in your home address and the distance you want the search to encompass—midway between home and work is ideal. Compare the results with your master list and scratch out anyone who doesn't fall in the target area.

ROUND 3: CHECK THE RECORDS

You're like a cop running a suspect's plates, except you're going to access the AMA instead of the DMV. The American Medical Association's online doctor finder contains basic background information on virtually every licensed physician in the United States. Log on to www.ama-assn.org/aps/amahg.htm and print the profiles for the remaining names on your list.

You shouldn't care so much *where* they graduated from medical school as *when*. Why? "You wouldn't want to establish a relationship with someone who's ready to retire," says Timothy T. Flaherty, M.D., a spokesman for the AMA. So cross out anyone who graduated before 1975—and, so you don't end up as someone's learning curve, after 2000.

Next, cut the candidates who aren't board certified by the American Board of Internal Medicine. To be board certified, an internist has to pass an exam that reflects real-world diagnosis and treatment situations.

Are there qualified doctors who haven't taken the test? Absolutely. But good luck figuring out who they are. Board certification is one tangible measure. Another is the AMA Physician's Recognition Award Certificate. A doctor needs to complete 50 or more hours of continuing education annually to earn one. Weed out those doctors who haven't taken the time.

ROUND 4: READ THE RAP SHEETS

Even doctors with the best of credentials can be health hazards. Go to www.ama-assn.org/ama/pub/category/2645.html; this AMA site provides links to the medical boards of all 50 states, from which you can directly access disciplinary and malpractice information.

Cut the doctors who have been disciplined. Lawsuits are a different matter, since one does not a quack make. "There are some physicians who are sued repeatedly, however. And in that case, where there's smoke, there's probably fire," says Robert A. Clifford, a past chairman of the American Bar Association's Section on Litigation. Cross out all smoldering names.

ROUND 5: BE PATIENT

You should be down to two or three doctors now. Make an appointment with each and note the following: How long was the wait? Was there a current *Men's Health* in the waiting room? Was the staff more Nightingale or Nurse Ratched? "The better doctor values staff members who work hard to please patients," says Mary Jean Schumans, R.N., N.P., director of nursing practice and policy for the American Nurses Association.

Your actual appointment should feel like an interrogation. As a new patient, you want to be grilled about your health before the doctor attempts to diagnose so much as a cold. "Your medical history, family history, allergies, habits, exercise, diet, smoking history—these are all very important," says Dr. Flaherty. Ask a few questions of your own, too: Do you offer phone or e-mail consultations? (Correct answer: "Yes.") Do you have hospital admitting privileges, and if so, where? (Correct answer: "Yes, at a teaching hospital.") Why wasn't this magazine in the waiting room? (Correct answer: "It was stolen.")

Finally, there's one last question: "Can I see myself trusting this person with my life?"

IN THE EVENT OF A TIE

Decide by word-of-mouth reputation. "The most important thing is to talk to other men," says Dr. Fleming. Gather votes until one doctor pulls ahead, and then congratulate the winner.

KNOW THIS

Profit Sharing

Drug companies aren't the only ones getting rich off of out-of-control prescription drug prices. According to data from the University of Minnesota, half a dozen other entities also take a cut of every single dollar you spend on prescriptions at the pharmacy.

The pharmacy 24%
Advertisers 22%
Manufacturing 17%
Research labs 15%
Drug company profit 13%
The government 6%
The drug distributor 3%

Best Time to Check Out

A new Canadian study reports that patients who are discharged from the hospital on a Friday are significantly more likely to die or be readmitted within 30 days than patients dismissed on any other day of the week. Sundays are best. "We're not sure why, but patients dismissed on Fridays may just be more unstable," says Carl van Walraven, M.D., a coauthor of the study. "Since more patients are discharged on Fridays, hospital staff could also be making slipups that affect the quality of people's recovery." Here's how likely you are to have problems with your recovery, compared with if you are released from the hospital on a Sunday:

Monday 16%
Tuesday 13%
Wednesday 19%
Thursday 19%
Friday 28%
Saturday 12%

PERCENTAGE OF AMERICANS WHO THINK PRESCRIPTION DRUG PRICES ARE JUSTIFIED BY RESEARCH AND DEVELOPMENT COSTS: 47

Keep Your Resistance Up

Beware the doctor who dispenses antibiotics as if they were Pez—75 percent of prescriptions for upper respiratory infections are unnecessary, according to a recent study. Doctors often prescribe because of patients' insistence, time constraints, and misconceptions about when antibiotics are necessary, says Vincenza Snow, M.D., the study's author.

Save Face

If you have to choose between lasers and freezing to remove a cancerous lesion from your face, don't opt for the laser. According to a new American Academy of Dermatology report, lasers don't always remove all cancerous cells from your skin. "Laser resurfacing doesn't eliminate a patient's risk of cancer entirely," says Jeffrey S. Dover, M.D., the study's author. "For many people, treatment with liquid nitrogen may be a much cheaper and more effective option."

Joint Decision

If you suffer from chronic knee pain, arthroscopic surgery may not be the answer. In an unusual 2-year study conducted at Houston V.A. Hospital, researchers found that men who had knee surgery actually had more knee problems after surgery than men who had placebo surgery—a "fake" surgery in which the knee is cut open but not actually repaired. "The study shows that for many men, arthroscopic surgery is simply not necessary," says Nelda Wray, M.D., a coauthor of the study.

A better option? Light, low-impact activities, like walking or swimming. When Dutch researchers in the Netherlands studied 100 people with arthritis of the knee, they found that active people had greater mobility and muscle strength than those who avoided activity.

Cut Your Healing Time

If you break a bone, ask your doctor about getting an ultrasound scan—not to examine the break but to help the bone heal faster. Canadian researchers

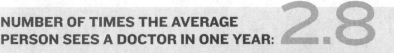

NUMBER OF TIMES THE AVERAGE PERSON SEES A DOCTOR IN ONE YEAR: 2.8

reviewed the records of 158 people with bone fractures and found that patients who had undergone ultrasound therapy healed up to six times faster than patients with similar breaks who didn't get the treatment.

Look the Other Way

Keep this in mind next time you're receiving a shot, having blood drawn, or even getting a tattoo: Looking away from the site really does make getting pricked with a needle seem less painful. In a British study, researchers found that levels of activity in the brain were much higher when people could see their arms being poked than when they couldn't. The more activity going on in your brain, the greater your body's pain-sensing capabilities become.

DOWN THE PIKE

Practice Makes Perfect

Young doctors will soon be able to practice abdominal surgery on lifelike artificial bodies rather than risk cutting into live patients. A British company is designing the first ultrarealistic latex teaching dummies specifically for medical students to learn to operate on. The dummies should help improve doctors' skills while lowering the cost of surgery and increasing surgical success rates.

Stuck on You

A form of laser-activated glue currently in development would allow doctors to attach a skin graft or suture a wound without the use of stitches, staples, or chemical-based adhesives. To bond tissue together using the new procedure, doctors coat the skin with a compound called rose bengal and then shoot it with green laser light. The resulting bond is twice as strong as that from other glues. The benefit for patients: less scarring and inflammation, and quicker healing times.

Eye-Opening Invention

Researchers at the University of New Mexico have designed a new product called a smart eye band that may be even better than glasses, contacts, or lasers for correcting common vision problems. The product consists of a band of artificial muscle that is surgically attached to the sclera—the white portion of the eye. Once activated, most commonly with an electromagnet worn behind your ear, the muscle contracts, adjusting the sclera. This changes the way light enters your eye so you can see more clearly. Although the device has yet to be approved by the FDA, researchers hope it will be available within a couple of years, at a cost of several hundred dollars per eye.

Better Hearing in a Pill

Go ahead and crank your stereo. A drug currently in development may be able to slow or prevent hearing loss caused by exposure to loud music or working in noisy locations. The medication works by bombarding cells in your ears with a compound that helps to prolong the cells' life span. That's important because you have only a limited supply of the tiny, hair-covered cells, which are responsible for converting sounds into signals your brain can process. When a cell dies, it isn't replaced, so every cell you lose is gone forever. Clinical trials for the drug could begin this year.

Take Two Chips and Call Me in the Morning

A new, implantable drug delivery chip will soon be able to release exact amounts of medication into your body, following a specific schedule set up by your doctor. The 3-centimeter-long, battery-powered chips are covered with hundreds of tiny pockets, each filled with a single dose of medication and sealed with a thin layer of gold. At a prescribed time, the chip's battery sends a burst of energy toward a seal, dissolving it and releasing the drug into the bloodstream. Once perfected, the chips may become the standard treatment for conditions such as Alzheimer's disease, diabetes, and Parkinson's disease.

Try This On for Size

Here's yet another way you may be taking your meds someday: by changing your underwear. European researchers are developing undergarments with medication woven into the fabrics. The drugs become active upon contact with the wearer's skin.

An Ulcer Test That's Easier to Stomach

Getting tested for an ulcer is no picnic: A doctor shoves a lighted probe into your stomach, hoping to spot the source of your pain. Fortunately, Scottish researchers have found a new breath test that detects up to 90 percent of ulcer-causing bacteria. It will need more testing before the office version reaches your doctor, though.

GAME PLAN

Manage Your Care

If you check in to a hospital, make sure you check out

Undergoing a "procedure," eh? Follow these tips and you'll reduce the amount of high-cost hell you'll face during your hospital stay. Even better, you'll cut your odds of being one of the 200,000 people each year who never make it back to the lobby.

Scrub before surgery. Two hours before your surgery, take a shower and use antibacterial soap to clean the area that's going to be cut, advises Leigh Neumayer, M.D., of the University of Utah in Salt Lake City. At least one out of every 20 hospital patients picks up an infection, so it's a smart precaution.

Cancel the wake-up call. Ask your nurse if she'll give you your medication at the start or end of her shift, advises Jeanne Burda, R.N., of Northwestern Memorial Hospital in Chicago. Otherwise, there's a good chance she'll rouse you at 3:30 A.M.

Check up on your surgeon. Ask the hospital pathologist if he would recommend your surgeon; this guy sees the results of surgeons' mistakes firsthand. The hospital's chief resident and operating room nurses are good sources of information, too.

Refuse the open-butt gown. Those gowns aren't mandatory, says Wayne Altman, M.D., of the Tufts–New England Medical Center. You just need light, loose-fitting clothes that won't hamper the orderlies if you start to croak. A pair of sweatpants and a loose T-shirt will work.

Mark the spot. Be certain that a nurse draws an X on the spot where the surgeon is supposed to cut you. We're not kidding. This is mandatory in many hospitals, says Dr. Neumayer. It's intended to prevent the lamebrain surgical mistakes that make headlines a dozen times each year.

Stay wired. Bring your laptop computer; many hospitals now offer in-room Internet access. After watching *General Hospital* for the third day, you'll be

NUMBER OF MEDICATION-PRESCRIBING MISTAKES THAT OCCUR EACH YEAR WITH THE POTENTIAL FOR ADVERSE OUTCOMES: 8.4 PER 100 HOSPITAL ADMISSIONS

giddy to do a little Web surfing. Have the nurses lock your laptop in a safe place at night.

Check your meds. Most errors result from mistaken identity, so be sure that your name is spelled correctly—including your middle initial—on your wrist ID, chart, drug labels, and test orders. Double-check that all medication is really meant for you.

Send the nurses pizza. Your water pitcher will never go unfilled. Go ahead and grab a slice or two for yourself. Unless you're a diabetic or a heart patient, or you're having surgery involving the stomach or intestines, you can probably eat whatever you like. (Ask first, though.)

TAKE ACTION

There are only two certain things in life, said Ben Franklin: death and taxes. But if Ben were alive today, he might add a third item to that list: rising health care costs.

In the past decade, the annual cost of health care has more than doubled, with the average family of four now spending roughly $16,500 a year. This includes out-of-pocket payments to doctors and hospitals, insurance premiums, medical equipment purchases, and federal and state tax money devoted to health care.

Sick of paying so much to be well? Here are some ways to cut your health care costs so that every backache, toothache, and cold won't be such a strain on your wallet.

Don't forgo health insurance. Even if you can barely afford it, take out a health insurance policy. While the cost of health insurance is undoubtedly high, the cost of being *uninsured* may be even greater. Just one hospital stay could clean out your bank account and leave you with a second mortgage.

One of the least expensive forms of health insurance is a high-deductible catastrophic policy, which usually covers major medical expenses and serious, long-term illnesses. These plans are best for relatively healthy people with low to average medical expenses. It's not cost-effective to have such a plan if you or a family member on the policy is chronically ill or if you can't meet your deductible in an emergency.

Open an account. Find out if your employer offers a medical spending account, and if so, open one. Such an account allows you to deduct money from your paycheck on a pretax basis to pay for most medical or dental expenses

PERCENTAGE OF WORKING FAMILIES
WHO DO NOT HAVE HEALTH INSURANCE: **11.6**

PERCENTAGE OF PEOPLE WHO SAY THE MOST IMPORTANT
HEALTH CARE ISSUE FOR THE PRESIDENT AND CONGRESS TO
DEAL WITH IS TO INCREASE THE NUMBER OF
AMERICANS COVERED BY HEALTH INSURANCE: **35**

PERCENTAGE WHO SAY IT'S TO HELP PEOPLE
AGE 65 AND OVER PAY FOR PRESCRIPTION DRUGS: **23**

that aren't reimbursed by your insurance company. Then every time you receive a bill that's not covered by insurance, you submit it to the account for reimbursement. Not only will this force you to save money to defray medical expenses; it will lower your taxable income and can therefore help you save on taxes. Just be careful how much you put into the account—you lose any money that's left over at the end of the year. So be conservative with your contributions the first year.

See your family doctor first. Before you go to a specialist, consult with your primary care physician. He knows you, can handle many problems himself, and is trained to look at your overall health, not just one part of your body. Specialists usually have higher fees and are not necessarily qualified to treat problems outside their specialty. There are some exceptions to this, however. If you suffer from a complex chronic disease such as rheumatoid arthritis, for example, you want your primary medical relationship to be with a rheumatologist.

Bargain with your doctor. A recent survey of more than 2,000 Americans found that 10 to 17 percent have tried to negotiate lower fees with their doctors, dentists, hospitals, or pharmacists—and half the time, they succeeded.

The time to bargain is at the beginning of the office visit or before you undergo a procedure. Tell your doctor in a sincere tone of voice that you feel he deserves the full fee, you want to give it to him, but you simply can't afford it. You could do it in a letter as well, if you prefer. Many doctors will work with you because they believe the cost of your going untreated is worse.

Some doctors will offer a discount if you pay with cash or check because it saves office staff the time and hassle of negotiating with insurance companies. Or your doctor may waive your co-payment or allow you to pay the bill in installments.

The first rule of haggling, however, is to be informed. Find out what Medicare or insurance plans are paying, and offer that amount. For a $42 annual subscription fee, www.myhealthcompass.com helps you determine hospital (and, in the near future, doctors') charges, as well as reimbursements by Medicare and health plans. The American Medical Association also publishes Medicare reimbursement rates on its website, www.ama-assn.org. Or simply use the 40 percent off rule. That's roughly the same discount managed care companies typically receive.

If you're too shy, you can even hire someone to do the haggling for you. Patient advocates, such as American Medical Consumers of La Crescenta, California, will act as a negotiator on your behalf for a fee of $50 to $90. To find an advocate, call them at (818) 957-3508. If you have a chronic debilitating condition or a life-threatening illness such as cancer, call the Patient Advocate Foundation at (800) 532-5274 for a personal advocate who will help negotiate fees with your doctors. Or check out the foundation's Web site, www.patientadvocate.org, which offers tips for negotiating medical fees and clearing up medical debt.

Before a test, know the score. Question the need for any test, be it an x-ray, MRI, or blood test. Find out why your doctor is recommending it and how the results will affect your course of treatment. Many medical tests are expensive and may not be essential to your care.

Ask about nonsurgical alternatives. Some experts estimate that 10 to 20 percent of all surgery is unnecessary. Make sure surgery is the best option, and seek a second opinion whenever possible. Also, learn about your condition on the Internet or in a library so you can make an informed decision.

Read the fine print. Your insurance policy may be as tedious as the tax code, but you need to know what it covers and what rules apply to your situation before you're admitted to the hospital for any kind of procedure. Some insurance policies require a second opinion before they'll pay for nonemergency surgery. Others require preauthorization from your insurance company before a scheduled hospital stay or a referral from your primary physician to see a specialist. If you're insured through a preferred provider organization, make sure all the doctors—including the anesthesiologists—are in the network.

Get an estimate. Ask the hospital in advance to estimate how much the procedure will cost. When you examine the bill, this will help you spot the most egregious errors.

Time it right. Hospitals are like hotels, charging for rooms by the day. Try to check in late in the day and leave early. Avoid checking in on weekends.

Recover at home. If you face a long recovery period, ask about home health services. It will be cheaper and, in many cases, better for you.

Leave it there. Don't assume that anything's free, and don't accept anything that you don't need. The best way to avoid being charged $15 for a pair of paper slippers is not to take them in the first place.

Save the ER for emergencies. The emergency room is an expensive place to be treated for a cut or sprained ankle. If you are having chest pains or are in a bad car wreck, you obviously need to go to an emergency room, but if your doctor's office is closed and your problem is relatively minor, go to a 24-hour urgent care center instead. Having a good self-care manual can be invaluable to help you know when you should seek immediate medical attention and when it can wait.

Pay less for prescription drugs. Prescription medications can be a significant part of your annual health care bill, especially when a family member has a chronic condition like high blood pressure or diabetes. Here are some ways to make your drug costs easier to swallow.

Choose your doctor wisely. You want a physician who uses medication sparingly, who discontinues them as soon as possible, and who uses the lowest possible dosage—not a doctor who spends 77.2 seconds with you and quickly scribbles a prescription as he heads out the door.

Sample the merchandise. Ask your doctor if he can give you any samples of the drug he has prescribed. Drug company salesmen often give doctors free samples just for this purpose.

Buy generic instead of name-brand drugs. On average, you'll pay about 30 percent less for generic drugs than you'd pay for their name-brand counterparts. Ask your doctor or your pharmacist whether there's a generic available.

If you're older than 60, ask for a senior discount. It's usually good for 20 or 30 percent off the list price.

Shop around. Even when buying generic prescription drugs, prices may vary from pharmacy to pharmacy. Call several pharmacies in your area to find the best price before filling the prescription. If you end up jumping from pharmacy to pharmacy, just remember to always tell the pharmacist about any drug allergies or other drugs you may be taking—doing so could avoid serious side effects from drug interactions.

Order by mail. You can save 20 to 30 percent on mail-order drugs. The savings can really add up if you have a chronic condition that requires regular medication.

Count 'em. With some drugs costing several dollars per pill, it's wise to count them and make sure they're all there before paying the bill.

Have a plan. Many insurers offer prescription coverage for a small additional premium that's well worth the price. Often you need pay only a few dollars for each prescription.

Spend less on OTC drugs. When buying over-the-counter drugs such as Tylenol, you can save as much as 40 percent by looking for the house brand of the same drug, acetaminophen. Many people are advised by their doctors to take a daily aspirin to prevent heart disease. In this case, buying in bulk

**THE PRINCIPLE AMERICANS FEEL
IS MOST IMPORTANT FOR INDIVIDUALS AND THEIR FAMILIES:**

ACCESS TO AFFORDABLE HEALTH CARE

**PERCENTAGE OF AMERICAN FAMILIES
WHO HAVE HAD AT LEAST ONE PROBLEM
WITH ACCESS TO HEALTH CARE IN THE PAST YEAR:** 44

**PERCENTAGE OF AMERICANS
WHO HAVE NOT SOUGHT MEDICAL ATTENTION
FOR A PARTICULAR PROBLEM BECAUSE OF THE COST:** 24

could save you several cents a pill. Just don't use this strategy for drugs you're not likely to use before the expiration date.

Save on dental care. Whether you need a new crown or Junior needs braces, keep in mind that you can save one-third to one-half by going to a dental school for your services. At more than 50 dental schools across the country, dental students who work under faculty supervision offer care at a fraction of customary dentist fees. To find a dental school near you, contact the American Dental Association Commission on Dental Accreditation, 211 East Chicago Avenue, Chicago, IL 60611.

Eye up savings on eyewear. If you wear glasses, shop around for affordable frames since their cost typically accounts for more than half the price of glasses. If you're a contact lens wearer, ask your eye doctor about rigid gas-permeable contact lenses. Over the long haul, this type of contact lens is the least expensive option. They can last several years. If they won't work for you, consider ordering your contacts in bulk from a mail-order firm like Lens Express. You'll pay 15 to 25 percent less.

ANY QUESTIONS?

Stick with the Old Standard

Are new prescription medicines necessarily better than old ones?

—D.W., Hadley, Massachusetts

No, they're not. In fact, Harvard researchers who tracked 548 new drugs for up to 25 years found that many showed major side effects *after* they went on the market. Older drugs have had more guinea pigs and thus have proven safety and effectiveness. So there's something to be said for the oldies but goodies.

Check Up on Your Doctor

How do I know if I'm getting a good physical exam?

—L.C., San Jose, California

Bad sign: You feel like a license applicant at the D.O.T. If your doc relies on questionnaires and assistants to gather info, you're likely not getting what you came for. The fix: Find a physician you trust, get to know him, and then stick with him for as long as you both shall live. That's right: Seek him out with the same attention you'd invest in finding a mate.

"Continuity of care is extremely important, and is underestimated by many patients," says James Martin, M.D., president-elect of the American Academy of Family Physicians. "When I really know you, the stresses you're under, your family history, previous hospitalizations, the medications you take, I can provide better care. But we need to talk to get that information."

After the chatter, a thorough physical should include abdominal, genital, skin, and reflex exams. The doctor should also check your circulation and listen to your lungs and heart. If you're over 40, rectal and prostate exams are—just relax, now—a must. Every 5 years, have blood work done, and make sure your doctor reviews the results.

PERCENTAGE OF DOCTORS WHO RECOMMEND OVER-THE-COUNTER DRUGS AS REMEDIES, PREVENTIVE MEASURES, OR SUPPLEMENTAL THERAPIES: 55

Now Hear This

Is there a quick test I can do to tell if my hearing is going?

—W.J., Oakdale, Tennessee

Place a hand directly behind one of your ears and rub your thumb and fore-finger together. Now test ear two. If you can hear the faint swishing sound, your ears are likely fine. Or hold a watch with a second hand about 6 to 10 inches away from each ear. You should be able to track the tick; if not, you could be losing high-frequency hearing. If you have trouble with either test, or if one ear is less receptive than the other, see an audiologist and get a baseline audiogram, says David Fabry, Ph.D., a past president of the American Academy of Audiology. It will likely cost $40 to $100, depending on how extensive the test is.

Wake Me When It's Over

I've been hearing a lot about so-called sedation dentistry. How safe is it?

—M.C., Stroudsburg, Pennsylvania

Sedation can be used for any dental work, but it's most commonly requested for Marathon Man–style procedures: wisdom tooth extraction and root canal therapy. The sedation part is nothing new, just increasingly popular. There are various levels of sedation, from Valium to nitrous oxide (a.k.a. laughing gas, with which you're giddy and awake), to general anesthesia (where you're out cold, dreaming of the hot hygienist). It can add hundreds of dollars to your bill, says Jeffrey Dorfman, D.D.S., an oral surgeon in New York City. There's also the slight chance you could develop nasty complications. You want a jaw-breaker who has adequate emergency equipment—a defibrillator, for example—and CPR-trained staff. Says Dr. Dorfman, "You don't want to have one doctor administering and monitoring the anesthesia while doing the procedure." No telling what he might yank out.

Protect Your Pearly Whites

My girlfriend complains that I grind my teeth in my sleep. Could I be doing irreversible damage?

—B.L., Bath, Maine

When you chew your food, you deliver a force of about 175 pounds per square inch (psi) to your teeth. But when you grind at night—the chop docs call it bruxism—there's no food to absorb the impact, so the force can amount to 300 psi. This means permanent damage, according to Maurice Ohayon, M.D., Ph.D., professor at the sleep epidemiology research center at Stanford University. "About 25 percent of teeth grinders end up needing dental work as a result of their nightly habit, which can cause inflammation of their gums and premature loss of their teeth," says Dr. Ohayon.

Your fangs might require crowning or reshaping, thanks to the erosion that grinding causes. Plus, you're more likely to experience morning headaches, jaw pain, and saliva-soaked pillows, which can be mighty annoying. Dr. Ohayon advises avoiding caffeine and alcohol after 7 P.M. and having your dentist check your bite. He may even recommend an acrylic night guard if your case is severe enough. You should also shed stress in your life. Start with a new girlfriend. The complainer sounds like somebody who just might cause teeth grinding.

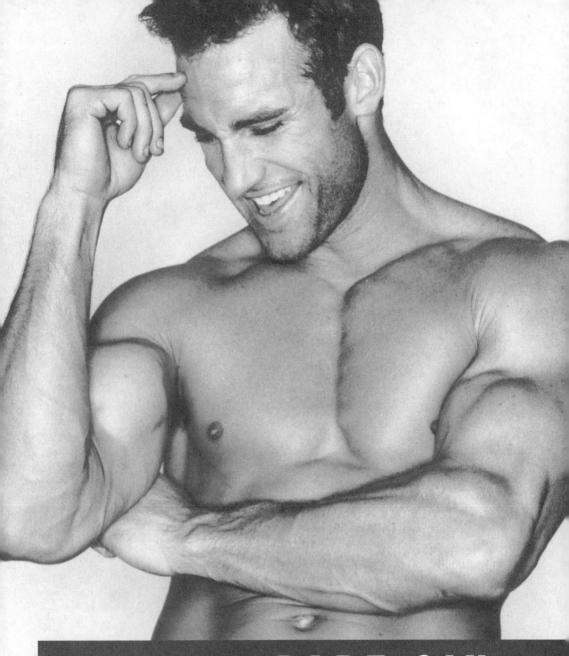

PART SIX
MEND YOUR
MIND

GAME SHOW

Who Will Get Alzheimer's?
One of these bright young guys—or you?

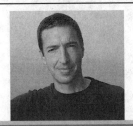

RON REAGAN
Age 43, 6'1", 170 lb
Television correspondent; taught himself to play guitar last year

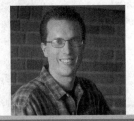

SCOTT MILLER
Age 34, 6'0", 185 lb
Former football player; now tackles tough legal issues

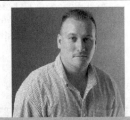

DAVID GLEASON
Age: 31, 6'1", 225 lb
Customer service rep; die-cast-car buff; eats ravioli for breakfast

WHY HE MIGHT
Reagan's father—former president Ronald Reagan—has Alzheimer's disease. The younger Reagan believes both of his grandmothers had Alzheimer's as well. Having one or more close family members with AD increases a person's risk twofold to threefold. One in 10 people over 65 and nearly half of those over 85 have the disease.

WHY HE MIGHT NOT
Reagan's life is not stress-filled. People with high stress are often forgetful and at risk of illnesses. He also reads a lot, mostly nonfiction books on natural history. Mental exercise like this may defend against memory loss and dementia, precursors to AD. He eats fresh fruit rich in antioxidants, which neutralize damaging particles in the brain (called free radicals) that could lead to Alzheimer's disease.

RON'S PREDICTION
"I hope that I have a few decades before I need to worry. I'm counting on some of the research that scientists are doing now to save me in the future."

WHY HE MIGHT
Miller has had three head injuries: a knock-out bicycle spill in second grade and two shots while playing football. Head injuries may increase the chance of Alzheimer's. He has no known family history of AD, but his father was adopted. Miller is somewhat forgetful—his wife makes sure he has a to-do list when he leaves the house. He's horrible at recalling names and is under considerable stress.

WHY HE MIGHT NOT
He has business and law degrees and works as an assistant attorney general. The more formal schooling a man has, the less likely he is to develop Alzheimer's. Miller exercises often, eats a balanced diet, and maintains a healthy weight. Keeping the body fit helps keep the brain in good shape.

SCOTT'S PREDICTION
"I may not know my entire family history, but at least my mother's side is okay. Further, my profession requires that I never stop learning."

WHY HE MIGHT
Gleason's blood pressure is 180/90, and his cholesterol is 225. His triglycerides are 462; under 200 is normal. A recent study in the *British Medical Journal* said systolic (the first number) blood pressure of 160 or greater during middle age doubles the risk of Alzheimer's later in life. Combined with high cholesterol, it makes the odds three and a half times as great. Gleason eats a high-fat diet, doesn't eat many fresh fruits or vegetables, and rarely exercises—all brain-punishing habits.

WHY HE MIGHT NOT
Gleason doesn't know of anyone in his family who has had Alzheimer's. While he doesn't have a college degree, he did take some college classes. He works on cars and computers as hobbies. He's never had a head injury.

DAVID'S PREDICTION
"So I'm not in peak condition. But I'm happy and stress-free. I think stress is what does it, and Miller has more of it than anybody."

And the Winner Is . . .
Ron Reagan

Gary Small, M.D., director of UCLA's center on aging and an expert in the early detection and prevention of Alzheimer's disease, helped us evaluate our contestants. Use the scorecard on the opposite page to gauge your own risk.

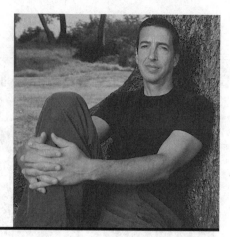

FINAL ANALYSIS

Dr. Small had a difficult time choosing a winner because all of the contestants' risk factors pose significant concern. Finally, he decided Gleason was out of the running. "The way he's going," Dr. Small says, "he may die of something else before he reaches an age when Alzheimer's may hit."

If other health risks don't nab Gleason, his high blood pressure and high cholesterol might. High BP can lead to decreased bloodflow to the brain and the death of brain tissue (stroke), and high cholesterol causes plaque formation in blood vessels and chokes off supplies of oxygen and nutrients.

Miller's head injuries do put him at increased risk. So does his forgetfulness, which generally precedes Alzheimer's disease, according to Dr. Small. Yet his high level of education might preserve his brain well into old age. Researchers are not yet sure why education may be protective. People who go to college may naturally have good brain genes. Or it could be because people who exercise their brains keep them healthy.

It's not a surprise that Reagan's family history of the disease is trouble—and that's ultimately what tipped the contest his way. His blood pressure and cholesterol are normal, and his diet is pretty healthy. However, he uses whole milk with his cereal every morning and has a weakness for cheese—both are high-fat habits. People who eat low-fat diets seem to have an edge against Alzheimer's, according to doctors. Reagan maintains a healthy weight by frequently hiking and swimming and by lifting weights. That's good because excessive body fat increases risk of illness.

Reagan should start taking vitamins daily as a simple preventive step, says Dr. Small. Doing so at a young age might prevent, or delay onset of, the disease. "It's never too early or too late to start protecting your brain," Dr. Small says. He recommends that all men exercise, eat a healthful diet, stay mentally active, reduce stress, and take vitamins C (1,000 milligrams) and E (400 milligrams) daily.

Mind Game

RISK FACTOR	POINT VALUE	RON	SCOTT	DAVID	YOU
AGE Incidence of Alzheimer's appears to double every 5 years after age 65.	Over 65? For every 5 years over: -2				
FAMILY HISTORY Having family members with AD increases risk.	One or more family members with Alzheimer's? -3	-3			
EDUCATION Higher education may be a protective factor.	Bachelor's degree or higher? $+1$		$+1$		
STIMULATION Staying mentally active appears protective.	Mentally stimulating career or hobbies? $+1$	$+1$	$+1$	$+1$	
HEAD INJURY Head trauma may increase risk, especially if you're knocked out cold.	Any minor head injuries, or blows causing unconsciousness? -1	-1	-1		
CARDIOVASCULAR SYSTEM Raised systolic blood pressure and high cholesterol during midlife may increase risk in later life.	Systolic blood pressure 160 or higher? -1 Cholesterol 250 or higher? -1			-1	
LIFESTYLE Keeping your body healthy also keeps your brain healthy.	High-fat diet? -1 No exercise? -1 Overweight? -1	-1		-1 -1 -1	
ANTIOXIDANTS Fresh fruits and vitamins C and E fight free radical damage to the brain.	Eat plenty of fresh fruit? $+1$ Take vitamin C and E supplements daily? $+1$	$+1$	$+1$		
OTHER Forgetfulness often precedes AD. People with high stress are often forgetful and prone to illnesses that can worsen memory.	Forgetful? -1 Under stress? -1	-1	-1 -1		
TOTALS		-4	0	-3	

▶ IF YOUR SCORE IS -2 OR LESS: Write yourself a note to see your doctor—you have a high risk of Alzheimer's disease.

▶ IF YOUR SCORE IS -1 TO $+2$: Your risk is moderate.

▶ IF YOUR SCORE IS $+3$ OR MORE: You'll be the sharpest old geezer on the block—*and don't you forget it!*

MUST READS

Mind over Matter

Use your head to heal your body with these six proven strategies

By Brian Reid

The man who walked into Dr. Herbert Benson's Boston office was a mess. He was a stress case at work, he suffered awful headaches, and his stratospheric blood pressure did not respond to high doses of prescription medicines. But rather than throw more drugs at him, Dr. Benson, an M.D. who works at a Harvard-affiliated health center called the Mind/Body Medical Institute, prescribed a 10- to 20-minute daily dose of what he calls the "relaxation response": a calming exercise of muscle relaxation and controlled breathing. "He found that, slowly and inexorably, the headaches became less profound," Dr. Benson says. "Eventually, they totally disappeared. His hypertension, which required relatively high doses of two medications, dropped so significantly that he needed only a fraction of the dose of one medication. This man gained a new perspective."

Stories of patients using meditation and positive energy to will themselves to health have been floating around since the days of leeches and bloodletting. For the most part, physicians have treated the mind-over-disease idea as an offshoot of voodoo medicine. Until recently, that is. Within the past 20 years, doctors and scientists have begun studying the mind–body connection in earnest, and now they're pinning down the science behind the brain's ability to influence healing. While you can't tell your immune system cells where to go, it's becoming increasingly clear that you *can* nudge them along.

"These aren't trivial effects," says Michael Irwin, M.D., director of the Cousins Center of Psychoneuroimmunology (that's 39 Scrabble points, not counting double word bonuses) at UCLA. He's testing what happens when people are taught to lighten up. "The effects we see with these behavioral interventions are bigger than those found with a placebo."

Here's proof: six scientific strategies you can use to think your way to better health.

I. CHANGE YOUR MIND

Stress is the number-one mental culprit in the delay of wound healing. Ohio State researchers studied 11 dental students, taking a chunk of flesh from the roofs of their mouths during summer vacation. Then, 3 days before the first exam of the next school term, they took a chunk from the opposite side of each student's mouth. On average, the wounds took 40 percent longer to heal during stressful exam time than during the carefree days of summer.

"You can become a victim of the environment or the mind," says William Malarkey, M.D., director of Ohio State's clinical research center and a member of the Center for Stress and Wound Healing, "or you can proactively change the environment of your mind."

What you can do: Take a deep breath. Hold it. Exhale slowly. Research has shown that relaxation techniques—such as controlled breathing with a focus on long, drawn-out exhalation—lower the effects of both stress and blood pressure. If you don't have the patience for relaxation methods or yoga training, try a Walkman-like device called Resperate, which guides you toward therapeutic breathing. It's available at www.drugstore.com for $300. (The yoga class sounds better and better, doesn't it?)

2. VISIT PLUTO

The best way to let your mind boss your body around is to enter a trance state, says Jim Nicolai, M.D., a fellow in integrative medicine at the University of Arizona in Tucson. Hypnosis is one technique you can use to hit that trance state, but you don't need a swaying gold watch to do the trick to yourself.

"Having a daydream is a good example," says Dr. Nicolai. "You can sense that there are things going on outside of you, but you just don't care. You're focused." When Harvard researchers used an MRI to examine what happens to the brain during meditation, they found that the practice activated parts of the brain involved in attention. And your cosmic voyage can do more than just help your body repair itself. Dr. Nicolai says trancelike states are ideal for working on your free throws.

Once your head is in the clouds, it's easier to tell your body what to do. Using techniques such as Dr. Benson's relaxation response cuts down on the level of stress hormones. Dr. Benson acknowledges that they play a role in revving men up to run or fight, but the hormones can be damaging when they leach into the rest of life. "What good is getting excited if you're not going to run or fight?" he asks.

What you can do: If you're up for seeing a hypnotist, look for a health care professional—such as a psychologist—who is licensed to perform hypnotherapy. (The American Society of Clinical Hypnosis directory is at

NUMBER OF YEARS OLDER A SMOKER'S BRAIN SEEMS, BASED ON COGNITIVE FUNCTION: 5

www.asch.net/certreferrals.asp.) A "certified" hypnotist doesn't necessarily have the medical background. If that's too Amazing Kreskin for you, just let your mind wander. Daydreaming isn't hard. Though Dr. Nicolai says that about 20 percent of us have trouble getting into a trance, he says it's a skill you can work on—starting with those breathing exercises.

3. RECRUIT A PLATOON

Friendships go a long way in helping a person on the mend. Decades of research suggest that support is a great way to improve coping skills in terminally ill patients, but new studies have shown that a good marriage actually juices the immune system even in those who aren't fighting for their lives.

"If we're isolated from those around us, we ourselves are at risk," says Dr. Irwin. "We need to have good social bonds."

Of course, the knife cuts both ways. Just as a strong bond with the buds or a happy marriage helps you bounce back more quickly, squabbling with your honey does a lot more than trigger depression and the urge to pour doubles of Johnnie Walker. For starters, it disrupts your immune system and your cardiovascular system, complicating more than just the healing of a broken heart.

What you can do: When it comes to social support, both quality and quantity count. A Carnegie Mellon University study found that people with the most types of social bonds are the least susceptible to the common cold. (The researchers didn't mess around, either. After evaluating the social ties of 276 healthy people, the scientists shoved cold-virus samples up the patients' noses.) As for quality, it pays to fight fair with your wife—couples who show "hostile behavior" in their relationships, whether they're newlyweds or they've been married for decades, have weaker immune systems than those in loving relationships who are good communicators. A healthy sex life gooses the mind's protective power over the body, too. Psychologists at Wilkes University in Pennsylvania recently discovered that sex improves your immune system by up to 30 percent by boosting levels of immunoglobulin A, your body's first defense against cold and flu germs. Get your flu shots, men!

4. MEET THE BEAST

Ignoring big problems will screw up your immune system as quickly as ignoring a big MasterCard bill will screw up your credit. If there are problems in other parts of your life, pushing them to the back burner isn't likely to lower your stress level, and it's almost certain to depress the immune cells that keep you operating at peak power.

A 2001 study by Ohio State researchers found that during periods of high stress, concentrations of immune cells were significantly higher in people who tackled their problems or emotions directly than in those who avoided them.

Especially at high stress levels, so-called active coping sparked the immune system to keep up its guard.

What you can do: When it comes to anxiety in your life, avoid whining, avoid hitting the bottle, and avoid avoidance. The active-coping mantra, which has been linked to lower rates of depression, requires changing or removing the source of stress and emphasizes long-term planning and patience. It worked for Lance Armstrong, whose desire to face his cancer head-on impressed doctors more than his will to live. "It was a bring-it-on attitude," says his doctor, Lawrence Einhorn, M.D., of the Indiana University School of Medicine in Indianapolis.

5. BEAT THE BLUES

Those with a tendency toward depression or anxiety also tend to have immune systems that aren't operating at their peak. Scientific models mimicking depression in mice have found that depressed mice are more susceptible to a form of the herpesvirus. And the data is clear that in humans, depression and the nation's number-one killer—heart disease—go hand in hand.

"We know that if you're depressed, you're at risk for cardiovascular disease," says Dr. Irwin. "You have a fivefold higher risk of having a heart attack."

Depression treatments are well-understood: See a therapist and talk to your doctor about antidepressant medications. The payoff can go well beyond emotional well-being. Return your mind to top form, and your body will follow.

What you can do: Sweat the blues away. James Blumenthal, Ph.D., professor of medical psychology at Duke University, assigned 156 people with major depression to one of three groups. Some took antidepressants, some were charged with exercising moderately for 45 minutes three times a week, and some did both. The results: Pills worked no better than pushups, and, 10 months later, those who exercised were least likely to have had their depression return.

Another study suggests that participating in sports like rock climbing or kayaking—anything that gets your adrenaline pumping—can have a significant impact on the body's ability to deal with stress. Texas A&M University researchers found that fit men experienced less psychological stress when doing challenging activities than did out-of-shape guys. And the better shape they were in, the better the men's bodies could react to mental stress.

Rock on: To find the best places to climb in your area, visit the Web site www.rockclimbing.com. For kayaking, check out www.americanwhitewater.org. If you're looking to combine a bunch of adrenaline boosters in one contest, go to the BALANCE BAR Adventure Race Series Events, at www.balancebaradventure.com.

For an even more powerful mood lifter and immune booster, exercise your social skills along with your body. If you're new to an area and want to make friends, try beach volleyball. "It's by far the most popular sport we offer,"

THE BEST MEDICINE

Laughter does your body good, inside and out. "Laughter affects many regions of the forebrain, and those regions regulate the hypothalamus, which sends out messages that allow your body to react in the appropriate way," says David Felten, M.D., Ph.D., executive director of the Susan Samueli Center for Complementary and Alternative Medicine at the University of California, Irvine, School of Medicine. And he's not just talking about peeing yourself. Here's what really happens when you start cracking up.

Heart. Laughter might protect you from a heart attack by preventing inflammation of the endothelium, the protective barrier lining the blood vessels in your heart. "Laughter improves blood pressure and heart rate, and may increase nitric oxide production," says Michael Miller, M.D., director of the center for preventive cardiology at the University of Maryland Medical Center in Baltimore. Nitric oxide is a naturally occurring gas that in the body acts as a vasodilator, relaxing the heart muscle and lowering blood pressure.

Respiratory system. Laughing brings more oxygen to your lungs, which can help ease chronic respiratory conditions. And Japanese researchers found that watching a funny video (they tested with Charlie Chaplin, but Johnny Knoxville should work, too) helped 26 people combat allergies for up to 2 hours.

Immune system. Laughter helps increase production of natural killer cells and T cells, which are the major antiviral and antitumor defenses of the immune system, Dr. Felten says.

Abdomen, diaphragm, shoulders, and face. When you laugh, your abdomen and diaphragm contract, your facial muscles stretch, and your back and shoulders unkink. It's kind of a half-day spa visit for your upper body.

says Jason Erkes, president of the Chicago Sport and Social Club. And, better yet, according to Erkes, the skill level is low, "so you don't have to worry about making a fool of yourself." Plus, you'll find lots of girls. In bikinis. If you live near a major city, go to www.sportandsocialclubs.com to find a program or league near you. Or check out your neighborhood YMCA, parks and recreation department, college extension program, or health club. Or just tear up your front lawn, fill it with sand, set up a volleyball net, and see who shows up. And hope they show up in bikinis.

6. PAGE DR. CARLIN

Voltaire, 2 centuries ago, said that medicine "consists of amusing the patient while nature cures the disease." Now science has proved it. In a 2001 study, a group from Loma Linda University School of Medicine took 52 men and showed them a goofy videotape for an hour, taking blood samples 10 minutes before, 30 minutes into, and 12 hours after the video.

The number of natural killer cells (they kill germs, not people) in the subjects' blood increased during the video, and remained high 12 hours later.

Though the men in the study were healthy, the researchers say that the immune boost seen in the patients helps explain the results of past studies, such as the group's 1997 finding that heart attack patients who watched 30 minutes of funny shows daily had lower blood pressures, needed fewer drugs, and suffered fewer additional heart attacks than their peers hooked on the History Channel.

What you can do: In the 1997 study, the Loma Linda heart patients saw results when they picked sitcoms. (Yes, all those *Seinfeld* reruns are doing you some good.) In the more recent study, the 52 healthy guys who had their blood drawn watched the tired watermelon-smashing shtick of the trapped-in-the-'70s comedian Gallagher. (Their fault—they chose the video.) But there was no difference in results. Research shows that humor—whether it's the laugh-out-loud kind or just a chuckle—reduces levels of stress hormones regardless of whether it's tasteful and sophisticated or slapstick and stupid. So, come next cold and flu season, leave the echinacea with Dr. Phil and make an appointment with doctors Moe, Larry, and Curly.

Shrink Rap

The guy who put De Niro in therapy tells how to get comfortable on the couch

By Harold Ramis

Sometimes I wish I could live in a constant state of denial. Guys do it all the time. Denial's so much easier. It's one of the biggest clichés in the realm of therapy, which is a kingdom of clichés. And those very clichés make it so easy for otherwise intelligent men to dismiss a process that could really help them.

Alas, denial has failed me. I've been in therapy for years, I'm 57 years old, and even now there are childhood issues I've just started dealing with—stuff about my parents that I had never thought of. Issues can sound pathetic when you talk about them outside the doctor's office, and that is part of the problem for some. But for me—revelatory. I embrace the clichés. That's the only way to break through, get something done. Maybe you've been thinking about therapy. Maybe your curiosity (or misery) is pushing you toward the clichés. Don't be afraid. You know 'em, but if you learn to love 'em, you might feel a whole lot better.

CLICHÉ #1: HAIRY MACHISMO

Someone once said that if you ask a man how he feels, he looks inside and sees a deep void. Someone else once said that men are numb from the neck to the crotch. Catchy phrases, but not really true. Men have feelings. We just ignore them.

Therapy? Hmm, this implies actually confronting something resembling a feeling. That's masculine heresy. That runs against the grain of what men are taught, beginning with that inevitable moment in every boy's life when an adult male—usually armed with a bat, some balls, and the best intentions—tells him, "Stop whining! Stop crying! Be a man!"

Well, while you're so busy being a man, you could be denying disorders like depression, bipolarity, and generalized anxiety, which are as medically real as cancer (and the basis of some great comedy material, of course).

From where I'm sitting, the "suck it up, be a man" argument doesn't have a lot of mileage left. Want proof? During *Analyze This*, we were shooting the scene in which Robert De Niro has his first full-blown panic attack. All of the other gangster extras were standing around while I was directing Bob on the textbook symptoms. As Bob was registering the information, one of the other gangsters piped up, "Ya know, when I have my panic attacks, I get very short of breath and I feel like I'm havin' a heart attack." Then another guy said, "For me, everything goes kinda white. I get dizzy, and I feel like I'm gonna die." All these tough guys were medicated! They were the last guys you would have expected to have panic disorder, let alone talk about it. They were also the last guys to whom you'd say, "Suck it up, be a man."

Face it. There are men out there tougher than you who are threatening to break the kneecaps of their problems. Is it a coincidence that they are also big and strong enough to break a real set of kneecaps? I don't think so.

CLICHÉ #2: THE THERAPY CULTURE

This is the flip side of male denial: dysfunctional overkill. These days, the couch is out of the closet—along with the skeletons canoodling on it. *Everyone* has depression. Everyone has a dysfunctional family. Everyone has antidepressants in his pocket. And everyone talks about it—or so it seems. People you just met will tell you that their family tree is in desperate need of pruning. In certain social circles, dysfunction is currency. Who had the worst childhood? Who's more screwed up? You could debate an 80-year-old man about his 10-mile, uphill walk to school and not have this much one-upmanship.

I don't want to be a part of that culture any more than you do. Don't think that by seeing a shrink you're joining some country club of despair. Competing with people who need to let you know how much they've suffered is not a requirement. The decision to seek therapy should be no more complex than simply saying, "I could use a little help here."

CLICHÉ #3: WOODY ALLEN SYNDROME

This is the idea that you can be in therapy your whole life without getting better. This cliché comes true only if you let it. I won't lie to you; long-term talk therapy is not a quick cure for an illness. ("Talk therapy" is the most simplistic way for me to differentiate one-on-one therapy from other kinds of drug, cognitive, or group therapies.) It's a philosophy, a point of view, a reality check, a confessional, and a way to process your story. You go in there and tell that story over and over until you begin to see things that provide insight. Repetition keys the breakthrough.

I've been in talk therapy for years, and I've gone in every combination. I've been married twice, so I went with both wives, with my parents, with my parents and my wives, with my children, with my children and my wives. But for the first time in my life, about 2 years ago, I decided to just go by myself, for the emotional and intellectual pleasure of talking about myself to someone who had to listen. It was a huge breakthrough. I actually got to issues that I should've tackled 30 years ago.

That's how the process works. I once gave a speech at the Chicago Institute for Psychoanalysis, and one of the shrinks asked me if my movie

AM I GOING NUTS?

Every day, pharmaceutical companies pummel you with drug ads suggesting that you just might be nutty (in a way treatable by their drugs). Even reasonably sane men have no choice but to wonder if their recent crappy moods are, in fact, rabid suicidal depression. Or something worse. Relax. Chances are you're right as Renfield (pre-*Dracula*). Still have doubts? For answers to those voices in your head, we consulted J. Alexander Bodkin, M.D., chief of the clinical pharmacological research program at McLean Hospital in Boston.

Am I depressed? You're in the clear if (1) you eat and (2) you sleep like a normal human being. (3) You still like to do all those things you've always liked to do. (4) You're not that cranky. And (5) you obsess about death less than Woody Allen. There are actually nine classic symptoms, and "clinical depression requires at least five of these symptoms to be present for more than 2 weeks," says Dr. Bodkin. For a detailed list, check out www.nimh.nih.gov.

Do I have a social phobia? Hey, a lot of people have pre-party jitters. After all, parties usually entail chatting up beautiful women who can smell fear. It's cool if you want a glass of wine to take the edge off so you can mingle. However, says Dr. Bodkin, if the anxiety is severe enough to keep you from enjoying yourself—or from showing up at all—you might have a clinical problem.

Do I have generalized anxiety disorder? Any guy who claims he doesn't worry is either lying or on the cover of *Mad* magazine. You worry. A lot. So what? Be worried (and seek treatment) if you worry so much that it takes over your life and is "clearly excessive for at least 6 months," says Dr. Bodkin.

Do I have obsessive-compulsive disorder? Maybe you're a man of habit. Maybe you get ticked off when something interferes with that habit. You're still okay, says Dr. Bodkin, if you don't have irresistible thoughts and behaviors. That is, the kind that take control of the cockpit and make you do things you don't want to do. If that's you, stop washing your hands and dial a shrink.

Groundhog Day was intended as a metaphor for psychoanalysis, because it seemed to be perfect for him in that sense. In the movie, Bill Murray repeats the same day over and over again, each time in a different psychological mode, and finally comes to a big insight and realization through the repetition.

That's psychoanalysis. You may want to buy the DVD, in fact.

CLICHÉ #4: THE THERAPIST

You know him. The overanalyzing, goateed, Freudian caricature who speaks in heavily accented tongues about cigars, trains, and tunnels. The great male fear? Your shrink tells you that your recurring nightmare about harvesting foot-long bananas with a penknife means exactly what you think it means.

Great results obviously depend on having the right therapist. A lot of people are turned off by therapy because they see the wrong person. You shouldn't be afraid to shop around—though that's a difficult concept for some. Finding the right shrink can be as much work as the therapy itself.

It takes time and money to find out you're going to the wrong person. Back in the 1980s, I saw a female therapist (cue the adult-film music) who wore see-through tops and chain-smoked through our sessions. It was kind of like having therapy with a barmaid. All I could think about was having sex with her. As you can guess, the experience was a failure on many levels.

The key to a short search is asking the right questions. By the time I moved to suburban Chicago 6 years ago, I knew enough about what I needed in a therapist to find the right guy on the first try. How? Because of my work, I'm surrounded by unusual people in extraordinary circumstances. So I needed a sophisticated shrink, someone a little worldly who could understand my life and where I was coming from.

Sure, you may not work in show business, but think about your job, your experiences, your family, your friends. Then seek out a shrink who is literate in your kind of life—or at least relates to you enough that you'd consider him for a jury of your peers.

CLICHÉ #5: "THE DOC WILL THINK I'M A FREAK"

Well . . . are you? The cops might think so, but your therapist won't. To whom would you rather explain yourself? A therapist must be totally nonjudgmental. Most of us feel guilty about everything. We don't want to tell anyone our negative thoughts because they're shameful, or wrong, or cruel. We really need a person who isn't passing judgment. That goes double for the dark secrets, the vices, the perversions.

I could confess my worst sin to a priest, and I'll burn in hell if I'm not absolved. I tell the same thing to a therapist, and he's completely neutral about it. There's no moral judgment attached. That's a big deal when you've got tough things to talk about.

Ultimately, a good therapist will help you realize that there's nothing shameful about it, and that you can be free of it. In the shrink's office, he's my advocate, and mine alone. He's not there to protect my wife or my kids. It's the one place where I can honestly and openly express myself without fear of hurting someone.

The Final Analysis. My shrink is like a voice in my head now—a good voice, mind you. Another cliché? Sure. But when I start feeling a certain way, I can call up that voice and remember, "Oh, yeah, that's why I feel this way. I was a lonely, miserable 12-year-old!" But I'm not anymore. None of us are. We're big boys now, and despite what you hear, big boys aren't afraid to face their problems—or ask for help to get them fixed. Rodney Dangerfield once said a great thing: "The only normal people are the ones you don't know very well."

That includes yourself.

Fear Not

Conquer stress by putting this primitive emotion in its place

By Robert Maurer, Ph.D.

Imagine a heavy barbell you've managed to bench-press off your chest. Your arms are extended, but the weight remains at arm's length, exerting pressure. Now that you've been holding it up for a while, it's starting to quiver, you're beginning to sweat, and there's no one around to spot you. It's that hopeless feeling you may think of as stress: that you're running out of strength and energy, and eventually the weight is going to crush you.

Been there?

There now?

As a clinical psychologist at the UCLA School of Medicine for the past 2 decades, I've treated hundreds of men who felt the weight of jobs, families, and financial responsibilities bearing down on them. And I've helped most of them relieve the pressure by convincing them of one thing: Stress doesn't exist.

PERCENTAGE OF DAYS OUT OF THE YEAR IN WHICH PEOPLE TYPICALLY EXPERIENCE AT LEAST ONE STRESSFUL EVENT: 40

PERCENTAGE OF DAYS THEY EXPERIENCE MORE THAN ONE STRESSFUL EVENT: 10

That's right. You read that correctly. Stress will one day take its place in medical history as a disease we couldn't cure because it didn't exist. The idea of stress was first floated by Dr. Hans Selye in 1936. (Rather strange that no one noticed this "disease" before then.) Since its "discovery," we have cured polio and made progress with almost every cancer, yet by all accounts stress remains in epidemic proportions. Those who suffer from it usually report one or more of the following symptoms: rapid heart rate, neck tension, lower-back pain, dry mouth, headache, loss of interest in sex, overeating, stomach distress, frequent urination, diarrhea, crying, insomnia, fatigue, sweating, and rapid breathing.

But these are not symptoms of that phantom disease stress. Rather, they are symptoms of an emotion that's far more primitive. An emotion that originates in a pea-size part of the brain called the amygdala. An emotion that causes our hearts to beat faster, our muscles to tense, our mouths to dry, and our digestive systems to shut down (is this sounding familiar?) as we prepare to either fight or flee. It is the age-old emotion of fear.

When highly successful men describe the challenges of life, they seldom use the word "stress." Instead they speak like this.

"When you are running an institution, you are always scared at first. You are afraid you'll break it. People don't think about leaders this way, but it's true. Everyone who is running something goes home at night and wrestles with the same fear. Am I going to be the one who blows this place up?"

—*Jack Welch, former CEO, General Electric*

" . . . Being scared to death was a condition of life in submarine warfare in the South Pacific. Being afraid is okay, if you are afraid with dignity. To a greater or lesser extent, fear is a part of the challenge."

—*Pat Riley, NBA coach*

"Going on stage is part catharsis for me, but it is always trying to work out my own fears."

—*Robin Williams, comedian/actor*

REACT LIKE A 3-YEAR-OLD

Why do these successful guys use the word "fear" rather than "stress" when describing the same emotional responses we all share? Being scared is the language of children, but they're not afraid to use it. This isn't immaturity or weakness; it's honesty.

Children never say they're "anxious about the bogeyman" or "stressed about thunder." Rather, they recognize they can't control the world, and they acknowledge the resulting anxiety for what it is: fear. To learn how to handle

SCARE TACTICS

Use these six steps to snuff the stuff that spooks you.

I. See fear for what it is. The next time you feel anxious, recognize that fear, not stress, is causing your anxiety. Identifying what's triggering your fear will help you handle it better.

2. Control your accelerator. As you approach a beautiful woman or prepare to speak at an important meeting, consciously slow your breathing. Respiration is the body's accelerator. Control your breathing and you control your fear.

3. Try a mental dry run. Imagine yourself in the stressful situation, then mentally create the tone of voice, attitude, and actions you want to display. Practicing the perfect response helps establish pathways in the brain that become self-fulfilling.

4. Practice out loud. Act out what you've been visualizing. Play the role of the confident, relaxed man. It'll help you learn new strategies for dealing with fear.

5. Bring the fear out in the daylight, where you can examine it. No matter how much training you do, if you wait for fear to present itself, it will always have the advantage of surprise. So it's better to confront it on your terms. Sign up for Toastmasters, then volunteer for that speech. Prod that quivering mass out of the shadows, to where you can deal with it.

6. Recruit help. A while back, some researchers surprised a bunch of wild gorillas with a fake leopard. The first thing these apes did was huddle together. Only from the security of their pack would they decide how to react. Take a lesson from them, you big monkey. It's doubly tough to face fear alone. Find someone (a wife, a buddy, a therapist) you can discuss your fear with, and ask for advice. A true friend will support your efforts to beat the fear that's bothering you, and tell you when you're being a misguided wimp. If there's no one like this in your life, no wonder you're so stressed.

fear better, they engage it by watching scary movies or dressing as monsters on Halloween. Rather than push the emotion out of their minds as adults often do, they learn to understand and, ultimately, handle it without being enslaved by the thing that scares them.

Successful men realize that the bigger the challenge, the more fear shows up. Like children, they accept fear as the price of being alive. Other men see fear as a disease or a sign of failure that's to be avoided at all costs. They don't think about it, talk about it, or even admit to having it. As a result, they end up depressed, angry, or fatigued or become abusers of food, alcohol, or other people. Or they may avoid pursuing their dreams just to avoid the essential emotion—fear—that they've labeled an enemy and are misinterpreting as stress.

In order to escape the symptoms of fear, you must admit to being scared. The more you desire in life, the more fear arises as the body's way of preparing itself for action. It's not a sign of weakness, but a signal of success and a call for courage. Assume that whenever you're upset or unhappy, there is fear underneath. There are only two basic fears: One is that you're not worthwhile or good enough to get the job, the woman, whatever; and the other is that you're going to lose control, such as in health or financial concerns. I'd wager that these fears underlie what many people think of as stress.

TURN OFF THE ALARM

But there's another facet to this. The fight-or-flight alarm system we all carry was designed to sound, create a response, and then shut down. When a deer is scared, it runs. When a lion is frightened, it attacks. But when a man is afraid, he obsesses about it and complains that he's stressed. He leaves his alarm system on, clanging. And the consequences can be deadly.

The healthy human response is, again, to do what children do. Reach to others for support. Men who do so live longer, have lower cholesterol, are more likely to endure crises without becoming ill, are more effective leaders, and have a greater chance of finding (and keeping) romance. Successful men have friends they can lean on in time of need.

Do you see the logic? The symptoms you're feeling are normal, healthful signals from a body faced with a life challenge (positive or negative). Our masculine culture values stoicism and independence, but what your body really craves is to draw strength from others.

So the next time you're feeling stressed, do two things: Identify your fear, and find people who can help you deal with it. You need emotional spotters, my friend.

Doing these two simple things will allow you to safely lower that quivering barbell and then push it back up many more times. You'll gain strength against the only enemy worth fighting: your fear.

Lighten Up

Raise your disposition from crappy to happy with these simple steps

By Laurence Roy Stains

You're eating the world's best pizza. With Heidi Klum. She's across the table, and she's looking particularly lovely in a little red tank top. She wants to play with your pepperoni tonight. Then, in the morning, you'll play Powerball and win $100 million.

You're totally happy, right?

Right—for a couple of months. After that, you'll go back to being your same old self. Studies show that people who are showered with fortune soon revert to the baseline of their genetic temperament, which may range from partly sunny to mostly cloudy with a 50 percent chance of rain on their own parade. Lottery winners, for example, aren't wildly happier than the rest of us—they're only a tiny bit happier.

Knowing that, however, won't stop the rest of us from the all-American pursuit of happiness. "Everybody wants to be a little happier than he is," says Ed Diener, Ph.D., a psychologist at the University of Illinois at Urbana-Champaign. And that would be okay if we knew what the hell we were doing. But we don't. "People are not very good at predicting the kinds of things that will make them happy," Diener says.

Which is why he and a few hundred other psychologists have started a little movement, with its own annual convention, called Positive Psychology. This sounds like a joke—most of psychology is hyperfocused on what makes people crazy and miserable. But Diener and his maverick band are trying to understand what they call subjective well-being. They have taken that big, squishy feeling called happiness and are dissecting it.

Diener himself has been studying happiness for the past 20 years. So he knows his stuff. He knows what doesn't make people happy. For instance, money won't do it—not unless you're living in a cardboard box. Good looks? Maybe a little. Bodily pleasures? Hmmm . . . you're getting warmer.

Diener's no hair shirt; "I don't think pleasure is a bad thing," he says. But it's overrated. Even if you do discover the world's best pizza, your senses are quickly sated, and the duration of the bliss is cut short by what psychologists call habituation. How about sex with a supermodel? Thrilling at first, but before long you find yourself on the "hedonic treadmill," and your mood adapts to the good life. To repeat this thrill, you'll have to start sleeping with Naomi Watts on the side.

So where, then, does happiness lie? Try friends. Family. Work. Goals. Values. Some happiness researchers believe that a winning combination of thought, action, and attitude will put us on an "upward spiral" toward bliss. All we have to do is train our brains to be happier. Does that really work? Diener himself is reserving judgment—he wants to see more studies done. But he's confident that "happiness is not solely genetic," he says. Accordingly, there are some steps people can take to ensure that they're as happy as they can be.

Diener's advice: Don't wait until you win the lottery. Right this instant, decide to bring a little more sunshine into your days and ways. Here are five steps on the stairway to seventh heaven.

CHANGE YOUR ACTIONS

Ken Sheldon, Ph.D., a psychologist at the University of Missouri in Columbia, has conducted four surveys of more than 1,000 college students; he measured their happiness over the course of a semester. The surveys provide dramatic evidence that a change of circumstances—such as moving to California, buying a new toy, or switching roommates—yields a happiness that is only fleeting. "Changing circumstances will give you a short-lived boost," he says, "but then you're right back where you started." On the other hand, he found that the students who took on new activities—they switched majors, joined a new club, or began a new exercise program—gained lasting joy.

DO THAT THING YOU DO

What do you do well? Whatever it is—snowboarding, building a deck, or accounting—you've probably felt the sensation of total involvement and pure mastery, when your training and skill are perfectly matched to the challenge, and time stops. Oddly, nobody ever came up with a good word for this peak experience until 1990, when a Czech-born psychologist, Mihaly Csikszent-mihalyi, wrote a bestseller titled *Flow*. These are some of the best moments in life; they happen "when a person's body or mind is stretched to its limits in a voluntary effort to accomplish something difficult and worthwhile." At the time, you may not say to yourself, Ha-cha-cha, I'm so happy. You're too full of

HAPPY HUNTING GROUND

Read our prescriptions for happiness in the accompanying story—then put them to the test. Here's a quick four-question quiz meant to measure your general level of happiness. It was devised by Sonja Lyubomirsky, Ph.D., psychology professor at the University of California at River-side. Take it again in a month or two to see if this "positive psychology" stuff actually works.

If it makes you happy just to take quizzes like this, there are 10 more good ones at the Web site www.authentichappiness.org. Enjoy.

1. In general, I consider myself . . .
   Not very happy >   1   2   3   4   5   6   7   < Very happy

2. Compared with most of my peers, I consider myself . . .
   Less happy >   1   2   3   4   5   6   7   < More happy

3. Some people are generally very happy. They enjoy life regardless of what is going on and get the most out of everything. To what extent does this characterization describe you?
   Not at all >   1   2   3   4   5   6   7   < A great deal

4. Some people are generally not very happy. Although they're not depressed, they never seem as happy as they might be. To what extent does this describe you?
   A great deal >   1   2   3   4   5   6   7   < Not at all

Total your answers and divide by 4. Two-thirds of adult Americans score between 3.8 and 5.8—above neutral, but by no means giddy.

seriousness and purpose. But afterward, when you look back, you say, That was excellent. That's the happiness that follows flow.

SET A GOAL—AND GET GOING

There's a lot to be said for knocking something big off your to-do list. Yet most of us are too easily frustrated by our lack of progress in the short term, so we miss out on achievements that require long-term commitment, according to David Myers, Ph.D., a psychologist at Hope College in Holland, Michigan, and author of *The Pursuit of Happiness*. "Although we often overestimate how much we will accomplish in any given day, we generally underestimate how much we can accomplish in a year," he says.

BE GRATEFUL

Psychologists Michael McCullough, Ph.D., and Robert Emmons, Ph.D., have done the pioneering work on gratitude. In a nutshell, they've found that being grateful makes people happier. They asked volunteers to keep daily diaries for 2 weeks; one group recorded daily hassles, another group jotted down events, and a third, the "gratitude group," listed up to five things they were thankful for each day. By the end, people in the gratitude group were so much happier, their spouses noticed a change. McCullough says that people who frequently experience gratitude also are more optimistic and helpful and have more determination and energy. "Every good trait you'd want for yourself or for other people seems to go along with being grateful," says McCullough, of the University of Miami.

MAKE TIME FOR FRIENDS

Not the television show—your real friends. Recently, Diener and Martin Seligman, Ph.D. (author of *Authentic Happiness*), of the University of Pennsylvania in Philadelphia, conducted a study of 222 Illinois college students. Then they zeroed in on the 22 happiest. "Every one of the happiest people had good social relationships," says Diener. They had at least two of these three associations: a romantic partner, a group of friends, and strong family ties. You now have Official Permission to tell your romantic partner that you're going out with the guys tonight.

Turn Your Luck Around

Make misfortune another opportunity to kick butt

By Laurence Roy Stains

It's been a rough year. Your stocks are way down. Your new boss is wack. Your biggest client disappeared in a corporate merger. Your new girlfriend went off to her high-school reunion, met an old boyfriend, and never came back. And, just this morning, you knocked the mirror off your car while backing out of the garage.

Blaming yourself for any of this would be very Presbyterian of you. "We all have a tendency to turn against ourselves when things happen that are painful," says David D. Burns, M.D., a Stanford psychiatrist and author of the classic bestseller *Feeling Good.* Dr. Burns says there's something narcissistic in that reaction. "We have this grandiose notion that things should go our way all the time. And when they don't, we either think we're losers or insist that life sucks."

Indeed it's common to feel responsible for events over which you have no control. It's so common, psychologists have a name for it: personalization. (It's one of the 10 major cognitive distortions—the standard list of stupid stuff we tell ourselves when we're being our own worst critics.) Personalization has a nasty edge to it. You don't just shrug and say, "I made a mistake." You look in the mirror and say, "I'm a loser."

That's why we happen to think that bad luck is a good idea. You see the benefit? You can stop beating up on yourself and blame bad luck instead . . . when appropriate, of course—felony convictions don't count. But bad stuff does happen to good people. There is such a thing as a bad break, in which case you need to give *yourself* a break.

You may think it sounds modern and smart to dismiss luck, but it's actually a little arrogant. And it can make you sick. Thinking you must always be in control can lead to high blood pressure and an early coronary. "That's the classic type-A personality," says James Blumenthal, Ph.D., a Duke psychologist who uses stress-reduction programs to treat cardiac patients. "Type A's are convinced that if they could just get everything under control, everything would be okay."

You can drive yourself crazy trying to micromanage the universe, or you can heed these pieces of advice:

Forget what you can't control. Let it go. Keep moving. When misfortune strikes, think, *Is there anything I could have done differently?* If so, learn from it without engaging in toxic self-blame. "Rather than use all of your energy feeling guilty, pinpoint the causes of your problems and solve them," advises Dr. Burns. "The Buddhists say our worst enemies are often our greatest allies in disguise. Have the philosophy that misfortune can be an opportunity for growth, even though it feels awful at the time."

Focus on what you can control. "Don't dwell on the terrible event," says Lawrence Perlmuter, Ph.D., a professor of psychology at Chicago Medical School. "What's done is done. Ask yourself, 'What choices do I have now?'" He recalls the advice at the end of Voltaire's *Candide*: Cultivate your own garden. If you're an ex-employee of a high-tech firm and your 401(k) is a tenth of what it was, you might say, "My garden used to be so much bigger." Well, guess what? "It ain't big anymore," Perlmuter says. "So let's figure out what you can grow in the garden that's left."

Be humble about luck. Credit it for at least some of your success. Do so and you'll walk in the footsteps of famous men from Julius Caesar to Warren Buffet. For softening the envy of others, it works like . . . well, a charm. As the architect Robert Venturi once said, "I find myself instantly liking people who credit their success to a lucky break."

Believe in luck and pluck. Without pluck, good luck is nearly worthless. After all, you have to know what to do with luck. And in some ways you make your own luck by creating opportunities for success. As the golfer Gary Player once said, "The harder I work, the luckier I get."

Be an optimist about bad luck. Think of optimism as a mental tool. With it, you build a wall between yourself and misfortune. Without it, you become fatalistic. You lose energy. You do less and less; you put off more and more. You sink into do-nothingism. "You become a passive sad sack," says the psychologist Martin E. P. Seligman, Ph.D. Seligman talks about the power of optimism in his new book, *Authentic Happiness*. Optimists are happier, that's for sure. But they also live longer and have better health habits, lower blood pressure, and stronger immune systems. At work, they're more productive and better paid. And they tend to see misfortune as temporary. Pessimists think of misfortune as permanent and pervasive: *I lost my job; I'll never get another one at my age.*

The key to being optimistic about misfortune is to remind yourself that it's temporary. Blaming bad luck is one way to achieve that. Here's why: Luck is fickle. That's the common theme about luck, across cultures and time. Two thousand years before you watched *Wheel of Fortune* on TV, the Romans thought of luck as a great wheel spun by the goddess Fortuna. According to the wisdom of the ancients, it's foolish to grow accustomed to good luck— and equally pathetic to think that fate is going to pick on you forever. (Unless you're a blues singer, or, worse, a bleacher bum at Wrigley or Fenway.)

If you say, "I'm just unlucky," you'll never change your luck. All you'll do is create a permanent rain cloud over your head. But if you say, "I was unlucky," that's good. You've got to believe what the Gypsies say: "Behind bad luck comes good luck."

"Then you're going to be resilient," says Seligman. "The more temporary the explanation, the more quickly you bounce back."

KNOW THIS

Cholesterol on the Brain

High cholesterol is bad for more than just your heart. A University of California at San Francisco study of 1,000 people found that having high cholesterol increases your risk of cognitive impairment—a precursor to Alzheimer's disease. Researchers found that patients with the highest blood cholesterol levels were nearly twice as likely to score poorly on concentration, memory, or language tests as men and women with lower cholesterol levels. Even more interesting: Patients who took a class of drugs called statins to control their high cholesterol tended to have the fewest overall problems remembering things and thinking clearly. "This suggests that taking statins may help reduce your risk of cognitive decline," says Kristine Yaffe, M.D., the study author.

Skip the Shellfish

Ingesting too much copper may contribute to Alzheimer's disease, causing cells in the brain to "rust," according to a new Italian study. Oysters, lobster, and liver are among the biggest sources of copper in most men's diets.

Forget These Herbs

Forgetting to take your ginkgo may not be such a bad thing after all. According to a report in the *Journal of the American Medical Association*, ginkgo has absolutely no beneficial effect on learning, memory, attention span, or ability to concentrate. In a study of 200 people over the age of 60 conducted at Southwestern Vermont Medical Center, researchers found that men who

NUMBER OF AMERICANS WHO HAVE ALZHEIMER'S DISEASE: 4.5 MILLION

NUMBER WHO ARE ESTIMATED TO HAVE THE DISEASE BY 2050: 16 MILLION

were given 40 milligrams of ginkgo three times a day for 6 weeks showed no improvement in memory compared with a similar group of men taking a placebo.

In related news, the latest research from Duke University suggests that St. John's wort is useless in the treatment of depression. After 8 weeks on the supplement, patients had no fewer symptoms of depression than if they'd been taking sugar pills.

Suicidal Tendencies

A study from the American Foundation for Suicide Prevention says suicide rates are down 14 percent—the lowest they've been in 15 years—primarily as a result of increased antidepressant drug use by people most at risk of committing suicide.

Remember to Study for This Test

According to a study at the University of Toronto, a common verbal memory test may be one of the best tools yet for predicting a person's Alzheimer's disease risk. Researchers studied the scores of a group of people who'd taken a test called the California Verbal Learning Test and found that people without Alzheimer's tended to score well on the test, while those with early stages of the disease showed lower scores. Visit a neuropsychologist if you're interested in taking the test. In the meantime, keep your memory sharp by reading, writing, or playing chess—and by taking a daily baby aspirin. A new multicenter study suggests long-term daily aspirin use can reduce your Alzheimer's risk by up to 45 percent.

Sleep Soundly

A new test may help your doctor determine whether or not you suffer from a hard-to-diagnose sleep disorder like sleep apnea, insomnia, or restless legs syndrome. In a study of 200 adults, researchers in Detroit found that the 11-question Global Sleep Assessment Questionnaire was more than 80 percent accurate in detecting most common sleep problems.

DOWN THE PIKE

A Shot of Da Gila

A little Gila monster spit may soon knock the cobwebs from your brain. Researchers found that the creature's deadly saliva contains a peptide that improves the brain's ability to learn and store information. Gilatide, a drug containing the substance, is currently in development.

Saved by a Scorpion

Doctors at hospitals in California and Alabama believe a new drug modeled after scorpion venom may be useful in the treatment of a deadly form of brain cancer called glioma. In animal trials, the drug successfully stopped the growth of hard-to-treat tumors caused by the disease.

GAME PLAN

Face-to-Face with 40

Handle midlife without a crisis

You thought adolescence was tough? Wait till it comes roaring back 25 years later—at least the sex, cars, and confusion parts. This time you have family and responsibilities, plus a little money. And you still don't have a clue. Here's how to keep cravings from becoming crises.

Get speed. Forget your old Mustang; it's gone. Test-drive the sneaky-fast Subaru Impreza WRX turbo sedan that's making car buffs giddy. It's safer, more reliable, and more comfortable than any of the old Detroit muscle. But even better, it's g-force quick and lots more fun to drive, says Larry Webster, of *Car and Driver* magazine. At $25,000, the Impreza is a match for much pricier Euro rockets. Your kids will fit in back. And yes, it comes in red.

Rock on, daddy-o. Yearning for lost cool? Sign up for guitar lessons. Playing rhythmic phrases on any instrument for 10 minutes can produce an endorphin high, says Steven Halpern, Ph.D., of San Anselmo, California, who wrote the book *Sound of Music* and studies the psychology of music. Plus, it keeps both hemispheres of your brain young and quick.

Get into leather. Your Ramones phase was cute, in '78. If you're going to relive the leather jacket, leave out the snaps and flaps. Or invest in "something classic with a bit of flair, maybe a three-button, charcoal striped suit," says *Men's Health* fashion director Brian Boyé.

Find a challenge. Midlifers often seek risks to prove they're still capable of doing things young men do. Try mountain biking for thrills and aerobic benefits. The ideal bike for new riders weighs less than 30 pounds and has a front and rear suspension with 3 to 4 inches of "travel."

Resist temptation. A coworker is the person with whom a middle-aged man is most likely to cheat. Put pictures of the family on your desk, in your wallet, on your dashboard. In a tight spot, do anything that'll force you to part company—like calling home.

Rekindle. An overture from another woman provides an ego boost and an addictive adrenaline rush. Avoid a lifetime of child support by boosting your wife's sex drive, too. Do the unexpected: Spoon her in the morning, not just after sex. Random acts of kindness on your part equal random acts of kinkiness on her part.

TAKE ACTION

When it comes to the part of your body that sits on top of your neck, we bet we know what's on your mind: Way too much. Allow us to take a few things *off* your mind with these strategies—eight easy ways research scientists have found to help you sleep better, feel more energized, reduce stress, and learn new things—not to mention keep you sharp into your seventies and beyond. We even threw in a recommendation to spend more time playing sports. We figured you wouldn't mind.

1. Don't work too hard. According to a new Japanese study, spending more than 5 hours a day in front of a computer screen may make you weary. Researchers analyzed data collected from 25,000 office workers over a 3-year period and found that individuals who crossed that 5-hour threshold daily were more likely to suffer from insomnia or fatigue or to feel lethargic, anxious, or "reluctant to go to work" than people who had less screen time.

2. Come out of your shell. Your personality could be weighing you down. According to a new study, shy, introverted people are more likely to feel drained on the job than people with more outgoing, extroverted personalities. Researchers at Tilburg University in the Netherlands made the discovery after questioning 700 people over a 2-year period. After analyzing the data, the researchers found that people who liked to be alone or who avoided public interaction often reported feeling more tired, stressed-out, and overwhelmed by their work than did their more sociable counterparts.

3. Chill out with Fido. Speaking of stress, when it comes to relieving it, nothing beats Bowser—not your buddies, not booze, not even your wife. In fact, spending time with your pet may be the *best* way to fight stress. Researchers at the State University of New York put people in stressful situations and measured changes in their blood pressures and heart rates. Sometimes the volunteers were alone, and sometimes they were in the presence of a friend or loved one or their favorite pet. "In almost all instances, the pet owners experienced the least stress and recovered from their stress the fastest," says Karen Allen, Ph.D., a research scientist at the State University of New York at Buffalo and the author of the study.

4. Stock up on Shakespeare. It turns out that poetry may be a powerful stress reliever as well. In a small Swiss study, researchers found that men who recited poetry for half an hour a day were able to lower their heart rates significantly, reducing their stress levels and possibly their risk of heart disease. Try reciting poetry to your pooch and your stress level should plummet.

5. Further your education. Studying for your master's? Call it a night and hit the sack. No matter what it is you're attempting to learn, you're better off practicing for a while and then going to bed, rather than staying up late to cram. A new Harvard University study found that getting a good night's sleep can improve your ability to master a skill by up to 20 percent. Cut your sleep short and you'll have a harder time improving your skills, cautions Matthew P. Walker, Ph.D., the study author.

6. Take a whiff. Speaking of sleep, here's how to get some easy Zzzzs. Researchers at Wheeling Jesuit University in West Virginia tested the effect of the scents of jasmine and lavender, compared with no scent at all, on the sleep patterns of 20 study subjects. Their finding: Those exposed to the jasmine fell asleep faster, tossed and turned less, and felt more refreshed in the morning than either of the other groups. Researchers aren't sure, but they suspect the scent has a calming effect on the central nervous system. Get your hit by placing a scented candle on your nightstand and burning it for about a minute before bedtime. (Don't worry; jasmine is more musky than girly-sweet.)

7. Keep your wits about you. Four and a half million Americans currently have Alzheimer's disease, but experts at the Rush Institute for Healthy Aging in Chicago estimate that by 2050, that number could jump to nearly 16 million. Bad genes can put you at greater risk of Alzheimer's, but making a few simple lifestyle changes can help reduce your risk.

Lifestyle Change	Risk Reduction
Eating more vitamin E–rich foods	67%
Eating a low-fat diet high in fruits and vegetables	55%
Getting a tetanus or diphtheria shot	60%
Taking ibuprofen or naproxen daily	14%
Lowering your systolic blood pressure	56%
Spending time outdoors or playing sports (just as we promised)	38%
Reading or doing crossword puzzles	47%

Make small talk. Another way to reduce your risk of Alzheimer's? Talk it up. A University of Michigan study reports that men who chat with friends and family often have better memories and are less likely to develop Alzheimer's than men who socialize less frequently. Why not make your next trip to the water cooler worth your while?

8. Don't grow old. Bob Dylan—who wrote the song "Forever Young"—must be a supplement popper. Studies from the University of California, the Henry

PERCENTAGE OF ADULTS WHO EXPERIENCE SYMPTOMS OF INSOMNIA AT LEAST A FEW TIMES A WEEK: 58

Ford Health System, and the Linus Pauling Institute found that elderly rats fed a supplement combo of acetyl-l-carnitine and alpha-lipoic acid stopped acting their age. They performed better on memory tests, had less age-related brain deterioration, held on to their hearing longer, and got around their cages quicker than untreated rodents. The theory? The supplements tune up the mitochondria, the cellular machines in all living things that convert food into energy. As we age, these little engines become less efficient at burning fuel (thereby slowing us down) and begin spewing out more free radicals (rusting us from the inside out). "Human clinical trials are still needed, but I'm optimistic that we're going to add years to people's lives," says Bruce Ames, Ph.D., a professor of the Graduate School of Biochemistry and Molecular Biology at the University of California in Berkeley, and one of the study authors. Want to start adding years now? Take 200 milligrams (mg) of alpha-lipoic acid and 500 mg of acetyl-l-carnitine twice a day, says Ames. Pick up a month's supply at GNC, Vitamin Shoppe, or www.juvenon.com for about $35.

ANY QUESTIONS?

20 Winks

Can I train my body to sleep only 4 to 6 hours a night?

—A.K., Skokie, Illinois

Scientists don't know why our bodies need between 7 and 8½ hours of sleep a night, but they do know that our mental performance and reaction times peak with at least that amount of rest, says Nancy Fishback, M.D., a spokeswoman for the American Academy of Sleep Medicine. If you try to get by on 4 to 6 hours regularly, you're going to weaken your immune system, and that's been linked to an increased risk of developing high blood pressure and heart disease. "People with high adrenaline may be able to function on little sleep, but that doesn't mean there's no long-term damage to their health," says Dr. Fishback.

While you can't train yourself long-term without any risks, you may have to pull an occasional late- or all-nighter. When you do, try to schedule an extra hour or two of sleep the following night. For the follow-up night, it's best to wake up naturally. You probably won't need the same number of hours that you lost, and your body will naturally judge how much makeup sleep it needs.

Pedal Power

I often hit the wall after lunchtime. How can I avoid that groggy feeling?

—B.T., Tucson

Cycle. Researchers at the University of Pennsylvania and the University of Georgia found that sleep-deprived men who cycled for 25 minutes at a mod-

PERCENTAGE OF ADULTS WHO GOT
8 OR MORE HOURS OF SLEEP A NIGHT IN 2001: 38

PERCENTAGE WHO GOT
AT LEAST THAT MUCH SLEEP IN 2002: 30

erate intensity perked right up. The effect isn't necessarily specific to cycling. "Doing virtually anything active, provided it's at a high enough intensity, will reduce your feelings of sleepiness," says James B. Crabbe, Ph.D., an exercise and sleep researcher at the University of Pennsylvania School of Medicine in Philadelphia.

Snack Attack

What's the best energy snack to keep in my desk drawer?

—E.L., Sacramento

A small (1-ounce) handful of nuts and dried fruit is a powerful mind/body booster, says Kristine Clark, Ph.D., director of sports nutrition at Pennsylvania State University in University Park. It provides the perfect mix of fat, protein, carbohydrates, and vitamins, Clark says. The protein in the nuts can improve your concentration, while the complex sugars in the fruit give your body a slow, steady energy boost. Plus, the monounsaturated fat from the nuts will keep you full till dinner.

Ecstasy or Agony?

My friends are bugging me to try X. I'm tempted but worried. Should I be?

—T.R., Delray Beach, Florida

Should you be tempted? Or worried? We'll answer the second question with a definite "yes." A new study at Johns Hopkins University found that using Ecstasy even once kills brain cells that produce dopamine, a neurotransmitter that helps control movement, emotional and cognitive responses, and the ability to feel pleasure. Worse yet, because X is synthetic, some guy could have cooked it up in his bathtub. Plus, it might just be the gift that keeps on giving. "Ecstasy affects the production of serotonin, a brain chemical involved in regulating mood and memory," says Jack Stein, Ph.D., a deputy director at the Office of Science Policy and Communications at the National Institute on Drug Abuse. "Short-term effects include depression-like feelings, anxiety, restlessness, and irritability, as well as sleep disturbances. Long-term use may result in memory impairment." That's not exactly a rave review.

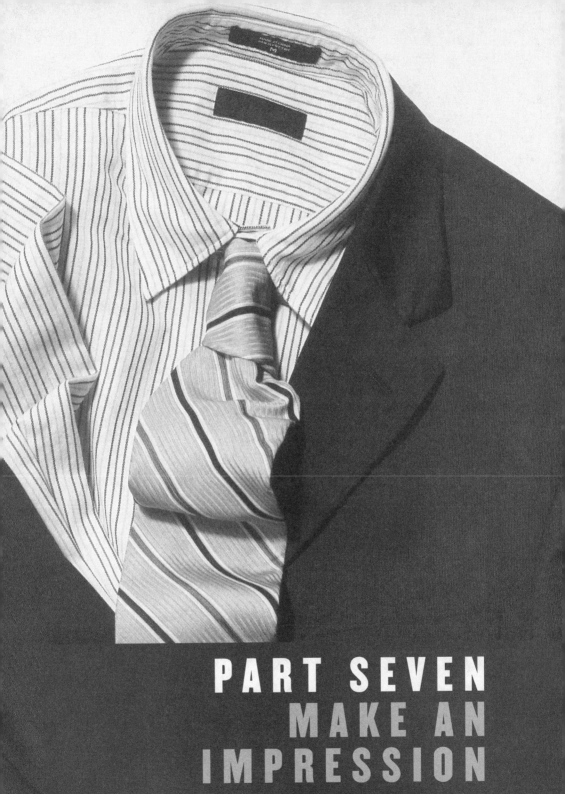

PART SEVEN
MAKE AN
IMPRESSION

GAME SHOW

Who Will Win Her Over?

Test your knowledge of women by predicting which flirt will get lucky

In this episode of the *Men's Health* Game Show, three readers will try to sweet-talk a beautiful young woman. The scenario: Grand Hyatt Boston, Ballroom C. Close to 300 people. The second day of a 3-day seminar called "Unleashing Personal Power and Fresh, Minty Breath." She's one row over, brunette, late twenties, short flowered skirt. Name tag: Tanya. When she's not taking extensive notes, she's sucking seductively on an Altoid. On her left ankle is a small tattoo, perhaps of a balloon or the severed head of Mario Lanza. The final break is in 10 minutes. Let's meet the contestants and see exactly what they do.

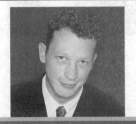

JEFFERY LINDENMUTH
Age 29, 5'11", 160 lb

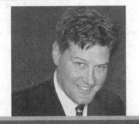

FRANK STARNER
Age 38, 6'1", 195 lb

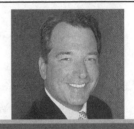

HAGEN DANISH
Age 40, 6', 180 lb

Job: Writer for www.drinks.com
Status: Single
Approach: Walks over with a smile during break; is polite, not pushy; won't climb over chairs to get to her
Opening line: "Hi. I ate those crab thingies over there, and I saw you have some Altoids. Can you spare one?"
Follow-up: "Thank you, Tanya. I'm Jeffery. Do you like the seminar?"
Body language: Considerable eye contact, inquisitive smile, rapt attention, no touching; won't scoop snacks into his briefcase in front of her
Personal info asked: "Have you been here before? Where are you from?"
Proposition: "I'm here alone, and I know a great place nearby for drinks and food. Care to join me later?"
Emergency maneuver: "What do you do for a living?" This will prompt her to ask him the same question, to which he'll reply: "I drink for a living." This always gets their attention.

Job: Business development manager
Status: Single
Approach: Picking up women isn't his style, so he's nervous; walks over and tries to make a joke—a feeble joke
Opening line: "Hi, I'm Frank Starner, president of the Well-Balanced People's Association. And you are?"
Follow-up: "At our next meeting, Anthony Robbins is going to speak. Would you like to attend as my guest?"
Body language: Handshake, respect for her space, eye contact, big smile
Personal info asked: "What do you do? What prompted you to attend this seminar? How long have you been focusing on a well-balanced lifestyle?"
Proposition: "If you have some time later, I'd like to discuss the details of the Robbins lecture with you."
Emergency maneuver: "Look, I admit I'm not very good at this. I just found you very attractive and wanted the opportunity to introduce myself."

Job: Casino supervisor
Status: Married 15 years
Approach: Confident that he understands women; removes ring; gets her to notice him by taking even more notes; nods intently at her; approaches later during break
Opening line: "Are you enjoying the conference as much as I am?"
Follow-up: Agrees completely with whatever she says (because that's the first step to getting anywhere)
Body language: Handshake, jaunty and eccentric air, a bon vivant
Personal info asked: "Where do you work? Ever been to Boston before?"
Proposition: "I've been dining alone these past few nights. Would you like to get out of here and eat some sushi? We could compare notes."
Emergency maneuver: "I'm not into sushi either. Let's see the town."

And the Winner Is . . .
Jeffery
Lindenmuth

Serving as our expert judge is Susan Rabin, author of *101 Ways to Flirt*. Here's how she rated the come-on strategies of each contestant:

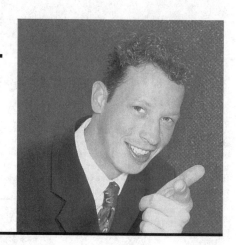

LINDENMUTH

What he did right: Was polite and gentlemanly; used Tanya's name (very important); opening line makes him appear considerate (women like that); expressed honest interest in her.

What he did wrong: Too much eye contact may make her feel uncomfortable (he may be a stalker—or, worse, an optometrist); a big smile is better than an inquisitive one (show teeth); admitting he drinks for a living is risky since he doesn't know how she feels about alcohol. She could be a teetotaler or a recovering drunk.

What he could have done better: "Hi. I ate those crab thingies over there, and I think they had garlic in them. I don't want to offend anyone. . . ." This shows

FIVE LINES THEY COULD HAVE USED

• During the seminar, slip her one of your business cards with this note scribbled on the back: "It's difficult to meet anyone in a place like this, but I'd really like to meet you." Don't sign with a smiley face.

• "I'm a stranger in town. Could you recommend a restaurant?" Even if she's a stranger, too, you'll have something in common. If she lives nearby, then she'll be happy to name names and give you directions, and perhaps a foot massage later. (Okay, we're exaggerating.)

• Fumble with an odd-looking utensil at the refreshment table and ask, "Do you know how this thing works?" (Vulnerability again.) This won't work with a fork.

• "What a great tattoo. I bet there's a story behind it." This also works with jewelry or anything else unusual that she's wearing or carrying. "Is that a birthmark?" will only get you into trouble.

• "I was really interested in (name a particular part of the lecture), but I missed some of it. I noticed you were taking notes. Could I look at them?" If you find doodles of monkeys riding rocket ships, you're in.

FIND YOUR FLIRTING STYLE

According to Susan Rabin, who runs a school of flirting in New York City, there are seven types of flirts. See where you fit:

I-Don't-Flirt Flirt

You have a negative attitude about flirting and probably consider it manipulative. Life is lonely, isn't it?

Insincere Flirt

You try to seduce women with hokey compliments. Instead, look for something nonphysical you genuinely admire about them. It's okay if it takes you a while.

Self-Centered Flirt

Every comment includes the word "I." Try asking more questions rather than giving replies.

Rejected Flirt

You're a negative thinker who never gives himself a chance. You can't be that ugly, can you?

Pressured Flirt

You rely on interrogation for conversation. Relax and ask fewer questions. Don't be afraid of silence.

Analytical Flirt

Your nervousness typically leads to indecisiveness. Stop thinking so much, and have the courage to follow your instincts.

Master Flirt

You don't need any help. You have the charm of God. In this instance, at least, your name is Jeffery Lindenmuth.

that he's considerate and vulnerable, a trait combination women find irresistible—which, of course, they later regret.

STARNER

What he did right: Introductory handshake. A professional one tells a woman she's your equal, which makes her feel better about all the cash she spent on the MBA.

What he did wrong: Tried too hard to be funny, which resulted in a weak joke she probably didn't understand; moved too fast (inviting her out in his follow-up); asked too many questions. Who does he work for—the Census Bureau?

What he could have done better: He needs to be himself, to stop overcompensating for his shyness; his emergency maneuver should have been his opening line (it's that vulnerability thing).

DANISH

What he did right: Respected her space (an arm's length).

What he did wrong: Self-centered opening line (dropping the last five words from "Are you enjoying the conference as much as I am?" shifts the focus from him to her); complete agreement with whatever she said (women loathe insincerity); asked her to leave in the middle of a seminar (that's arrogant and rude).

What he could have done better: Keep the ring on and phone his wife. And don't be surprised if a man answers the phone.

MUST READS

Rebound like the Best of 'em

They had their hands on the brass ring—and watched it slip from their grasp. Let these former sure things teach you how to bounce back from failure

By Bruce Schoenfeld

IMAGINE THE DOWNSIDE OF SUCCESS
Dan O'Brien, 36, athlete

The High: The ad campaign kicked off during the 1992 Super Bowl. Two American decathletes, one named Dan and one named Dave, were primed for a showdown at the Barcelona Olympics. Reebok sponsored both.

Over 6 months, the company spent $25 million promoting the greatest made-for-advertising rivalry since breakfast cereal's Quisp versus Quake showdown. The barrage was scheduled to peak at the Olympics, where it was assumed that either O'Brien or Dave Johnson would earn Olympic gold in the grueling 10-event competition. The winner would get fame, fortune, and the unofficial title of world's greatest athlete. Reebok would win either way.

O'Brien, then 26, was cocky, primed for success. On the day of the pole vault competition during the Olympic Trials, O'Brien was so confident he didn't bother securing a couple of easy jumps; he started right off with a challenging height: 15 feet, $8^3/4$ inches, a height he'd equaled or exceeded dozens—no, hundreds—of times. And yet on his first, then second, then third and final try, he failed to clear it, earning a score of zero for the event. O'Brien didn't make the team. His failure became a national joke.

The Low: After drowning his disappointment on Bourbon Street, O'Brien staggered in a daze through the weeks that followed, wondering how he'd managed to blow the opportunity of a lifetime in three sprints down the pole vault runway. "I remember feeling really alone, with nobody to turn to," he says now. "I'd never failed before. I had no idea how to deal with it."

When O'Brien is asked how much money he lost by simply failing to clear

"The first draft of everything is sh-t."   **—Ernest Hemingway**

"When you find yourself in a hole, stop digging."   **—Will Rogers**

the bar, the answer comes quickly. "Five million dollars," he says. "It didn't hit me right away because I wasn't thinking about it in those terms, but in the days that followed, I read that figure over and over again in the papers. 'Dan O'Brien just blew $5 million.' It hit me then."

The Rebound: O'Brien hit back with a two-part strategy. First, he extrapolated out into the future. If he'd made the team and won the gold, he would have had instant wealth and fame. But where would he have wound up after that? O'Brien came to believe that failure at 26 saved him from the inevitable self-destruction that would have followed. He was a free spirit and a drinker. He'd had a difficult childhood, battled with issues brought on by his racially mixed heritage, flunked out of college. He'd been making up for past troubles with a vengeance. And $5 million would have bought a lot of vengeance.

The second part of his strategy was to envision a different kind of future—a path that would lead him to the same wealth and fame, but without the pitfalls. Failure had provided a reality check.

In 1996 in Atlanta, O'Brien exorcised his demons with an emotional performance on his native soil, winning the gold. He might have been headed for a second gold in Sydney in 2000 when an injury sidelined him before the Olympic Trials. And he's still competing now, pushing himself toward one last Olympics, in Athens in 2004.

The difference in perspective gained with such a spectacular blunder has changed the way O'Brien considers his own achievements. Just making the team in 2004 will mean more to him, it's fair to say, than a gold medal would have in 1992. "Had I won the first time, I would have accepted it as my due and learned nothing from it," he says. "Now I know I can fight off adversity. I realize that I have to keep working for success. That's a lesson for life."

FOCUS ON THE WORK, NOT THE REWARDS
Michael Dukakis, 69, professor, politician

The High: George Bush was scared. And why not—the handpicked successor to the most popular president of the past generation was losing, badly, to the opposing candidate, a diminutive Democrat named Dukakis.

Michael Dukakis's claim to fame was the Massachusetts Miracle, the historic economic turnaround the state had enjoyed under his governorship. "Then I win the nomination, and the Red Sox are doing well, and the place is jumping!" Dukakis recalls. Holding a 17-point advantage over George Bush following his party's national convention, he seemed destined to succeed Ronald Reagan as the leader of the free world.

> **"I'd rather be a failure at something I love than a success at something I hate."**   —George Burns

And yet destiny ran aground somewhere along the path to the White House. Dukakis ran what is generally considered the worst presidential campaign by a major candidate in modern history. He refused to respond to attack ads, showed no emotion when a television commentator hypothesized about his wife being raped and killed, and was photographed driving a tank in an outfit that made him look like Snoopy. On Election Day, he was trounced.

The Low: When he returned to Boston following the tempestuous 1988 campaign, Dukakis found a decade of statewide accomplishments beginning to unravel. He announced he wouldn't run for a fourth term in 1990. But even leaving office didn't feel like liberation. "If you're as deeply invested in what you're doing as most of us are, you develop a kind of proprietary feeling about it," he says. "So there was no feeling of joy or relief to leave a situation that was not what I'd hoped it would be when I left."

The Rebound: People try to tell Dukakis that he should be grateful to have been spared the stress and strain. After all, presidents seem to age a decade for every term in office. Dukakis is 69 today but could pass for a decade younger. "What they don't understand is, we want pressure, those of us who get into this," he says. "We want to be in the middle of the fight. We want to be making decisions."

Still, Dukakis acknowledges that if anyone is suited to making a life for himself after having the presidency in his sights, he's the man. He wasn't in politics for the trappings of the offices he held; even his detractors acknowledged that. As governor, he lived in a modest house, with no security detail. He took the subway to work. Nowadays, he believes that modesty is what keeps him happy and productive: He focuses on enjoying the work he does, not the rewards that work brings him. As a professor of political science at Northeastern University in Boston, Dukakis-the-policy-wonk gets to enjoy talking politics for a living. As vice chairman of Amtrak, Dukakis-the-public-servant ("If I'd been president, you'd see a national rail system that would knock your socks off," he says) gets to fight for an enterprise that desperately needs his help.

RECLAIM CONTROL—SLOWLY
Deborah Norville, 44, news anchor

The High: From the day Deborah Norville was hired as a reporter by the CBS affiliate in Atlanta while still an undergraduate at the University of

Georgia, she was on the fast track to television stardom. At 19, she deftly handled a live interview with President Jimmy Carter. She became an anchor weeks after her summa cum laude graduation in 1980. She advanced from Atlanta to Chicago to the network. She was the golden girl.

In 1989, while working as a newsreader on NBC's *Today* show, she was promoted to coanchor beside Bryant Gumbel, succeeding Jane Pauley in one of the most visible jobs in America. From almost her first week at *Today*, Norville was savaged by the media. They dismissed her as a dumb blonde, or whispered that she'd orchestrated Pauley's departure.

Norville was too focused on work to treat the criticism seriously, but viewers did. Ratings plummeted, and she was out.

The Low: "I didn't think I would ever work in broadcasting again, I had been so thoroughly tarred," she says.

She was 33, and television was all she knew. Set for success, she was utterly unprepared to fail. "I spiraled totally down," she says. "I did not get dressed; I literally wore out a bathrobe. I was completely nonfunctional. Fat, unemployed, paralyzed by depression."

The Rebound: Like an alcoholic, Norville had to overcome failure one step at a time. "I realized one day that I'd given my career control over my life, and now I wanted the control back," she says. "So I swore to myself that I would get out of bed and take a shower, which was a big deal for me at the time."

From showering once, she resolved to do it every day. She'd get dressed, put on makeup, and get herself out the door. Ultimately, she landed a job in radio, 3 hours each weekday on the ABC network. The nature of the medium helped resurrect the self-confidence of this former beauty pageant contestant. "For the first time in my career, nobody could say, 'She got the job because she's blue-eyed and blonde,'" she says.

After a year, Norville was ready to try television again. She signed on as a correspondent for an obscure CBS show called *Street Stories*, which ran for a year and a half in the early 1990s. "I knew what people were saying," she says. "'Oh, that Deborah Norville, how far she's fallen.' I was just happy to have the job."

The show often took her out of town, away from her two young sons. Before the *Today* show, she would have made the schedule work by sacrificing family time. But Norville had come to understand that television was capricious, while family endured. She sacrificed the job for one that would keep her close to home, though it meant leaving the network.

"The greatest mistake you can make in life is to be continually
fearing you will make one." —**Elbert Hubbard**

Since 1995, she has been host of *Inside Edition*, and she recently spent a week as a substitute anchor on CBS's morning program *The Early Show*, competing against *Today*. "There's an inevitability to falling into a pothole somewhere along the way," she says. "Either it has happened to you and you've learned from it, or you really need to be reading this. Because it will happen, believe me. I understand that now."

LIVE WITH FAILURE—FOR A LITTLE WHILE
Barry Minkow, 36, businessman, pastor

The High: At 16, Barry Minkow started ZZZZ Best carpet cleaning service out of his parents' garage. He knew the industry, having worked at carpet cleaning jobs after school, and he had a mind for business. With the help of a $1,600 loan from a friend, he saw ZZZZ Best begin to grow.

Minkow was a nerdy kid who couldn't get a date, but making money made him feel important. He guessed that the business might make him rich eventually, but he didn't want to wait. He started padding profits with stolen money orders, graduated to falsified credit card slips, stole and fenced his grandmother's jewelry, fell in with the Genovese crime family. Minkow's self-esteem grew as ZZZZ Best's paper profits skyrocketed. Before long, he took the company public. He bought a Ferrari.

At one point, he employed 1,400 people. *People* magazine wrote a feature. The mayor of Los Angeles declared a Barry Minkow Day. He was 19.

The Low: By then, his legitimate company had become a fraud. Valued by Wall Street at $280 million, ZZZZ Best was primed for collapse. When the Los Angeles Police Department's OCID (Organized Crime Investigation Division) followed known mobsters to his house, Minkow was indicted in January 1988 on 54 counts of wire, mail, and stock fraud and found guilty in December of that year.

His time in prison, however, was marked not by anger or remorse but by reflection. "The road to compromise is really kind of interesting," he says now. "One thing comes up, then another. You tell a lie here, and then you don't just have to lie to the accountant; you have to lie to the lawyers and the banker. You think, 'I'm going to make good on the money. I'm just doing what everybody does.' Next thing you know, you're millions of dollars down, and it's out of control."

The Rebound: Minkow came to terms with his failure on a cold night in a prison in Colorado. The warden told him and the rest of the new inmates that their requests for a transfer to a less onerous site weren't going to work. They were stuck there, he said, so they might as well unpack their bags and their minds.

"Ever tried. Ever failed. No matter. Try again.
Fail again. Fail better." —Samuel Beckett

"We're going to turn this team around
360 degrees."   —**Jason Kidd, when drafted by the Dallas Mavericks**

"I thought, 'What great advice!'" Minkow says. "Slow down. Figure out what went wrong. If you're newly divorced, don't rush into another relationship. If you fail in business, don't start a new business the next day. Go through the process of failure. Unpack! And that's just what I did."

Beginning his studies while in prison, Minkow earned a college degree and overturned his old philosophy of life.

Today Minkow is the senior pastor of a church in San Diego. He spends much of his time preaching against fraud in American business. He has vowed to pay back every dollar he defrauded from investors. That's where his speaking fees and other ancillary income go. It's been an arduous process, and he's barely halfway home. "That's the hardest part for me, that I can't make it all happen overnight," he says. "But truth plus time equals trust. It's the only way you get there; you can't speed up the process."

TAKE A DIFFERENT PATH TO GLORY
Randy Pfund, 51, NBA executive

The High: All Randy Pfund ever wanted to do was coach basketball. The son of a coach, he spent 18 years preparing to lead a team of his own. He apprenticed under some of the profession's best minds as an assistant, starting at a high school and progressing to college and the National Basketball Association. He paid his dues riding buses and driving vans. He worked his way up the ladder.

It paid off. In 1992, having never served as a head coach on any level, Pfund was named head coach of the Los Angeles Lakers, pro basketball's marquee job. "I started at the lowest coaching rank you can start at, the freshman 'B' coach at a high school," he says. "I ended up with what people consider to be one of the dream jobs in all of sports."

He had been mentored by former Lakers head coach Pat Riley, who won four championships with the team. Pfund arrived at the top with the perfect résumé, prepared to do a perfect job. "I don't think there's one chance in 100 that I didn't have a good idea how to run an NBA team," he says.

But the scoreboard seemed to indicate otherwise. Pfund's Lakers won 66 games and lost 80 during his tenure. Nobody else has ever coached the nine-time NBA champions for a full season and managed a losing record. With 18 games left in Pfund's second season, Lakers owner Jerry Buss came into his office and fired him.

The Low: Despite his perfect background, Pfund was out of work. His professional reputation was in tatters, his unusual name a punch line in a Jay Leno monologue.

"I have learned throughout my life as a composer chiefly through my mistakes and pursuits of false assumptions, not by my exposure to founts of wisdom and knowledge." —Igor Stravinsky

"No one had ever given up on me before," Pfund says. "I'd always been a success. Now here were (Lakers GM) Jerry West and Jerry Buss looking me in the eye and saying, 'We're going to try something else.' It was tough. This was all I knew."

The Rebound: Pfund sat down alone "in a dark room," he says, and did a lot of thinking. "I took the time—and without a job, I had the time—to ask myself what I did well. Should I think about other professions? Instead, I came out thinking that I do have a sound basis for coaching. But I also understood that a new challenge would be good."

Then Pfund did a smart thing. He found someone who believed in him, and went to work for him. In his case, it was Riley, who was starting over as head coach and president of the NBA's Miami Heat.

Riley wanted him on board as an assistant, but Pfund wasn't ready to walk that path again. "I'd been pushing, pushing, pushing for 20 years, trying to move up the ranks and get that opportunity," he says. "Then I had it, and I was knocked off the block. I figured a new challenge would invigorate me more than the same old thing."

Pfund began as player personnel director of the Heat. Later he was promoted to president of basketball operations. While Riley still runs the team, Pfund is in on every decision.

After 2 decades, Pfund doesn't necessarily have coaching out of his system, but if he never gets the chance to prove his talents as a coach, he won't feel unfulfilled. And if he does, succeeding in Miami has given him his confidence back. "I'd be ready tomorrow," he says.

Shake on It

14 ways to make an impressive first impression

By Hugh O'Neill

A man needs a firm grip, son." In hindsight, it was clearly a blunder to build our professional lives around Dad's handshake tip for making a good first impression. We probably should have expanded the old skill set a tad, mastered something in addition to the fake-sincere double pump. But hey, the old man meant well, and besides, though our careers are pretty much kaput, there's still hope for you.

According to Roger Ailes, president of Fox News and the architect of Ronald Reagan's campaign media message, in the first 7 seconds of a first meeting we make no less than 11 judgments of each other, assessing in a flash everything from the other man's educational level and competence to his wealth and political stripe. Given the speed at which first impressions are formed, it's no snap to control how you're perceived. Nonetheless, you can tip the first-meeting odds in your favor by avoiding a few common mistakes and keeping some key concepts in mind.

Polish thyself. We know, you know. Neat, clean, impeccable, shined = respect. When in doubt about the proper level of formality in dress for a first meeting, opt for the more formal.

Scan the news. The morning of your meeting, check out the headlines. "Current events often come up in the course of business meetings," says Ailes. If you arrive for an 11 A.M. meeting unaware that Elvis has returned to Earth to save us, it's not likely you're up to speed on the changes roiling your industry, either.

Watch the clock. Being early is nearly as bad as being late. "Besides looking like you have nothing better to do than wait," says Ailes, one of the shrewdest image makers in the country, "you risk making the other person feel rushed." If necessary, kill some time in Mature Cinema around the corner. But don't show up and announce yourself even 5 minutes early.

Give yourself a speech. If you set your mind just right, your brain will steer you through most situations. Moments before the meeting, give yourself a quick pep talk, reminding yourself of your ambition: to convey, first, your enthusiasm about and mastery of your initiative, and second—and this is the part men often overlook—your respect for what the person you're meeting with has to offer. Lots of us are good at outlining our plans for world conquest, but less good at honoring the other guy's importance to the scheme. He has to feel he's getting his props.

Walk tall. Good posture makes you look proud, open, and trustworthy, instead of sneaky, ashamed, and on the lam.

SEX CAN POWER YOUR CAREER

People with higher testosterone levels make better first impressions than folks lower on the he-hormone scale, according to a recent study published in the *Journal of Research in Personality*. "High-testosterone people are less hesitant, less nervous, and more focused," says the study author, James Dabbs, Ph.D., a psychology professor at Georgia State University. Though the study makes no such claim, we believe that even a brief testosterone spike—caused by, let's say, a home-cooked quickie right before you dress for an interview—gives you a job-getting edge. But don't forget to zip up. High testosterone rarely overcomes an open barn door.

Flash teeth. Before you're even greeted, smile. People feel more confident when they're smiling, according to Ailes. You're upbeat, warm, delighted to be here. "Don't use a closed-lip smile," says Mary Mitchell, a communications expert and author of *The First Five Minutes*. "It can look smug."

Worship Covey. We have no advice better than Habit #5 from Steven Covey's book, *The Seven Habits of Highly Effective People*: "Seek first to understand, then to be understood." Pair that with the immortal words oft credited to Yogi Berra: "You can observe a lot just by watching." People aren't impressed by the self-absorbed. So ask questions. Find out his issues.

Let him see through you. "Many executives believe a poker face is a strategic advantage," says Ailes. "But often, you gain credibility only when you're com-

MAXIMIZING MESSAGE MACHINES

Your actual first impression is often on voice mail. Far more mistakes are made trying to be folksy than are made being too formal. Remember these strategies for recording the message others hear on your voice mail.

Warm up. Before you make the recording, talk for a minute or so to tune the squeaks out of your voice, says Thomas Hand, CEO of Infrastructure Support Services. "Have a glass of water," he suggests. "A dry throat can sound raspy." As you record, have a smile in your voice. Consider the old salesman's trick of keeping a mirror by your desk to monitor your expression as you talk.

Review yourself. Make a clear-eyed assessment of the recording. Better yet, ask a friend to listen to it and fire away with criticism. "Ask yourself, 'Does this sound like a person with whom I'd want to do business?'" says Hand. Do it over until it does.

Hire a stand-in. One of our guys convinced one of our women to record his voice-mail greeting, as in, "You've reached the office of Mr. Hot-Shot Who Has This Personal Assistant Who Is Clearly Both Competent and a Smokin' Babe." Now, our man doesn't have an assistant. But this trick evokes an image of a man with a staff at his command, instead of a guy trying to jam a stack of paper into the fax machine.

When you leave a message, leave your mark:

Keep it simple, businesslike. Don't congratulate a Microsoft guy on yesterday's stirring Seahawks win. Just "Good morning, Bill, this is [insert your name here] from [insert your company here]." No long, detailed messages. Most voice mails over 20 seconds long get cut off before they've run their course.

Get like Brando. Not morbidly obese, but, like a method actor, in the moment. Beware of sounding formulaic, as though you're just going through the paces of leaving a message. There's nothing routine about this. You're sorry you've missed this guy, and you're looking forward to talking to him.

Pepper some pauses. Take barely perceptible pauses at key points in the message: right after your introduction, before and after giving your phone number, and just before the send-off. Take it slow and easy. Speaking hurriedly makes you seem nervous.

Resist the slangy sign-off. Just "I'll look forward to speaking with you, Lars," not "Later, 'gator."

pletely open." You want to achieve transparency, a sense that you're confident enough to be self-critical. If he accurately cites a shortcoming of your proposal or your company, cop to the flaw, but in a positive way: "You're right about that, and we're committed to improving our company softball team." Awareness of both your strengths and your weaknesses makes you seem mature and ambitious, even if you're juvenile and lazy.

Slow down just a bit. "When we're nervous, we tend to talk faster than when we're relaxed," says Thomas Hand, CEO of Infrastructure Support Systems, a consulting firm. Make a deliberate effort to speak just a little more slowly than you normally do. Also, modulate your voice, changing its pitch and volume, and vary your talking pace.

Expose yourself. Don't sit with your arms crossed. It can come across as defensive or, even worse, judgmental, says Mitchell.

Look, but don't stare. Eye contact shows that you're interested and, further, that you're not afraid he'll recognize you from the wanted posters. But holding his gaze too long can come across as intimidating. Every 5 seconds or so, break your glance off and peek quickly at the photo of his suh-weeeet 17-year-old daughter on the shelf behind his desk. Do not ask, "Is she legal?"

Settle for simple. This is not the meeting where you explain your theory of exactly how marketing has been transformed forever by Eminem. Go for clear. Save your fascinating, paradigm-busting insights for later.

Get out of there, gratefully. Be sure the meeting ends before the first awkward silence tells you it's been over for 5 minutes. Your exit sentence is built around a "thank you" sentiment, but you are not grateful because he's such a great man and you're such a nothing (unless he's 30 years older than you). You're grateful because you've enjoyed exchanging ideas with another smart, busy guy.

Become a correspondent. "In this e-mail era, the power of a handwritten follow-up letter is dramatic," says Anne Marie Sabath, president of At Ease, a firm that teaches protocol and etiquette. A letter conveys professionalism and thoughtfulness. "E-mail feels like a hasty attempt to cross something off a to-do list."

Stand and Deliver

Master the power of public address

By Steve Calechman

"I will make an ass of myself."

That's the bottom line, isn't it? The fear of public speaking captured in a single sentence. The size of the crowd may vary—could be a ballroom, could be a living room—but the fear is the same: "I will suck." Followed by the real kicker: "Everybody will see me suck and adjust their opinion accordingly."

Public speaking is destiny for all of us. You will eventually be made to stand. Will you deliver? You'd better. "Public speaking is synonymous with leadership," says T. J. Walker, a speech trainer in New York City with clients as diverse as the Charles Schwab corporation and the Osmond family. "Nothing shouts out 'girlie man' more than a guy who's afraid to speak in front of an audience."

Good communicators win friends. Win debates. Win accounts. Here, veteran speech makers do some talking about talking. Heed their words and you won't worry about dying in the spotlight. You'll be too busy killing.

Deaden your nerves. Realize that the pre-show shakes happen, no matter how long you've been speaking and no matter how much you prepare, says John Kasich, a former U.S. congressman from Ohio and host of the Fox News show *From the Heartland with John Kasich*. "Don't freak out about a speech. You're not being asked to talk about an issue foreign to you. Tell people what you know. Tell people what you care about. Just *tell* them."

Nail the opening. When facing a roomful of businesspeople, remember the Wisk commercial, says Walker. The company's got ring around the collar. Show them how you're going to remove it. For less formal occasions, go with Jon Miller's approach. The play-by-play man for ESPN's *Sunday Night Baseball* is also a veteran of the banquet circuit. "I start out real loud and try to get an immediate laugh," usually at his own expense, he says. But his best attention-grabbing trick? He opens with "I'm going to tell you a story that's never been told before."

Suck 'em in. The worst speakers Alan Dershowitz knows are "verbal masturbators," who talk without engaging the audience. "Speaking is like lovemaking," says the Harvard law professor and veteran wooer of juries. "It's interactive at its best." His solution: "I tell them at the beginning that I'll be taking questions. It makes them listen."

Obstruct abstractions. Some words are like a warm breeze—they feel good but are still just hot air, says speaking coach Michael Sheehan, who trains executives from NBC and Microsoft. "Full-service agency," "state of the art," and "integrated business solutions" mean nothing. Here are six better words: "Let me give you an example."

Set it, then forget it. If you know your subject, you're invincible, says Tony V, a stand-up comedian and semiregular on *Late Night with Conan O'Brien*. Knowledge allows you to "update every minute. If you don't get a good reaction, turn it up a notch. Go right to a strong part, and then you can come back. That's why you can't get locked into an outline. Just know your info, and things logically find their place."

Jack up your act. Consider two Als: Pacino and Gore. Which one would you rather listen to for 30 minutes on the environment? Our former Godfather would grab us by our lapels. But our former VP? "People think they're more animated than they are," Sheehan says. If you need proof of your own

Gore-ness, videotape yourself. Sheehan recommends shooting for "10 percent over the top." That guarantees liveliness.

Screw up on purpose. If you're unknown and trying to impress, this might not be the best move. But if you're the big boss man and are coming in with a daunting reputation, don't be humble—they won't believe you. Just show some vulnerability. "I'll deliberately make a mistake to become human," Dershowitz says. It doesn't need to be a factual error. Just a pause or stammer. "I don't want to seem like I'm winning them over with glibness."

Beware momentary lapses (and crib notes!). In the early 1980s, Miller was speaking at a sportswriters' dinner in New York City, and he was getting good

STAND UP FOR YOURSELF
By Steve Calechman

Last year I made my debut on the comedy club circuit. It was also my farewell performance.

I won't repeat the first joke I told, but you aren't missing anything: The response was . . . silence. Not pin-drop quiet, but pretty darn close. I didn't get a new career out of the experience, but I did get something more valuable: a lesson in fear.

See, sometimes the best way to gain traction on a fear is to face an exaggerated version of it. If you're afraid of heights, bungee-jump. If you're terrified of flying, take piloting lessons. And if you have the most common phobia in America—fear of public speaking—do stand-up comedy. The perspective gained often makes the original fear seem inconsequential. I know. I swallowed my anxiety about public speaking and got up in front of a Friday-night crowd at the Comedy Cabaret in Philadelphia. With no experience as a gag slinger, and with material I'd mainly written myself, I persevered for 5 minutes. Overall, I got two laughs, and a fight broke out at the bar afterward. (It was unrelated to my act, I think.) Now whenever I have to talk to a large audience, I reflect on my open-mike experience. It's made all other types of public performance seem like singing in the shower.

To find comedy clubs near you, visit the Web site www.comedyhome.com. Most clubs have an open-mike night. There are also numerous comedy coaches and schools offering professional instruction, culminating with an "appearance" at an area club. Check your local community college's schedule or try one of these more renowned programs:

Humber School of Comedy, Toronto. Summer workshops and weekend seminars in selected cities. (416) 675-6622, www.comedy.humberc.on.ca/index.html

Comedy Cabaret Humor Workshop, Philadelphia. $200 for 6-week clinics. (215) 322-6642, www.comedycabaret.com/classes.html

American Comedy Institute, New York City. $425 for an intensive 5-day workshop. (212) 279-6980, www.comedyinstitute.com

Comic Belief Program, Calgary, Alberta. $400 for 20-plus hours of instruction designed specifically for people with a fear of public speaking. Online instruction also available. (403) 244-1430, www.cheersproject.com

Greg Dean's Stand-up Comedy Workshop, Santa Monica, California. $350 for a 5-week course or $13.27 for Dean's book. (310) 285-3799, www.stand-upcomedy.com

laughs. Then he noticed people in the back standing up and talking. He figured he was losing them and had better get right to his big finish (another thing that's good to have). He wrapped, said g'night, and sat down. By then, the whole crowd was standing and turning to the back of the room. Why? Joe DiMaggio had walked in. Miller realized how lucky he was. If DiMaggio had entered and Miller had been buried in notes, he would've missed the moment and plodded on to total embarrassment. "Notes are the anti–'staying in the moment,'" he says.

Go short. "If they ask for 45 minutes, I'll say that I'll do 25, and then expand if it's going well," Dershowitz says. "It's better to plan short and go long than the other way around."

Serve well-done toasts and roasts. Tony V does a lot of both, and his rules are simple. For toasts, "keep it clean and end with something heartfelt. Anything longer than a minute is way too long." For roasts: Everything's fair game; just make it personal. "Underlying it is love. You care for the guy, and it works when you can talk about the truth." Pile on all you want. Just shut up after 4 minutes.

Let them figure it out. Whether it's a speech or a closing argument, "I never say, 'Therefore you must conclude,'" says Dershowitz. "They have a greater investment in the conclusion if you let them reach it."

Watch the masters. Years ago, Kasich listened to the Reverend Billy Graham address a packed stadium and realized one of the great secrets of public address: "Fifty thousand people, and everyone thinks Graham is speaking just to him." Dershowitz concurs. You want your speech to seem like a conversation between you and each audience member, he says. For an object lesson, he recommends watching some David Mamet—specifically, *Glengarry Glen Ross*. "(Mamet's) the master of interactive conversation," Dershowitz says. "He invites response." You're not watching Alec Baldwin's speech to find ways to drop more F bombs; you just want to get the back-and-forth.

And remember, it ain't brain surgery. No matter how nervous you are, odds are you won't suck. "The bar is horribly low," says Sheehan. "The audience will be so relieved you're not terrible. It's easy to be acceptable."

There's a Price on Your Head

Millions of American men are losing their hair. Thanks to one company, many of them are also losing their shirts

By Bill Gifford

This woman has me by the short hairs. The short, fine, about-to-fall-out-and-never-grow-back hairs. "Are you thinning, balding, or both?" the telemarketer, a young woman evidently, asks pertly.

"Um, thinning," I say.

"Have you heard of DHT?" she asks.

"I think so," I reply. "What is it again?"

"DHT is dihydrotestosterone," she says, sounding a lot like she's reading from a script, "a bad body chemical that is the reason you are thinning and balding."

Luckily, she has the answer. "Avacor," she informs me, "has a clinically proven 90 percent success rate." *Ninety percent?* The two FDA-approved hair loss treatments—Rogaine (a.k.a. minoxidil) and Propecia—claim only 33 and 67 percent regrowth rates respectively. All I have to do is buy the three-part "hair care system"—an all-natural "DHT blocker," a "physician's topical solution," and a "scalp-detoxifying shampoo." The cost: $220 for a 3-month supply.

I hesitate at the price. "Can I see the study?"

"You'll get it with your order," she says.

I hem some more. "Well, then can you tell me what's actually in Avacor?"

"We don't just give out our formula over the phone," she says. She can tell me, however, that it is "all natural" and has no side effects.

"It's definitely worth a try if you want to keep your hair," she adds, beginning to sound noticeably impatient. "We have a money-back guarantee, so there's nothing to lose."

"START REGROWING YOUR HAIR TODAY!"

I'd heard the ads, of course. If you're a guy and you own an AM radio, there's almost no escaping the Avacor spots and their ubiquitous narrator, a man who identifies himself only as "Dr. Gordon." From morning drive time to the wee hours of the night, sports talk to contemporary Christian, Dr. Gordon rules the airwaves, the balding man's medical savior.

One typical radio ad goes, "I'm Dr. Gordon of the Hair and Skin Treatment Center in New York. Here's what my patients have to say about the revolutionary new hair care system Avacor." There follows a stream of testimonials from formerly shedding guys—age 39 or 26 or 42—who've miraculously sprouted full crops of hair. "Avacor is all natural," Dr. Gordon says in some of the ads, "and completely safe and effective. Stop your hair loss and start regrowing a full, healthy head of hair today."

In the TV ads, Dr. Gordon recounts his own miraculous results: Well into his fifties, he sports a healthy shock of white hair, which he says he's regrown thanks to 6 years on Avacor. (According to the telemarketer I talked to, Dr. Gordon invented Avacor, but he doesn't mention this in the ads.) His voice is kind of high-pitched, almost geeky—how could this guy lie to you?

Apparently, the ad barrage is working; according to *Response*, the magazine of the direct marketing industry, Avacor was the third-best-selling product on the Internet in April 2002, beating out such as-seen-on-TV giants as the Turbo Cooker and the Juiceman II.

"I get asked about Avacor more than anything else," says Spencer Kobren, a consumer advocate, author of *The Bald Truth*, and host of a nationally syndicated radio talk show of the same name. And almost every man with a molting mane asks Kobren the same $220 question: Does Avacor live up to its claims?

Wilma Bergfeld, M.D., doubts it. As director of dermatology at the Cleveland Clinic and one of the country's leading baldness experts, she knows hair loss treatments, and when I told her about Avacor's supposed success rate, she scoffed, "Oh, pooh! Nothing's 90 percent."

Okay, but what about the too-funny-to-be-fake testimonials posted on Avacor's Web site by its manufacturer, Global Vision Products? (After experiencing ¼ inch of hair growth, Jim writes, "Thinking I could accelerate the growth, I had my wife shave off all the new hair.")

"Much of healing is in the mind of the healed, and a patient using magic foo-foo lotion on his hair may actually feel it is helping," notes Douglas Altchek, M.D., clinical professor of dermatology at Mount Sinai Medical Center in New York City. "Very often, particularly in something like hair growth, state of mind is quite important." (Case in point: In the clinical trials of Rogaine, 16 percent of the *placebo* group had measurable new hair growth.)

Which is why, if you're using Avacor and still want to believe, you should stop reading now.

I GET THE GOODS

A few days after my chat with the phone rep, my shipment arrives. And what's this? As promised, it contains a glossy medical study.

The study looks impressive. Grandly titled "The Biological Effects of Combined Herbal Oral and Topical Formulations on Androgenetic Alopecia," it lists as authors R. Ortiz, M.D.; D. J. Carlisi, M.D.; and one A. Imbriolo, Global Vision's president, identified here as an "herbal medicine consultant." Although the study is formatted like a reprint from some august medical journal, it appears on closer inspection to be unpublished.

It's also a bit short on specifics. It doesn't list any ingredients of the "herbal-based topical formulation" or the "herbal oral medication" used in the study. Normally, scientists tell you what it is they're testing. And although the heading describes this as a "controlled study," there is no mention of any control group. At the end, the authors sum up their results: "The overall outcome of this therapeutic modality has proved to be an extremely beneficial

NUMBER OF AMERICAN MEN WHO ARE LOSING THEIR HAIR: MORE THAN 33 MILLION

treatment approach in the management of androgertic (sic) alopecia."
(Alopecia is hair loss.)

Accompanying the study is a small graph that at first glance appears to chart the number of patients reporting hair growth over time. But a closer look by Ken Washenik, M.D., Ph.D., former director of dermatopharmacology at New York University, reveals that this isn't the case: "You can't conclude this from the graph. It lacks hair-growth measurements. What it seems to show is that over time, more people bought Avacor."

Dr. Altchek's assessment of the Avacor study and its methodology isn't any more favorable: "Yet another non-peer-reviewed, non-double-blind, seemingly scientific study subsidized by the makers of the product."

I turn to the bottles. The "All Natural Herbal DHT Blocker" contains, among other things, "maidenhair tree, vaccinium murtillus, equisetum, sabal serulate." As it turns out, these are ancient or obscure (and in a couple of instances, misspelled) names for common herbs like *Ginkgo biloba*, horsetail, and bilberry. But according to the *German Commission E Monographs*—the bible of herbal medicine—none are known for their hair-growing properties.

The last ingredient on the list stumps me for a while, until I figure out that "sabal serulate" is actually *Sabal serrulata*, or saw palmetto. Bingo: Saw-palmetto-berry extract has been used for years to treat prostate enlargement, which like baldness is linked to overproduction of DHT. A number of studies have suggested that saw palmetto somehow inhibits the production of DHT—which is how Propecia works—but it's never been proven to halt or reverse hair loss.

"After Propecia came out, companies selling dubious hair loss remedies latched on to the science behind it," says Spencer Kobren, who has also been investigating Avacor and its claims. "The fact that we understand what causes baldness gives these guys a lot of ammunition."

"Do I have patients who are on saw palmetto? Yes," says Dr. Bergfeld. "Have I seen changes in some of them? Yes. But it's been one patient, two patients. It's not 90 percent."

Then there's the topical formula. The label lists "adenophorae, chanomelis, lobellae, notoptcryll, tarakaci," and a few chemicals with long, complicated names. I draw a near total blank on the herbs, although "lobellae" seems to be a variant spelling of lobelia, commonly known as "puke weed" or "gag root."

Hmmm.

And what's this? While the telemarketer had assured me that Avacor does not contain minoxidil—"There are no chemicals or drugs in Avacor; this is all natural," she'd said—there it is: 2,4-Diamino-6 piperidinopyrimdine 3 oxide.

When I call up the Global Vision offices in New York City, I'm transferred to Henry Edelson, M.D., who identifies himself as "director of research."

"It is minoxidil," confirms Dr. Edelson. (He adds that the sales rep "was

AVACOR ISN'T THE ONLY ONE TRYING TO GET INSIDE YOUR HEAD

Folliguard Extra by Jungle M.D. ($200 for a 3-month supply)

What it is: A 2 percent minoxidil solution; a saw palmetto–based supplement; and a shampoo containing capsicum—the hot stuff in peppers—and peppermint, among other ingredients.

What they claim: "Helps reactivate hair growth."

What you should know: It's basically marked-up minoxidil and an unproven "DHT blocker" containing saw palmetto and *Pygeum africanum*, two herbs used to treat enlarged prostates. As for the "Scalp Volumizing Shampoo," the capsicum and peppermint will make your scalp feel tingly; but according to Ken Washenik, M.D., Ph.D., former director of dermatopharmacology at New York University, "tingling does not equal hair growth."

Hair Advantage by Daniel Rogers Laboratories ($180 for a 3-month supply)

What it is: Shampoo; a "nutrient serum" containing something called Loniten, as well as tarakaci, notoptcryll, and other herbs; and a supplement spiked with saw palmetto, maidenhair tree, *Vaccinium murtillus*, and equisetum.

What they claim: "You'll begin to see new growth after about 3 months."

What you should know: It's nearly identical to Avacor—Loniten is another name for minoxidil (the original version, once taken orally to control high blood pressure). Also, Daniel Rogers Laboratories has an "unsatisfactory" rating from the Better Business Bureau and has received a warning from the FDA for claiming that one of its earlier products, Natural Hairs, could promote hair growth.

Nu Hair by Biotech Corp. ($60 for a 1-month supply)

What it is: A supplement containing the Chinese herb *he shou wou*, saw palmetto, and other ingredients. Also, a "Thinning Hair Serum," which contains horsetail, henna, rosemary, saw palmetto, progesterone, *he shou wou*, and nettle.

What they claim: "Thickens hair naturally; 'energizes' follicular growth."

What you should know: Biotech received an FDA warning letter in 1999 for claims related to the now discontinued Shen Min with Minoxidil. Marketing for Nu Hair has been toned down, but not all the way: The supplement is labeled "Hair Regrowth Tablets," but the ingredients are still unproven.

Thymuskin by Biotechne Complex ($70 for a 1-month supply)

What it is: A shampoo containing, among other things, extract of calf thymus glands.

What they claim: Thymus extract supposedly boosts immune function, the decline of which is (the company says) a cause of hair loss. "Clinically proven" in Germany.

What you should know: While the German studies seem to show some effectiveness with hair loss caused by autoimmune problems and also with male pattern baldness, the product needs more rigorous testing, say Jerry Shapiro, M.D., and Marty Sawaya, M.D., coauthors of a University of Miami study on hair loss treatments.

giving out inappropriate information. Thanks for calling that to our attention.") During our conversation, I press Dr. Edelson for the exact biological mechanism behind Avacor, but he simply says, "When it all works together, it works."

No surprise there: Minoxidil has been shown—"clinically proven," in fact—to help grow hair. So it stands to reason that a product containing minoxidil would regrow hair in some users.

On the other hand, drugstore minoxidil costs about 10 bucks a month, and saw palmetto gel caps are another $10 to $15 from CVS. Subtract that from the $220 I'd spent on Avacor, and I've just paid Global Vision about $150 for three 6-ounce bottles of almond-scented shampoo. Dr. Gordon played me for a sucker.

THE MYSTERY MAN

Who is Dr. Gordon, anyway? New York City dermatologists who specialize in hair loss don't know. "Neither my colleagues nor I know him professionally," says Dr. Washenik. "And the dermatologic community here is kind of small."

The good news: Dr. David L. Gordon did go to medical school. He is a doctor (a radiologist). State records show that he graduated in 1975 from the Autonomous University of Guadalajara, Mexico (also the alma mater of study author Dr. Ortiz).

Now the bad news: Dr. David L. Gordon is also a graduate of the Queensboro Correctional Facility in New York, where, according to the New York State Department of Health, he did time for Medicaid fraud in the mid-1990s. As a result, the medical board stripped him of his license in 1995.

This raises all sorts of questions, but my calls to Global Vision are now going unreturned. So I decide to pay the company an unscheduled visit. My first stop is the office of the New York Hair and Skin Treatment Center, located on the second floor of the same building in New York City where Global Vision is housed.

The center appears to consist of two rooms: an outer waiting area with a few chairs (but no receptionist) and an inner office, where I find Dr. Gordon sitting behind a desk. One wall is covered in framed diplomas, for him as well as for Dr. Robert Ortiz and Dr. Henry Edelson, whose names are on the plaque outside the office door.

He's the same man in the ads, 50-ish, with white hair, only without the white lab coat. His hair clings to his head in a disheveled mop cut (perhaps he would have looked better bald). When Dr. Gordon stands up, I see that he has a hunchback. I introduce myself, and his face falls. "Go," he says, shutting the door. "I'm not talking to you."

Moments later he comes back out and waves me inside.

"The reason I lost my license was because I was entrapped by my scumbag brother into a Medicaid treatment scam!" he shouts. "I had no idea what was going on!"

Dr. Gordon admits that he had agreed to review and sign off on bogus sonograms taken by his brother and his cronies at sonogram centers on Long Island. "I was having trouble keeping my practice open," he says. He helped his brother find other doctors to sign off on the sonograms as well—and only later did he learn that the sonograms were fake, he says. The claims were submitted to Medicaid, and the doctors and the sonogram centers would split the payment. According to the New York Medicaid fraud control unit, the ring scammed more than $1 million. Dr. Gordon blamed his brother for the scheme, but the state medical board didn't buy it and permanently revoked his right to practice medicine.

Oddest of all, he vehemently denies any link to Avacor or Global Vision. He claims he has had no role in developing the product, and no financial interest in the company. "I'm just like Mr. Whipple, who did the toilet paper commercials," he says. "Tony is my friend," referring to Anthony Imbriolo, president of Global Vision. "He knew I was having problems, and he tried to help me. That's as far as it goes."

I would like to stay and talk with Anthony Imbriolo, but a man who introduces himself as Dr. Edelson enters the room and urges me in quiet but serious tones to leave.

Turns out in 1987 Imbriolo was sued by Upjohn, the maker of Rogaine, for patent infringement. He was accused of creating his own version of minoxidil, the active ingredient in Rogaine, and selling it under another product name. In his defense, Imbriolo claimed that he wasn't making minoxidil but simply buying Rogaine, mixing it with other ingredients, and reselling the result as "Minoxidil Plus." That would have been perfectly legal—at least as far as patent law goes—because Upjohn would still have been paid for its product. But Imbriolo couldn't produce invoices for his Rogaine purchases, and when a federal judge ordered him to take a bottle of Rogaine and whip up some "Minoxidil Plus" in the courtroom, he couldn't do it. In a letter to the judge, his own lawyer described him as a "bucket chemist."

Finally, in 1995, he was found in contempt of court. In her opinion, the judge wrote that Imbriolo "willfully has sought to evade the Court's authority through an illusive trail of feigned ignorance, faulty recordkeeping, questionable documentation, and hidden overseas purchases." Imbriolo was fined and ordered to pay attorneys' fees to Upjohn.

By that point, it didn't matter much: Upjohn's patent expired the following year, which meant that Imbriolo could now make his own minoxidil without fear of being sued. Global Vision was incorporated, and Avacor went on the market in 1999.

THE CONTROVERSY CONTINUES

In 1989, the FDA banned the marketing of all over-the-counter hair growth products, except those approved under the agency's New Drug Application process. Rogaine went through the process and was approved, as were the generic versions you see on pharmacy and supermarket shelves. Avacor? It hasn't passed the scrutiny of the New Drug Application process, let alone been approved. Bottom line: Global Vision is in violation of FDA regulations.

"We are aware of this product," one FDA official told me. "We do follow-up on products that are in violation of the law." Well, eventually they do. The official added that unapproved products are the agency's second priority, after risks to public health.

The FDA might also want to look into the discrepancy between Avacor's advertising, which claims that it is completely safe, and the fine print on the bottles. It warns that users should discontinue using the product if they experience symptoms such as "chest pain, rapid heartbeat, faintness, dizziness,

HOMEGROWN HAIR

Skip the snake oil and save your failing follicles with this three-step plan.

Step 1. Buy cheap minoxidil. It doesn't matter if it's CVS brand or Walgreens, generic minoxidil is FDA-approved to help grow hair. Pick up the 5 percent Extra-Strength variety, but trash the enclosed spray applicator. "You'll end up spraying most of your dosage on your hair instead of your scalp, and it won't have its full effect," says Ivan Cohen, M.D., professor of dermatology at Yale University. "The medicine dropper allows you to get the product directly onto your scalp." And if you fertilize post-shower, towel your head off first. "If there's too much water, the solution will be diluted, and it won't work as well," says Dr. Cohen.

Step 2. Pretend you have dandruff. We know; you need hair to have dandruff. But a study cited in *Dermatology Times* magazine showed that balding men who lathered daily with I percent zinc pyrithione dandruff shampoo for 26 weeks grew about six times more hair than men using regular shampoo. The theory? A significant number of balding men have inflamed scalps. "Low-grade inflammation can speed up the rate at which you lose your hair," says Dr. Cohen. "Using a zinc pyrithione shampoo could help reduce the inflammation." Generic dandruff shampoo with zinc pyrithione will run you $3.

Step 3. Ask your doctor about Propecia. Also known as finasteride, this prescription pill blocks testosterone from being turned into dihydrotestosterone (DHT), a hormone that causes hair follicles to become dormant. And unlike minoxidil, which grows hair only on the top of the head, popping a daily dose of Propecia can also put the brakes on a receding hairline—if you start taking it now. "The most important thing with Propecia is that the earlier you start taking it, the better it will work," says Dr. Cohen. "If you wait, you'll never get back to where you could have been."

sudden unexplained weight gain." (Not coincidentally, these are the same warnings that appear on all bottles of minoxidil.)

It seems the Federal Trade Commission (FTC) may join the fray, too. Last November, the National Advertising Division (NAD) of the Better Business Bureau sent a letter to Global Vision, asking it to substantiate its advertising claims. When the NAD didn't get a satisfactory answer, it referred Global Vision to the FTC. (The agency doesn't comment on its investigations.)

Meanwhile, Avacor is still on the radio several times a day in major markets such as New York City, Philadelphia, and Los Angeles.

All this was terribly discouraging; so much for the placebo effect. I called, and after a little guff from customer service, I got a return authorization. (A month or so later, I received a check.)

And yet some users of Avacor—and umpteen other unproved baldness cures—continue to hope. These are the men who count the hairs in their combs or shower drains, the guys who exercise upside down to stimulate bloodflow to their scalps, the men who can't walk past a mirror without rating themselves on the Norwood Scale for male pattern baldness. For them, every disappointed-looking blind date is a potential Avacor saleswoman.

I'm talking about guys like Darin Schneider, a 30-year-old software engineer from Denver. He ordered Avacor about 5 months ago, even though he had his doubts. "I almost sent the stuff back because I was so disappointed with the 'statistical' analysis."

But he tried it anyway. At first, his hair loss accelerated. But after 2 months, it slowed and stopped. "I don't really expect to grow new hair, although that would certainly be nice," he says. If some product out there could regrow his hair, or allow him to keep it, with a 90 percent chance of success, he says, he'd be more than happy to pay $70 a month for it. "I spend that much on stupid stuff each month anyway."

That should be music to Dr. Gordon's ears.

Saving Face

Zits, sores, flakes, bumps, rashes (and worse) are sharing your mirror. Here's how to stare 'em down

By Bill Gottlieb

Imagine how incredibly ugly you would look without your face. There you'd be, casually sitting at a bar, flashing your big rictus grin, and then, right before your exposed eyeballs, the other patrons would run out in drunken horror.

Of course, simply *having* a face is no guarantee that you won't produce the same results when you show up on ladies' night. There are all sorts of bumps, blemishes, and dermatological baddies that can keep a man's mug from being a kisser.

We know, a pimple here or an age spot there might not seem like a sentence of celibacy, but remember that you're working with only about 30 square inches of epidermis. We're talking valuable real estate. This means anything that isn't an eye, a nose, a mouth, or a mustache is a squatter. Match up what you see in the mirror with this ID guide, and we'll tell you how to serve up a few eviction notices.

YOU KEEP BLUSHING

Your problem isn't psychological; it's dermatological. An estimated 5 percent of men over 40 have rosacea—a condition in which hyperactive blood vessels produce a sporadic red-in-the-face effect. If the condition is left untreated, the blush lasts longer, and bumps and pimples start to pop up.

To get a new face: Get the heck out of the sun; ultraviolet A radiation is a common rosacea trigger. And when you do venture out, slather on sunscreen that includes Parsol-1789, a.k.a. avobenzone, as an ingredient, says Leonard J. Swinyer, M.D., clinical professor of dermatology at the University of Utah in Salt Lake City. Sunscreens with Parsol-1789 do the best job of blocking UVA rays. Note: Make sure the sunscreen is also labeled "noncomedogenic," to keep your pores from getting clogged.

While you're protecting yourself from a solar flare-up, watch the wine, too. According to Manjula Jegasothy, M.D., director of the Miami Skin Institute, red wine is most likely to produce a matching face. "People with rosacea are particularly sensitive to tannins, chemicals found in red wine," she says.

Exercise, another trigger, keeps rosacea sufferers flushed for as long as 3 hours after cooling off. Keep your body temp under control throughout your workout by draping a cool, damp towel around your neck, chewing on ice chips, or periodically misting your face with cool water.

And if that doesn't work: Ask your dermatologist about Noritate, a prescription anti-inflammatory cream that treats the bumps caused by rosacea, says Coyle Connolly, D.O., a dermatologist at Philadelphia College of Osteo-

NUMBER OF MEN WHO HAD SOME SORT OF COSMETIC
SURGERY LAST YEAR: MORE THAN 1 MILLION

NUMBER OF MEN WHO HAD
COSMETIC SURGERY 5 YEARS AGO: 286,000

pathic Medicine. Your doctor will probably also give you a vitamin C cream to reduce the reddening. The alternative: a ski mask.

YOU'RE SEEING SPOTS

Who put them there? You did, by going SPF-less one too many times. Commonly known as age spots, these brown marks are actually little piles of sun-damaged dermis that clump together over the years.

To get a new face: Once a day at bedtime, apply a skin cream that contains the spot-erasing ingredient kojic acid. "It's just as effective as popular over-the-counter skin-bleaching agents containing hydroquinone, but causes much less irritation," says Jeanette Jacknin, M.D., author of *Smart Medicine for Your Skin*. Check your drugstore for ProCyte Kojic Complex gel. Can't find it? You can order a product called Skin Whitening Cream for $25 at www.skinlightening.com. And to prevent new age spots from forming, start basting your face with sunscreen *now*.

And if that doesn't work: Have someone shoot you with a laser. The painless pulses from an alexandrite laser will turn a brown age spot into a grayish white scab that will eventually fall off and leave behind unmarked flesh. Expect to pay $500 per session, or more if you're well-spotted.

YOU LOOK LIKE A 17-YEAR-OLD

You're oily and pimple-prone. It's those raging hormones again; testosterone can trigger an overproduction of sebum, a pore-clogging oily substance. Throw in some bacteria, and the clog may turn into an attention-grabbing red pustule, known better by the unscientific name "zit."

To get a new face: Put the Brillo pad down and use Benzac AC, a water-based, 2.5 percent benzoyl peroxide cleanser. It'll limit oil production, flush your pores, and kill bacteria without irritating your skin the way 10 percent peroxide solutions can, says Dr. Jacknin. Wash with the stuff once or twice a day (waiting 30 seconds before rinsing) and you'll knock out existing pimples and prevent new ones from forming. Benzac AC is available by prescription only, so you'll need a note from your doctor.

Pores still pumping more oil than Kuwait? Complete the mop-up job by wiping your face with an over-the-counter astringent that contains witch hazel, says John Bocachica, M.D., director of the division of dermatology at Loma Linda University in California. "Witch hazel cleanses the skin and has anti-inflammatory properties." Of course, it also has that cool, evil-sounding name.

And if that doesn't work: Rub on a prescription retinoid cream to open up your pores and push out debris before they get completely clogged. Just make sure you ask your dermatologist for 0.1 percent Retin-A Micro or Avita; both are gentler than standard preparations.

YOUR FACE IS, UH, SHEDDING

Red, itchy, flaking patches along your eyebrows, around your nose and mouth, and underneath your beard spell seborrheic dermatitis. The ol' snake face is thought to occur when the skin fungus pityrosporum starts multiplying out of control.

To get a new face: Realize that you basically have dandruff on your face. And the best way to handle dandruff? Wash your mug with an antifungal dandruff shampoo, like Nizoral. Lather up the affected areas, wait a few minutes, and then rinse. "It may clear up the problem in 7 to 10 days," says Dr. Jegasothy.

And if that doesn't work: Shave off the mustache and the goofy goatee. "It's rare to see seborrheic dermatitis on a man who is smooth-shaven," says Dr. Bocachica. But before you move your Mach3 up to your eyebrows, ask your dermatologist for a stronger, prescription version of Nizoral to be used along with an antifungal cream, like Lamisil. This tag-team treatment should stop you from flaking out.

YOUR LIP IS TINGLING

If your lips had lips, you'd hear them tell you a cold sore was coming. Instead, you get a tingling sensation when the normally dormant herpesvirus that causes cold sores is awakened by sunlight, stress, or trauma.

To get a new face: Go to the drugstore and pick up a tube of Abreva. A study published in the *Journal of the American Academy of Dermatology* showed that using a docosanol-containing cream like Abreva five times a day can speed up healing of cold sores by 18 hours. Next, hit the health food store and buy Herpilyn, a cream that contains allantoin (a skin-softening ingredient) and the herb lemon balm. Six German studies have shown that Herpilyn can help cold sores heal faster. Alternating between the two creams throughout the day seems to work best. (If time becomes an issue, quit your job.)

And if that doesn't work: Talk to your dermatologist about a prescription for the antiviral drugs Valtrex and Famvir. "If you have breakouts six or more times a year, taking one of these oral medications may help," says Dr. Bocachica.

YOU NOTICE THESE LITTLE RED BUMPS

Your hair is so curly that every time you bring steel to stubble, the hair that's left behind grows back into your skin instead of growing out. The result is pseudofolliculitis barbae—hard, red, infected bumps that make your face look like mosquito fodder.

To get a new face: Wash with an antibacterial face soap and follow with a witch hazel–based astringent. The soap will kill the germs hanging out on your ingrown follicles, and the astringent will help close your pores to keep new germs from getting in.

WORST-FACE SCENARIOS

Don't see your reflection in any of the conditions described above? Keep reading; you may be one of the unlucky few with a faceful of something rare.

You've been visited by a Godzilla-size pimple. It's a boil. Get rid of it with a warm compress, says David Leffell, M.D., professor of dermatology at Yale University. Soak a washcloth in warm water, wring it out, and put it on a dish in the microwave. Now nuke the cloth for 15 to 30 seconds, then (after making sure it's not too hot) take it out and apply it to the boil for a few minutes. Repeat until the boil ruptures. Apply an antibiotic ointment like Neosporin and slap on a bandage; you should be completely healed in 3 to 5 days.

You have cracked red sores at the corners of your mouth. It may be a condition called angular cheilitis, which can be caused by an overpopulation of yeast. The best treatment: the antifungal cream Lotrimin (clotrimazole), applied two or three times a day, says Leonard J. Swinyer, M.D., clinical professor of dermatology at the University of Utah in Salt Lake City.

There's a honey-colored oozing crust on your cheek. Chances are it's impetigo. It's caused by either a strep or a staph infection, so use an antibiotic ointment twice a day. Expect it to clear up in 2 to 3 weeks. If it doesn't heal by then, see a dermatologist to rule out skin cancer.

To prevent future bumps, give up handheld razors—the closer the shave, the sharper the edge of the hair, and the more likely it will be to pierce the skin. Instead, use an electric razor with round heads, like a Norelco. "A square or angled head puts more pressure on the hair, bending it so that it's more likely to grow back into the skin," says Dr. Bocachica.

And if that doesn't work: Have even more fun with lasers. Diode laser treatments are able to destroy the hair follicles in problem areas, like the sides of the neck and along the jawline. "Ninety to 95 percent of men treated with diode lasers never have ingrown hairs again," says Bruce Katz, M.D., director of the JUVA Skin and Laser Center in New York City. You'll need three to five treatments 6 weeks apart. Figure on paying about $400 for each zap session.

KNOW THIS

Clear Up Acne

A new procedure recently approved by the FDA may provide a longer lasting, more effective form of treatment for acne. The ClearLight therapy system is like a tanning bed for pimples. A doctor zaps your skin with high-intensity beams of light, destroying zit-promoting bacteria. A single $150 treatment can kill up to 70 percent of the bacteria on your skin. Results last for several months. For more information, visit www.lumenis.com.

Stop Being So Sensitive

Whitening your teeth could leave you in pain. According to a study done at the University of Southern California in Los Angeles, 50 percent of all people who use dentist-prescribed kits to bleach their teeth experience temporary pain and tooth sensitivity. The cause: a bleaching agent called carbamide peroxide gel. However, "the longer you use the kit, the less sensitive your teeth become," says Michael Jorgensen, D.D.S., the study author.

Stop the Stink

Put on your antiperspirant at night, before you go to bed. Why at night? "Even after you dry off from your morning shower, your pores still hold enough water to dilute the antiperspirant," says Marion Buschbaum, M.D., a dermatologist at Boston Medical Center. By comparison, your skin is completely dry by the time you're ready to hit the sack, allowing the antiperspirant to concentrate in the pores. If you need extra peace of mind, you can still apply antiperspirant in the morning, but it really isn't necessary; the active ingredients—aluminum chloride or zinc chloride—are good for 24 hours, says Dr. Buschbaum.

ROUGH AMOUNT OF MONEY YOU'D SAVE BY USING
A PEROXIDE-BASED, AT-HOME TEETH WHITENER
RATHER THAN A DENTIST'S TREATMENT: **$200**

Do Away with Dandruff

Right before you go to bed, dampen your dome with a little warm water and then rub a quarter-size dollop of baby oil into your scalp. When you wake up, shampoo as usual. "Many times, people have thick, scaly dandruff that flakes off in large pieces throughout the day," says Andrew Pollack, M.D., director of the Philadelphia Institute of Dermatology. "Baby oil penetrates and helps soften up the dandruff scales, loosening them so they fall right off in the shower the next morning."

Get a Smoother Shave

Splash your stubble with warm water, slather on the shaving cream—but don't shave. Wait about 3 minutes, then bring blade to face. "Exposure to water causes hair to expand 34 percent in volume, making it softer and easier to cut," says Karen Burke, M.D., a dermatologist in private practice in New York City. "But we found in our study that this doesn't happen until after 2 minutes and 50 seconds."

Try This On for Size

When buying jeans, see if you can easily slide your wallet out of your back pocket. If not, they're too tight; have the saleswoman remove them immediately.

Make Your Clothes Last

Before you dump last week's wardrobe into the washing machine, turn all of your dress shirts, knit shirts, chinos, and slacks inside out. Besides reducing the chances that a button will get snagged on the metal drum and pop off, you'll also cut down on the beating the outside of the fabric takes. "It keeps the clothes from getting wear marks where they bang around in the washer and dryer," says Linda Cobb, a.k.a. the Queen of Clean, author of *How the Queen Cleans Everything*. "They'll look newer longer."

PERCENTAGE OF WOMEN WHO HAVE "STOLEN" A GUY'S SHIRT BECAUSE THEY LOVED THE WAY IT SMELLED: 62

Iron It Out

We hate ironing. Or we would, if we ever actually tried it. But now we might. A company called Reveal All sells ironing board covers with a photo of a babe in a bikini. Start ironing and the heat makes the bikini disappear. You can purchase the cover for $24 from www.ironingfun.com.

DOWN THE PIKE

No Sweat

Microbiologists in the United Kingdom have developed a deodorant that's 90 percent more effective than existing brands at stopping the stink. The active ingredient keeps bacteria from absorbing iron in your sweat. Without iron for fuel, the bacteria starve—leaving you odor-free. No marketing plans yet. Know anybody at Procter & Gamble?

A Healthy Tan

Someday you may be able to look like a bronzed god even in the dead of the winter. Scientists are developing an implantable drug that tans your skin without any help from the sun. The product, called Melanotan, works by increasing levels of the pigment melanin in the skin. The higher the levels, the darker the skin and the less likely you'll be to get a sunburn or develop skin cancer.

"Melanin is like natural sunscreen," says Wayne Millen, Ph.D., chief executive of the Australian company making the prescription drug. Melanotan could be available in the United States by 2005. A single implant contains enough pigment to keep you tan for at least 90 days.

**PERCENTAGE OF MEN WHO
WEAR COLOGNE AT LEAST 4 DAYS A WEEK:** 36

GAME PLAN

Make a Big Deal over Dinner

Negotiate your way from cocktails to a signed contract

Hosting a successful business dinner takes more than springing for the large shake. You have to do all you can to make sure the contract ends up in your hand and not in the soup.

Make him drool. Negotiating is about making impressions. Before you pick a place, call his personal assistant and find out his favorite food. Choose a restaurant that serves it (find good restaurants at www.zagat.com).

Feed her wallet. A week before the meeting, make two reservations—one for that night and one for the big dinner. At your first dinner, tip more than 30 percent; then tell the server how important the next dinner is.

Mingle at the bar. Order a drink that shows you're confident and knowledgeable, like Maker's Mark bourbon on the rocks, says Raymond Foley, publisher of *Bartender* magazine. Stick to one.

Position yourself. Sit directly across from the decision maker, and keep your shoulders up. Leaning back or slumping shows disinterest—or superiority. He won't take kindly to either.

Come in under budget. You have a spending limit; he wants to blow it. To keep your job without looking cheap, have the place design a special wine list within your price range. He'll never know.

Order meat. Filet mignon is a power dinner, says Dana May Casperson, author of *Power Etiquette*. It's also a moist cut—meaning you won't splash him with bloody juice when you slice it.

Make the deal over dessert. Arrange a "stay away" code with the server—like tugging on your ear. That'll give you 15 uninterrupted minutes to close the deal. Offer your client chocolate; it'll improve his mood.

Negotiate smart. When he makes a good offer, don't give in. Grunt an inquisitive "Hmm?" This negotiation tactic subconsciously makes people sweeten the deal.

TAKE ACTION

Behold, if you will, the tragedy that is split pants. There you are, cruising through another perfectly fabulous day—making deals, making money, making women swoon—when you innocently bend over to pick up a pen on the floor. Rrriiiip! Instantly, the conference room falls silent, every eye in the meeting turns your way, and your young, way-too-attractive assistant stifles a girlish giggle.

Day over, Mr. Big Shot? Not if you know how to overcome those split pants—or any other little problem that can turn a man's day from amazing to appalling in the blink of an eye. When small stuff is throwing you, land on your feet with these simple but ingenious solutions.

Problem: You're at work and you split your pants. Take them off. Turn them inside out. (Have you closed your office door, Mr. No Pants?) Now staple along the inner seam. There's extra fabric where the stitching is, so your handiwork won't be seen and, more important, won't be felt, says Courtney Kilmartin, a makeup artist and wardrobe stylist in Boston.

Problem: You sit on gum on the bus. Ice it. Once the gum hardens, scrape it off with a credit card. If ice doesn't work, put some peanut butter on the spot and let it sit for 5 minutes—the gum will come off in pieces, says Laura Dellutri, owner of America's Cleaning Connection in Kansas City, Kansas. Finish up with a damp cloth to pull up the residue. You risk an oil spot, but then, that's probably preferable to Bazooka.

Problem: You eat garlic for lunch, then learn there's an unexpected meeting. Before you leave the restaurant, go to the bar and dip a lemon twist in a pinch of salt and chew on it, says Peter Kelly, a chef instructor at Johnson & Wales University in Providence, Rhode Island. The lemon oil and salt will help break down the garlic. The tequila's optional.

Problem: You have food on your tie. If the spot is crusty, scrape off as much as you can with a credit card, Dellutri says. Then dab the stain with your tongue—saliva breaks down the food, as it would if you had actually gotten it into your mouth. For oil or grease stains, sprinkle baby powder on the spot; cover it with several paper towels and put a book on it, says Clare Spiegel, an image consultant in Coral Springs, Florida. The paper towels will absorb the stain.

Problem: You can't stop laughing during a meeting. Breathe deeply from your diaphragm and squeeze a pen with your fingers. The former will help you relax, and both will give you something else to focus on, says Leslie Shapiro, a behavior therapist at the OCD Institute at McLean Hospital in Belmont,

Massachusetts. Need something else to think about? Your parents making out. You're welcome.

Problem: The pen you're squeezing to stop laughing breaks, and you get ink on your shirt. Best tip: Go straight to the dry cleaner. Can't leave work? Then put a paper towel underneath the fabric and shoot the spot with hair spray (someone in the office will have some). Then wet another paper towel and press it against the ink, Dellutri says. The ink will go into the paper towel that's underneath.

Problem: Your hair is inexplicably sticking up in one spot. Hit the men's room and dab a little liquid soap on the roots of the flyaway hair, says Leslie Baumann, M.D., director of cosmetic dermatology at the University of Miami School of Medicine. It will coat the hair and prevent static electricity—the cause of your problem.

Problem: You can't remember somebody's name, and he's heading your way. Just say, "I'm sorry. It's been one of those days. Would you tell me your name again?" says Jacqueline Whitmore, of the Protocol School of Palm Beach, Florida. Don't say you don't remember—it looks as if you don't care. You might not; just don't look that way.

Problem: You forgot it's your girlfriend's birthday—and you don't have time to go to the mall. Hop online and make a weekend reservation at a hotel, inn, or B-and-B since they're open 24 hours. (Expedia.com and Orbitz.com can help with hotels.) Then make a card that looks like a coupon for the trip, says Paul Joannides, author of *Guide to Great Dates*. She'll actually think you're romantic.

Problem: You overcooked the pasta—and your guests are getting hungry. Sauté it with some olive oil. It'll remove excess moisture, Kelly says. You can also throw the pasta in a baking dish, cover it with sauce and some cheese, and nuke it for 5 to 7 minutes, or use the oven for 15 minutes at 350°F.

Problem: The cork breaks and falls into the wine bottle. Pour the wine into a decanter (a glass or ceramic pitcher will do) and the pieces will float and stick to the sides of the original bottle, says Cat Silirie, wine director at No. 9 Park restaurant in Boston. If the cork turns into dust, pour the wine through a coffee filter.

Problem: You can't fall asleep and you don't want to be late for work again. Make two columns on a pad of paper. On one side write down what's bothering you, and on the other write down what you'll do about it, even if it's "I'll deal with it tomorrow," says Edward O'Malley, Ph.D., director of the Sleep Disorders Center at Norwalk Hospital in Connecticut. Now you've been productive and gotten the thoughts out of your head. Then go watch a rerun of a sitcom. You'll be distracted without becoming too engaged. Finally, UPN has a purpose.

PERCENTAGE LESS MONEY A SHORT MAN EARNS COMPARED WITH A MAN WHO STANDS 6 FEET OR MORE:

ANY QUESTIONS?

Stench Warfare

Sometimes my sweat reeks and sometimes it doesn't. What's up?

—P.P., Tulsa, Oklahoma

It depends where you're sniffing. You have two types of sweat glands—eccrine and apocrine—among the 2 to 4 million that riddle your skin. Fortunately for you, and the rest of us who have to share an elevator, the vast majority are eccrine glands, which are found on the biggest parts of your arms and back and chest. These produce a scent-free brine of mostly water, sodium, and chloride. (Ever notice how the sweat drenching the front of your workout shirt doesn't smell nearly as bad as your pits?) Apocrine sweat glands, on the other hand, are found mostly in your underarm and groin areas, which are hotbeds for bacteria. When the secretions expelled by your apocrine glands mix with the bacteria, you smell like Swamp Thing.

"Stress, especially, can cause an excess of apocrine excretions, making your armpits really stink," says Lisa Kates, M.D., a dermatologist at Cook County Hospital in Chicago. You've noticed, right? And on those days when your pits don't seem to stink? Either you're very calm or your antiperspirant is working great, she says. The active ingredient—either zirconium or aluminum chloride—temporarily plugs apocrine sweat glands, effectively damming the odor-causing brew.

Save Your Breath

Is mouthwash a scam?

—D.D., Provo, Utah

That depends on your expectations. If you want fresher breath, a swish of any brand will temporarily improve your kissability. "But that's like putting cologne over sweat," says Van B. Haywood, D.M.D., professor at the Georgia School of Dentistry in Augusta. To put down germs, too, get Listerine Antiseptic or a generic knockoff that lists the same ingredients: thymol, eucalyptol, salicylate, and menthol. According to the American Dental Association, this is the only proven over-the-counter formula for nuking mouth germs.

Get It Off Your Chest

I see they now make rub-on hair removers for men. Do they work?

—P.M., Trumbull, Connecticut

One-third of all men shave hair from their chests and backs, say the makers of Nair, who hope to cut into that number by selling Nair for Men. We found that it works okay on our monkey-rug backs and chests, but it can leave a monkey-rug-burn rash. To see how you'd react, try it on a small patch first. If you see any redness, scaling, or blisters, go back to the razor. If nose or ear hair is your problem, Nair isn't your product. Try round-tipped scissors, or go electric: The Remington Precision trimmer ($15) worked for us.

Trim Your Bushes

I have bushy eyebrows. How can I keep them trim?

—W.B., Guilford, Connecticut

First, comb your brows straight up with a fine comb. Then use a small scissors or a sideburns trimmer to cut the hairs that extend above the brow line. Third, thin the eyebrows by laying the comb flat against your skin so that the brow hairs stick up through the teeth. Cut them down to the comb. It will keep you from giving your brows a buzz cut. And finally, find another barber. Brow trimming should be part of every proper haircut.

Keep 'em, for Pleats' Sake

Have pleated casual pants gone out of style?

—S.O., Carlsbad, California

While flat-front casual pants are currently all the rage, our fashion experts advise us not to pitch the pleats. "We're in the middle of a flat-front pants craze, but that doesn't mean that pleats are out of style," says Brian Boyé, *Men's Health* fashion director. "Just as men are starting to grasp the idea of a slimmer, pleatless pant, the designers who led the flat-front frenzy—Prada,

PERCENTAGE OF MEN WHO BOUGHT PLEATED PANTS IN 2001 : **52**

PERCENTAGE WHO BOUGHT PLEATED PANTS IN 2002: **62**

Gucci, and the like—are starting up with the pleats again." That means our designer knockoffs will soon start sporting them, too. If you wear them, look for slacks that have one or two pleats at most ("More than two looks tacky," Boyé says). And make sure the pleats lie flat when you put them on, or your paunch will look puffier. Yep, that means breaking out the iron.

Here's a Tip

Do I have to tip bathroom attendants? What's the etiquette?

—G.K., New York City

If you can afford to dine in posh restaurants that provide attendants, you can afford to tip them at least a dollar, says Letitia Baldrige, an etiquette expert and author of *The Complete Guide to Executive Manners.* As for protocol, one tip is sufficient for one or two whiz visits. On long nights with several encores, tip after your first and last trips. If you make any kind of mess while you're in there—we'll spare you our sordid scenarios—fork over a ten-spot. Only have plastic? Offer a sincere smile and a warm "Thank you." "They're used to dealing with so many rude people that sometimes they'll settle for your sympathy," Baldrige says.

Index

Underscored page references indicate boxed text. **Boldface** references indicate illustrations.

A

Abdominal fat, reducing, 36, 38
Abdominal muscles, building, 5, 35
Abreva, 283
ACE inhibitors, 148
Acetaminophen, 166
Acetyl-l-carnitine, 252
Acid reflux, smoking and, 111
Acne, 282, 285
Activase, 141
Actos, 148
Acupressure, for
  nausea, 109
  headaches, 118
Acupuncture, for insomnia, 92–93
ACVI, 114
Addictions
  sex and love
    characteristics and signs of, 56, 57, 60
    masturbation as, 55
    recovery from, 58–63, 60
    substitution in overcoming, 90
Adult-onset asthma, overweight and, 201
Advil. See Ibuprofen
AEDs, 168
Affairs, erectile dysfunction and, 75–76
African-Americans, prostate cancer rates
    and, 166
Age spots, 282
Aging
  of brain, smoking and, 229
  dietary supplements to combat, 252
  muscle loss due to, 39
AIDS
  measles and, 73
  risk of, with unprotected sex, 54
Ailments. See also specific ailments or
    conditions
  in common among couples, 71
  foodborne, number of people contracting,
    106
  risk of, from exposure to blood, 96
Air travel, deep vein thrombosis and, 97
Albuterol, 197, 200
Alcohol, 91–92, 111

Allantoin, 283
Allergies
  foam mattresses and, 118
  to pets, 88
  pollen-trapping nose plugs for, 113
Allerpet D, 88
Alopecia. See Hair loss
Alpha amylase, 29
Alpha-lipoic acid, 252
Alzheimer's disease
  aspirin for preventing, 158–59, 247
  cholesterol and, 246
  dietary copper and, 246
  lifestyle changes to reduce risk of, 251
  risk factors for, 226, 227
  verbal memory test for predicting, 247
Amends, in cure for sex addiction, 56–62
AmLactin 12 percent, 120
Anchorage, Alaska, impotence rate in, 73
Anger
  controlling, 93–94
  risk of heart attack and, 143
Angina, acetaminophen for, 166
Angioplasty, 142, 142
Antibacterial soaps, 112, 113, 120, 283
Antibiotics
  for fevers, 121
  unnecessary, 209
Antidepressants, for
  back pain, 105
  weight loss, 34, 135
Antihistamines, for
  nausea, 109
  colds, 117–18
Anti-inflammatories, for
  rosacea, 281–82
  colds, 117–18
Antioxidants
  garlic and, 166
  for reducing risk of heart attack, 143
Antiperspirants, 285
Anxiety
  generalized disorder, 235
  risk of stroke and, 151
Apomine, 163

Apomorphine nasal spray for erectile
    dysfunction, 73
Appetite
  control of, with
    bupropion, 34, <u>135</u>
    monounsaturated fats, 254
    third-helping hormone, 29–30
  food cravings, 9–2, 26
  high-fructose corn syrup and, 6–9
  insufficient sleep and, 26
Arms, supersets for enlarging, <u>13</u>
Arteries, measuring inflammation of, 146–49
Arthritis, back pain and, 104
Arthroscopic surgery, 209
Aspirin
  bleeding from, <u>157</u>
  health benefits of, 157–59
  during heart attack, <u>141</u>
  purchasing, <u>158</u>
  for reducing risk of diseases
    Alzheimer's, 247
    heart attack, <u>143</u>, <u>145</u>, 158
Asthma, 200–201
Atridox, <u>199</u>
Atrovent, 200
Automated external defibrillators (AEDs),
    168
Avacor
  effectiveness of, 274
  ingredients in, 275, 277
  marketing of, 273, 280
  promoters of, 277–78
  side effects of, 279–80
Avandia, 148
Avelox, <u>197</u>
Avita, 282
Avobenzone, 281

B

Baby oil, for dandruff, 286
Back pain
  best sleeping positions for, 121
  chiropractic care for, 84
  factors in, <u>85</u>
  heat treatments for
    heat wraps, 104, 119
    intradiskal electrothermal therapy,
      111–12
  listening to music to soothe, 105, 119
  medications for
    antidepressants, 105
    chondroitin sulfate, 104
    ibuprofen, 84, <u>85</u>, <u>199</u>
  posture while driving, to relieve, 119

  strategies to cope with, 102–5
  stretching to ease, 84, <u>85</u>, 90, 104
  surgery for, <u>103</u>
Bacteria
  antibacterial soaps for, 112, 113, 120,
    283
  streptococcus, oral sex and, 71
  on towels, 123
Baldness. *See* Hair loss
Band-Aid Liquid Bandage, 122
Basketball, avoiding injuries from, 22–23
Benadryl, <u>109</u>
Bench press, 16, **16**, 35–36
Benign prostatic hyperplasia, 199–200
Bent-arm cable shrug, 18, **18**
Benzac AC, 282
Benzoyl peroxide, 282
Beta human chorionic gonadotropin (beta
    hCG), 48
Biosafe home cholesterol test, <u>179</u>
Blacks, prostate cancer rates among, 166
Bleeding, 94–97
  caused by aspirin, <u>157</u>
  wearing bandages for, 122
Blood pressure
  high
    aspirin for reducing, 157
    as cause of nosebleeds, 95
    dietary controls to stop, 198–99
    drug-free treatment for, 86–87, 198–99
    epinephrine dental anesthetic and,
      115
    reduced frequency of sex and, 71–72
  ideal range for, <u>179</u>
Blood sugar
  erectile dysfunction and, 72, 76
  migraine headaches and, 89
Blue balls, 78
Blushing, 281–82
BMI, ideal range for, <u>179</u>
Board certification of doctors, 206
Body fat. *See also* Overweight
  abdominal, 4, 38
  on chest, 39
  effect of leptin on, 8
  as fuel, 38
  monitors, 34–35
  supersets for reducing, <u>13</u>, 15–16, **16**
Body mass index, ideal range, <u>179</u>
Body odors, 285, 288, 292
Body temperature, lowering, 29
Boerhaave's syndrome, 107–8
Bone fractures, ultrasound therapy for,
    209–10

BPH, 199–200
Brain cancer, scorpion venom for, 248
Brave Soldier Antiseptic Healing Ointment, 119–20
Breakfast
  cravings, 9–10
  weight loss and, 33
Breasts on men, 39
Breathing
  controlled, for relaxation, 229, <u>239</u>
  difficulty, drug-free remedy for, 200–201
Brushing and flossing teeth, 165
Bruxism, 221–22
Bupropion, for
  smoking cessation, <u>199</u>
  weight loss, 34, <u>135</u>
Business meetings
  dinners, 289
  first impressions in, 267–69
Bypass surgery, 144, <u>144</u>, 163

C

Cabbage, lung cancer and, <u>134</u>
Cable incline triceps extension with rope attachment, 19–20, **19**
Cable side stepup, 20, **20**
Caffeine, false sense of energy from, 10
Calcium
  kidney stones and, <u>100</u>
  supplements, 171
  for weight loss, 34
California Verbal Learning Test, 247
Calories
  average consumption of, 8, <u>8</u>
  from high-fructose corn syrup, 6
  sources of, 201
Cancer. *See also specific types of cancer*
  radiation exposure from CT scans and, 204–5
  running for reducing risk of, 27–28
  St. John's wort and, 160
  screening for, 116, <u>137</u>
  vitamin D for reducing risk of, 166–67
Capsaicin, effect of, on blood pressure, 87
Carbohydrates
  for breakfast, 10, 33
  effect of insulin on, 8
  high-fructose corn syrup, 6
  migraine headache and, 88–89
  mood and, 10
Cardiovascular fitness and strength, exercise program for, <u>25</u>
Cardura, <u>197</u>
Cat allergies, 88

Catecholamines, 160
Celebrex, 194, <u>199</u>
Centrum Silver, 171
Cetaphil soap, 120
CETi-1 vaccine for cholesterol control, 162
Chemotherapy for testicular cancer, 51
Chest
  pains, 169
  tightness or fullness in, <u>140</u>
Chicken for weight loss, 33–34
Chiropractic care, 84
Chitosan fat blockers, 26
Chlamydia, 54
Chlorhexidine, <u>199</u>
Chocolate
  for coughs and sore throats, 113
  cravings for, 11
Cholesterol
  Alzheimer's disease and, 246
  Biosafe home test for, <u>179</u>
  CETi-1 vaccine for, 162
  factors affecting, <u>177</u>
  niacin and, 148, 176
  as predictor of heart attack, 147
  psyllium for, 89
  soy foods and, 176
  statin drugs for reducing, <u>145</u>, 148, 166, 177
  testing for, <u>136</u>
  users of vitamins for, <u>91</u>
Chondroitin sulfate for back pain, 104
Cigarettes. *See* Smoking
Cipro
  as alternative to Avelox, <u>197</u>
  for gonorrhea, 54
Cisplatin for testicular cancer, 51
Cities, health in
  best, 135–38
  rankings, <u>132–33</u>
  worst, 131, 134
Claustrophobia, self-treatment for, 87
ClearLight therapy system, 285
Close-grip chinup, 14
Clothing, care of, 286, 290, 291
Cognitive function
  Gila monster saliva and, 248
  statin drugs and, 246
Cold compresses for conjunctivitis, 94
Colds and flu
  drug treatment for, 117–18, <u>118</u>
  foods to combat, 121–22
  users of vitamins for, <u>91</u>
Cold sores, 120, 283

Colonoscopy, virtual, 204
Colorectal cancer (CRC)
  acetaminophen for preventing, 166
  adenoma-carcinoma sequence in, 128
  aspirin for preventing, 158
  calcium for combating, 171
  colon scan for, 204
  risk factors for, 128, <u>129</u>
Complexed prostate-specific antigen, <u>130</u>,
  156
Compulsions. *See* Addictions
Computers, work at, 250
Condoms, sexually transmitted diseases and,
  53–54
Conjunctivitis, cold compresses for, 94
Controlled breathing, 229, <u>239</u>
Cordase, 73
Cosmetic surgery, <u>281</u>
Coughs, 113
Couples, diseases common in, 71
CPR, <u>168</u>
CPSA, <u>130</u>, 156
Cravings, for
  foods, 9–12, 26
  smoking, 89–90
CRC. *See* Colorectal cancer
C-reactive protein level, 146–49
Crunch with a plus, 17–18, **17**
C6 peptide test for Lyme disease, 112
CT scans, 202–5
Cycling, avoiding injuries from, 24

D

Dandruff, 283, 286
DASH diet, 198–99
Deadlift, 16, **16**, 37
Deep vein thrombosis (DVT), 97
Defined contribution health plan, <u>179</u>
Dental care
  flossing and brushing, 165
  saving costs of, 219
  sedation dentistry and, 221
  suggestions for, 115–16
  teeth grinding and, 221–22
  teeth whitening, 285, <u>285</u>
Denti-Patch, 115
Deodorant, 288
Depression
  insomnia and, <u>92</u>
  participating in sports for, 231–32
  St. John's wort and, 247
  symptoms of, <u>235</u>
DHT, 200, 273
DiaBeta, 201

Diabetes
  erectile dysfunction and, 72, 76
  high-fructose corn syrup and, 7
  impotence and, <u>131</u>
  smart tattoo glucose monitor for, 162
  snoring and, 160
  type 2, preventing, 201
  weight training and, <u>27</u>, 201
Diet. *See also* Food
  Alzheimer's and, 246
  colorectal cancer and, <u>129</u>
  DASH, 198–99
  fads, <u>29</u>
  Mediterranean, <u>145</u>
  muscle gain and, 41
  for preventing diabetes, 201
  for reducing risk of heart disease, 165
  supplements, 26, <u>91</u>, 170–71, 252
Digital rectal exam (DRE), 152–53
Dihydrotestosterone (DHT), 200, 273
Dimenhydrinate, <u>109</u>
Diseases. *See also specific diseases or
    conditions*
  common among couples, 71
  foodborne, number of people contracting,
    <u>106</u>
  risk of, from exposure to blood, <u>96</u>
Docosanol, 283
Doctors
  average number of visits to, <u>209</u>
  choosing
    American Medical Association online
      doctor finder, <u>179</u>
    primary care physician, 205–7, 220
    surgeon, 213
  credentials and certification of, 206
  emergency room, overwork of, 178, 180
  emphasis on specialization by, 182,
    185–86
  lack of family doctors, 181
  manipulation of, by drug companies
    American Medical Association position
      on, 196
    prescribing decisions and, 188–89, <u>189</u>,
      190
    questions to ask that will reveal, <u>194</u>
  negotiating fees with, 216–17
  No Free Lunch organization, 189
  primary care physician vs. specialist,
    216
Dove soap, 120
Doxycycline, <u>199</u>
Dramamine, <u>109</u>
DRE, 152–53

Dress, formality of, in first impressions, 267
Dribble, postvoid, 80
Drinking
   alcohol abuse, 91–92
   occasional, 111
Driving
   distractions from, 167, _167_
   head restraint position for, 119
   posture during, to ease back pain, 119
   using seat belts while, _139_, 167, _167_
   Subaru Impreza WRX, 249
Drug companies
   competition among, 191
   fostering of drug dependence by, 192
   manipulation of doctors by
      American Medical Association position
         on, 196
      prescribing decisions and, 188–89, _189_,
         190
      questions to ask that will reveal, _194_
   spending on marketing and
      administration, 188, 193, _193_
Drug-free remedies for common conditions,
      197–201
Drugs. _See also specific drugs; specific
      illnesses or conditions; specific types of
      drugs_
   generic, 218
   prescription
      costs of, to patient, 195, _208_, 217–18
      delivery systems for, 212
      errors in prescribing of, _213_
      FDA approval of, 191, _193_, _195_
      free samples of, 192, 218
      generic, 218
      inappropriate, 189, 190, 195
      low-cost alternatives to, _197_
      new vs. old, 220
      numbers of, _196_
      profits from, 208
      unnecessary, 209
Dumbbell squat jump, 15, **15**
DVT, 97

E
Ecstasy, 254
Ego, curbing, in lovemaking, 64
Ejaculate, blood in, 96
Emergency rooms
   average wait in, _178_
   financial issues faced by, 180
   nonemergency use of, 181, 217
   overcrowding and overworked physicians
      in, 178, 180

for primary care, 181
   uninsured users of, 180
   using, 164
Epididymitis, 78
Erectile dysfunction
   apomorphine nasal spray for, 73
   cities with highest and lowest prevalence
      of, _73_, _131_
   Korean ginseng for, 72
   preventing, 75–77
   risk factors for
      diabetes, 72, _131_
      obesity, _131_
      penile trauma, 76
      prostate cancer surgery, 154–55
      smoking, 75
Erections
   firmer, normal blood pressure and, 72
   nocturnal, 77
   pelvic crunch exercise for, 79–80
   in Peyronie's disease, 73
Esophageal artery, damage of, 107
Exercise
   for abdominals, 35
   aerobic, 152, 200, 201
   for back pain, 84, _85_, 104
   to combat sleepiness, 253–54
   for controlling anger, 93–94
   for depression, 231
   for difficulty breathing, 200–201
   for fat loss, 15–16, **16**
   fitness log for, 35
   during illness, 41
   for larger muscles, 13–14, **14**
   muscular soreness from, 40, _138_
   for overcoming addictions, 90, 92
   for preventing sports injuries, 22–25
   raisins and, 34
   for reducing risk of heart disease, _143_, _145_,
      165
   rosacea and, 281
   for small muscles, 17–20, **17**, **18**, **19**, 20
   specific
      bench press, 16, **16**, 35–36
      bent-arm cable shrug, 18, **18**
      cable incline triceps extension with rope
         attachment, 19–20, **19**
      cable side stepup, 20, **20**
      close-grip chinup, 14
      crunch with a plus, 17–18, **17**
      deadlift, 16, **16**, 37
      dumbbell squat jump, 15, **15**
      incline dumbbell bench press, 14, **14**
      military presses, 25

Exercise (cont.)
  specific (cont.)
    pelvic crunch, 79–80
    pullups and negative pullups, 36
    pushup, 14, **14**
    running, 27–28, 39–40
    squat, 15, **15**
    stepup variation, 36–37
    stretching, 90
    swimmer's backstroke, 19, **19**
    warmup, 22
    weight lifting (see Weight lifting)
    wide-grip lat pulldown, 14
  strength and power, 14–15, 24
  on treadmills, 35
  vision, 91
External obliques, 18–19, **19**
Eyebrows, trimming, 293
Eye contact, correct use of, 269
Eyesight, exercises for, 91

F

Facial features, women's attraction to, 4
Facial skin, conditions of
  age spots, 282
  blushing, 281–82
  cold sores, 283
  pimples, 282, 285
  pseudofolliculitis barbae, 283–84
  seborrheic dermatitis, 283
Failure, methods to rebound from
  changing path, 265–66
  envisioning success, 260–61
  focusing on work, 261–62
  living with failure, 264–65
  reclaiming control, 262–64
Famvir, 283
Fantasy during masturbation, 70
Fat. See Body fat
Fat blockers, 26
Fats, monounsaturated
  in satisfying hunger, 254
  for weight loss, 33
Fear
  coping with, 238–40, _239_
  of public speaking, 269–72, _271_
Feet, 35
Fever, when to treat, 121
Fiber, dietary, for
  controlling cravings, 10
  preventing diabetes, 201
  reducing cholesterol, 89
Figure-eight tongue technique, 66
Finasteride, 200, _279_

First impressions, making favorable, 267–69
Fish, eating, _143_, _149_
Fitness log, 35
Flavonoids, protective effect of, _143_
Flaxseed, 166
Flirting, 258–59, _258_, _259_
Flomax, 80, 200
Flu and colds
  drug treatment for, 117–18, _118_
  foods to combat, 121–22
  vitamins and, _91_
Flu shots, to reduce risk of stroke, 152
Folic acid, 11–12, _143_, 151–52
Folliguard Extra, _276_
Food. See also Diet
  associating, with relaxation, 11–12
  cabbage, _134_
  cravings for, 9–12, 26
  fiber in, 10, 89, 201
  for fighting infections, 121–22
  fish, _143_, _149_
  flaxseed, 166
  folic acid in, 11–12, 151–52
  fructose in, _7_
  illnesses from, _106_
  lycopene in, _143_
  mood and, 10, 11
  niacin in, 148, 176
  pectin in, 166
  protein in, 10, 33
  snacks, 33–34, 254
  soy, _100_, 176
  for weight loss, 33–34
Framingham Risk Assessment, 176
Free radicals
  lycopene to reduce, 87
  raisins to minimize damage from, 34
Friendships
  happiness and, 243
  immune system and, 230
  in overcoming fear, _239_, 240
Fructose, 7, _7_
Full-body scans, 202–5

G

Garlic, 165-66, 290
Gastric bypass surgery, 27, 30
Generalized anxiety disorder, _235_
Generic drugs, 218. See also Drugs,
  prescription
Genetic traits
  abdominal fat, 38
  food cravings, 26
Genital warts, 53

Geodon, <u>197</u>
Germ-free surfaces, 113–14
Gila monster saliva, 248
Ginkgo, 246–47
Ginseng, Korean, 72
Gleason score, 154
Glioma, scorpion venom for, 248
Global Sleep Assessment Questionnaire, 247
Global Vision. *See* Avacor
Glucose level, normal, 201
Golf, as alternative to softball, 23
Gonorrhea, 54
Grooming, to attract women, 64
G-spot, stimulating, 65
Gum, removing, from clothing, 290
Gum disease
   PerioChip treatment for, <u>199</u>
   risk of stroke and, 165
Gym, choosing, 31–32
Gynecomastia, 39

H

Hair Advantage, <u>276</u>
Hair loss, 272–80, <u>276</u>, <u>279</u>
   Avacor treatment for
      effectiveness of, 274
      ingredients in, 275, 277
      marketing of, 273, 280
      promoters of, 277–78
      side effects of, 279–80
   products for, <u>276</u>
   testosterone and, 200
   three-step plan for, <u>279</u>
Hair removers, 293
Haldol, <u>197</u>
Hands as sex toys, 64–65
Happiness, 240–43, <u>242</u>
HDL. *See* Cholesterol
Headaches
   acupressure for, 118
   migraine, 88–89, 111
Health, optimal number of orgasms for, <u>76</u>
Health care. *See also* Doctors; Health
      insurance; Hospitals
   access to, <u>218</u>
   costs of, 215–19, <u>218</u>
   managed care, 183–86, <u>183</u>
   responsibility for own, <u>179</u>, 185
   socialized medicine, 186–87
   status of, in United States, 179–82, <u>186</u>
   using primary care physician vs. specialist,
      216
Health insurance, <u>179</u>, <u>183</u>, 184, 186-187,
   215, 217

Hearing loss
   medication for, 211–12
   self-test for, 221
Heart attack and heart disease
   C-reactive protein level as predictor of,
      146–49
   diagnosing, 162
   Framingham Risk Assessment for, 176
   risk factors for, 140, <u>140</u>, <u>177</u>
      dental work, 115
      depression, 231–32
      excess iron, 171
      waist size, 160
   role of plaque in
      artery inflammation and, 147
      blood clots and, <u>145</u>, 163, 202
      detecting, 163
      measuring, 202
      vitamin E and aspirin to reduce, <u>143</u>
   strategies for preventing, <u>143</u>, <u>145</u>
      aspirin, 158
      calcium, 171
      frequency of sex, <u>71</u>
      intense exercise with improvement in
         diet, 165
      laughing, <u>232</u>
      weight training, <u>27</u>
   symptoms of, 140, <u>140</u>, 169
   treatments for
      angioplasty, 142, <u>142</u>
      aspirin during attack, <u>141</u>
      bypass surgery, 144, <u>144</u>
      garlic to limit damage caused by, 165–66
      saunas, 165
      statin drugs, 166
      timeliness of, <u>141</u>, 146
Heartburn, 169
Heart scan, 202–3
Heat treatments for back pain
   intradiskal electrothermal therapy, 111–12
   wraps, 104, 119
Height, earnings and, <u>291</u>
Hematospermia, 96
Hematuria, 94–95
Hepatitis B virus, 54
Hepatitis C virus, 161
Herpes, 53
Herpes simplex virus, 120, 283
Herpilyn, 283
HFCS, 6–9
High blood pressure. *See* Blood pressure,
   high
High cholesterol. *See* Cholesterol
High-fructose corn syrup, 6–9

HIV
  measles and, 73
  risk of, from unprotected sex, 54
  trichomoniasis and, 55
HMOs. *See* Health insurance
Homocysteine, risk of stroke and, 151–52
Hospitals, 208, 213–14, 217. *See also*
      Emergency rooms
Hot tubs, sperm count and, 79
Housework as physical activity, 28
Human papillomavirus (HPV), 53
Hunger
  bupropion to control, 34, <u>135</u>
  food cravings, 9–12, 26
  high-fructose corn syrup and, 6–9
  insufficient sleep and, 26
  third-helping hormone and, 29–30
Hydrodiuril, <u>197</u>
Hydroquinone, 282
Hypertension. *See* Blood presure, high
Hypnotism, 229–30

I

Ibuprofen
  for back pain, 84, <u>85</u>, <u>199</u>
  vs. Celebrex, 194
  before dental work, 115
  liquid gel capsule form of, 119
Ice cream, cravings for, 12
IDET, 111–12
IGS, 30
Illnesses. *See also specific illnesses or
      conditions*
  in common among couples, 71
  foodborne, number of people contracting,
      <u>106</u>
  risk of, from exposure to blood, <u>96</u>
Immune system, boosting of, 28, 230–32,
      <u>232</u>
Implantable Gastric Stimulator (IGS), 30
Impotence. *See* Erectile dysfunction
Incline dumbbell bench press, 14, **14**
Incontinence, prostate cancer surgery and,
      155
Infidelity, resisting, 249
Inflammation of artery wall, measuring,
      146–49
Ingrown hairs, 283–84
Inguinal orchiectomy, 49–50
Insomnia. *See also* Sleep
  acupuncture for, 92–93
  depression and, <u>92</u>
  diagnosing disorders causing, 247
  overcoming, 291

  sufferers of, <u>251</u>
  users of vitamins for, <u>91</u>
Insulin, function of, 8
Insurance, health. *See* Health care; Health
      insurance
Insurance industry
  administrative costs of, 186
  cost cutting and denial of coverage by,
      183–85
  impact of, <u>183</u>, 184
  questions to ask of, <u>179</u>
Interferon, in treating colds, 117–18
Internists, 205
Interviews, first impressions in, 267–69
Intradiskal electrothermal therapy (IDET),
      111–12
Ipratropium, 200
Iron, risk of heart disease and, 171
Irritable male syndrome, <u>79</u>

J

Jasmine, for better sleep, 251
Jock itch, 120
Jogger's bladder, 94

K

Kidney stones
  preventing, <u>100</u>
  recurrence rate of, 102
  scan for, 203–4
  symptoms of, 97–98
  treatments for, 101
Knee pain, surgery for, 209
Kojic acid, 282
Korean ginseng, 72

L

Lamisil, 283
Laser-activated glue vs. sutures, 211
Laser treatments, for
  age spots, 282
  ingrown hairs, 284
  lesion removal, 209
Latin-style thrusting, 66
Laughter, <u>232</u>, 290–291
Laurent-Perrier Brut NV, 74
LDL. *See* Cholesterol
Legs, stepup variation exercise for, 36–37
Leptin, 8, 34
Lesions, skin
  laser vs. freezing for removal of, 209
Letters, follow-up, 269
Levator scapulae, 18, **18**
Libido, irritable male syndrome and, <u>79</u>

Lidocaine, 115
Lifestyle for reducing risk of heart attack, 145
Lines, opening
　in flirting, 258
　for public speaking, 270
Lip balm, 120
Lipitor, 148
Lipton, 145
Listerine Antiseptic, 292
Liver disease, hepatitis B virus and, 54
Loniten, 276
Love addiction. *See* Sex and love addiction
Lovemaking, 64–66
Luck, 244–45
Lung cancer, cabbage for protection against, 134
Lungs
　difficulty breathing, 200–201
　laughter to improve, 232
　pleurisy in, 169
　scan of, 203
Lycopene, effect of, on free radicals, 87
Lyme disease test, 112

M

Magnesium in chocolate, mood and, 11
Mallory-Weiss syndrome, 107
Malpractice, finding information about, 207
Managed care. *See* Health insurance
Marijuana, gynecomastia and, 39
Martial arts as alternative to tennis, 25
Massage, precoital, 65–66
Masturbation, 55, 67–70, 67, 68, 69
Measles, AIDS and, 73
Medical care. *See also* Doctors; Health
　　insurance; Hospitals
　access to, 218
　responsibility for own, 179, 185
　status of, in United States, 179–82, 186
　using primary care physician vs. specialist, 216
Medical errors, 180, 213
Medical insurance. *See* Health insurance
Medical spending accounts, 215–16
Medical tests. *See* Tests, medical
Medications. *See* Drugs
Meetings, first impressions in, 267–69
Mega-One Iron Free, 171
Melanoma deaths, 163
Melanotan, 288
Men's Health weight-loss challenge, 33
Mental disorders, 235
Mepivacaine, 115

Message machines, using, 268
Metamucil, 89
Micronase, 201
Midlife, dealing with, 249
Migraine headaches, 88–89, 111
Milk compress for cold sores, 120
Million-Pound Challenge, 33
Mind, healing power of, 274
Minoxidil, 275, 276, 277, 279
Misfortune, dealing with, 244–45
Moisturizing cream, 120
Monogamy, masturbation and, 70
Monounsaturated fat, for
　satisfying hunger, 254
　weight loss, 33
Moods, food and, 10, 11
Mosquitos, risk of infection from, 96
Motrin. *See* Ibuprofen
Mountain biking, 249
Moves during lovemaking, 65–66
Muscles
　abdominal, 5, 35
　loss of, with aging, 39
　pubococcygeus (PC), 79–80
　soreness in, 40, 138, 169
Musical instruments, 249
Music, for back pain, 105, 119

N

Nair for Men, 293
Nasal spray
　apomorphine, for erectile dysfunction, 73
　saline, for stuffy nose, 118
Nausea, combating, 109. *See also* Vomit(ing)
Near infrared spectroscopy, 163
Neck, woman's, 64, 66
Negative pullups, 36
Nerves, pinched, 169
Neuropeptide Y, increase in appetite and, 9
Niacin, 148, 176
Nipples, bleeding, 95
Nitric oxide
　effect of carbon monoxide on, 151
　erection strength and, 77
　laughter and, 232
Nizoral, 283
Nocturnal erections, 77
Nonseminoma cancers, 50
Nonsteroidal anti-inflammatory drugs, 105
Norelco razor, 284
Noritate, 281–82
Nosebleeds, 95
NSAIDs, 105
Nu Hair, 276

Nuts
as snack for energy, 254
for weight loss, 33

O

Obesity. *See* Overweight
Obsessive-compulsive disorder, 235
Omega-3 fatty acids, 143, 166
Online doctor finder, 206
Opening lines
in flirting, 258
for public speaking, 270
Openness in business meetings, 268–69
Optimism, 168, 245
Oral cancer, screening for, 116
Oral sex
danger of, during pregnancy, 71
figure-eight tongue technique for, 66
Orchiectomy, inguinal, 49–50
Orgasms, 68–69, 76
Osteopaths, 206
Overweight
cities with highest and lowest prevalence
of, 135
high-fructose corn syrup and, 6–9
insufficient sleep and, 26
risks posed by
adult-onset asthma, 201
diabetes, 76
heart disease, 143, 160
impotence, 131
sleep apnea, 89
Oxalate, kidney stones and, 100

P

PaceMaster ProElite, 35
Pain, muscular, 40, 138, 169. *See also* Back
pain
Panic attack, 169
Parasol-1789, 281
Partial-body-weight-support system, 105
Patient advocates, 216–17
Paxil, 105
PBWS, 105
PC muscle, 79–80
Pectin, 166
PEG Interferon, 161
Pelvic crunch exercise, 79–80
Penicillin for syphilis, 54
Penis. *See also* Erectile dysfunction
Peyronie's disease of, 73
trauma to, impotence and, 76
Peppermint for nausea, 109
Perdue Short Cuts Chicken Strips, 34

PerioChip, 199
Periodontal disease
risk of stroke and, 165
treatment for, 199
Perrier Jouet Brut NV, 74
Personalization cognitive distortion, 244
Petroleum jelly lip balm, 120
Pets
allergies to, 88
stress and, 250
PET scan, 144, 144
Peyronie's disease, 73
Phase 2 weight-loss pill, 29
Phobias
self-treatment for, 87
social, 235
Physical activity. *See* Exercise; Sports
Physicians. *See* Doctors
Physician's Recognition Award Certificate,
206
Pimples, 282, 285
Pinched nerves, 169
Pinkeye, 94
Plantar fasciitis, 35
Plaque, coronary
artery inflammation and, 147
blood clots and, 145, 163, 202
detecting, 163
measuring, 202
vitamin E and aspirin to reduce, 143
Plavix, 148
Pleated pants, 293, 293
Pleurisy, 169
Poetry for stress relief, 250
Pollen-trapping nose plugs, 113
Polluted air, colds and, 118
Polyps, colorectal. *See also* Colorectal cancer
as risk for colon cancer, 128
scan for, 204
smoking and, 161
Positive Psychology, 241
Positron emission tomography (PET) scan,
144, 144
Posture
during business dinners, 289
in first impressions, 267, 269
while driving, to ease back pain, 119
Postvoid dribble, 80
Potato chips, craving for, 11–12
Pot smoking, gynecomastia and, 39
Poultry, risk of infection from, 96
Power and strength, supersets for, 13, 14–15
dumbbell squat jump, 15, **15**
squat, 15, **15**

Prandin, 201
Pravachol, 148
Precoital massage, 65–66
Pregnancy
  anxiety about, 75
  danger of oral sex during, 71
Prescription drugs. *See* Drugs, prescription
Primary care physician
  choosing, 179, 205–7, 220
  as gatekeeper, 183
  vs. specialist, 216
Privinil, 145
ProCyte Kojic Complex gel, 282
Prolapsed gastropathy, 108
Propecia, 279
Proscar, 200, 279
ProstActive, 80, 200
Prostate
  biopsy of, 154
  complexed prostate-specific antigen and,
    130, 156
  enlarged, 199–200
  prostate specific antigen and, 153–56
Prostate cancer
  aspirin for preventing, 157–58
  among Blacks, 166
  digital rectal exam for, 152–53
  flaxseed for, 166
  Gleason score for aggressiveness of, 154
  pectin for, 166
Protein
  for breakfast, 10, 33
  snacks for weight loss, 33–34
Protexa, 113
PSA, 153–56
Pseudofolliculitis barbae, 283–84
Psyllium for high cholesterol, 89
Public speaking, 269–72
Pubococcygeus (PC) muscle, 79–80
Pullups and negative pullups, 36
Pulmonary rehabilitation, 200–201
Punctuality, in first impressions, 267
Pushup, 14, **14**

R
Radiation therapy, for testicular cancer,
  51
Raisins, to reduce free radical damage, 34
Refractory period, 79–80
Relaxation
  associating, with food, 11–12
  mind techniques for
    controlled breathing, 228–29
    facing stress, 230–31

  humor, 232–33
  social ties, 230
  trancelike states, 229–30
orgasms for, 68
pets and, 250
poetry and, 250
Relenza, 197
Religious services, health and, 170
Remedies, drug-free, for common
  conditions, 197–201. *See also specific
  illnesses or conditions; specific
  remedies or types of remedies*
Remington Precision trimmer, 293
Resistance training. *See* Weight lifting
Resolutions, New Year's, 36
Retin-A Micro, 282
Retroperitoneal lymph node dissection
  (RPLND), 51–52
Rezulin, 195
Ribavirin, 161
Rib injuries, 169
Robot-assisted surgery, 30, 163
Rock climbing, for back pain, 90
Romantic escapes, 74
Rosacea, 281–82
RPLND, 51–52
Ruinart 1990 Brut, 74
Running
  avoiding injuries from, 21–22
  combined with weight lifting, 39–40
  jogger's bladder from, 94
  jogger's nipples from, 95
  for preventing cancer, 27–28

S
St. John's wort, cancer and, 160
Saline nasal spray, 118
Salt, bitter medications and, 118
Saunas, 165
Saw palmetto, 80, 200, 275, 277
Scans, full-body, 202–5
Scorpion venom, for brain cancer, 248
Seat belts, 139, 167
Seborrheic dermatitis, 283
Secondhand smoke, 143, 151
Sedation dentistry, 221
Seduction, of women, 64–67, 65
Self-examination, for testicular cancer, 50
Seminoma cancers, 50
Serratus anterior, 17–18, **17**
Sex
  frequency of, risk of heart attack or stroke
    and, 71
  immune system and, 230

Sex (*cont.*)
   seducing women and, 64–67, <u>65</u>
   unprotected, risk of disease from, 53–55
Sex and love addiction
   characteristics and signs of, 56, <u>57</u>, <u>60</u>
   masturbation as most common form of,
      <u>55</u>
   recovery from, 56–63, <u>60</u>
Sex and Love Addicts Anonymous, <u>60</u>
Sex toys, 64–65, 78
Sexually transmitted diseases, 53–55
Shaving, 284, 286
Shoes, 35
Shoveling snow safely, 170
Sickness. *See also specific illnesses or
      conditions*
   in common among couples, 71
   foodborne, number of people contracting,
      <u>106</u>
   risk of, from exposure to blood, <u>96</u>
Silica in toothpaste, 165
Silver dental fillings, 115
Single-scull rowing as alternative to
      swimming, 24
Skin conditions
   age spots, 282
   blushing, 281–82
   cold sores, 283
   injuries, 119–20
   pimples, 282, 285
   pseudofolliculitis barbae, 283–84
   seborrheic dermatitis, 283
   injuries, 119–20
   protecting from, 120, 122
Skin cancer, <u>163</u>, <u>137</u>, 163, 209
Skin Whitening Cream, 282
Sleep. *See also* Insomnia
   activity and, 253–54
   apnea, headaches and, 89
   aroma conducive to, 251
   deprivation of, among emergency room
      doctors, 180
   diagnosing disorders of, 247
   hours of, 253, <u>253</u>
   insufficient, weight gain and, 26
   mastering skills and, 251
   positions to ease pain
      in back, 121
      of kidney stones, <u>100</u>
   susceptibility to flu and, 117
   teeth grinding during, 221–22
   tryptophan and, 12
Smart eye band for vision correction, 211
Smiling, in first impressions, 268
Smoking
   acid reflux and, 111
   brain aging and, <u>229</u>
   colorectal cancer and, 128
   colorectal polyps and, 161
   impotence and, 75
   pot, gynecomastia and, 39
   quitting, 89–90, 161, <u>161</u>, <u>199</u>
   risk of heart attack and, <u>144</u>
   risk of kidney disease and, 161, 203
   secondhand smoke and, <u>143</u>, 151
Snacks, 33–34, 254
Snoring, risk of diabetes and, 160
Snow shoveling safely, 170
Soaps, antibacterial, 112, 113, 120, 283
Soccer as alternative to cycling, 24
Socialized medicine, 186–87
Social phobia, <u>235</u>
Social support
   happiness and, 243
   immune system and, 230, 231
   in overcoming fear, <u>239</u>, 240
Soda
   caffeine-free, 10
   high-fructose corn syrup in, 7, 8
   risk of stroke and, 151
Softball, avoiding injuries from, 23
Soreness. *See also* Back pain
   of muscles, 40, <u>138</u>, 169
   in throat, 113
Soy
   cholesterol level and, 176
   kidney stones and, <u>100</u>
Speech and voice, in first impressions, 269
Sperm
   health of, <u>67</u>, <u>69</u>
   hot tubs and, 79
Spinal surgery, <u>103</u>
Sports
   avoiding injuries from
      basketball, 22–23
      cycling, 24
      running, 21–22
      softball, 23
      swimming, 23–24
      tennis, 24–25
   for stress relief, 231–32
Sports drinks, kidney stones and, <u>100</u>
Squat exercise, 15, **15**
Statin drugs
   cognitive function and, 246
   for C-reactive protein levels, 148
   for reducing cholesterol, <u>145</u>, 148, 166, 177
STDs, 53–55

Steak, rare, and risk of infection, <u>96</u>
Stepup variation, 36–37
Steroids, gynecomastia and, 39
Stomach stapling, 27, 30
Stool, blood in, 96–97
Strength
   cardiovascular fitness and, exercise
      program for, <u>25</u>
   power and, supersets for, <u>13</u>, 14–15
      dumbbell squat jump, 15, **15**
      squat, 15, **15**
Streptococcus bacteria, oral sex and, 71
Stress
   body odor and, 292
   fear as, 238–40, <u>239</u>
   frequency of, <u>237</u>
   relief from, 250
   serotonin and, 10
   symptoms of, 238
   techniques to reduce
      controlled breathing, 228–29
      facing stress, 230–31
      humor, 232–33
      social ties, 230
      trancelike states, 229–30
Stretching, for back pain, 84, <u>85</u>, 90, 104
Stroke
   reducing risk of, <u>71</u>, 150–52, 159, 165
   risk posed by aspirin, <u>157</u>
   testosterone level and, 27
Subaru Impreza WRX, 249
Success, envisioning downside of, 260–61
Sucrose, 9
Suicide rates, 247
Sunlight, for reducing risk of cancer,
      166–67
Sunscreen, 167, 281, 282
Supersets, 12–13
   for bigger muscles, 13
      close-grip chinup, 14
      incline dumbbell bench press, 14, **14**
      pushup, 14, **14**
      wide-grip lat pulldown, 14
   for fat loss, 15–16
      bench press, 16, **16**
      deadlift, 16, **16**
   for strength and power, 14–15
      dumbbell squat jump, 15, **15**
      squat, 15, **15**
Supplements, dietary, 26, 170–71, 252
Surgery
   arthroscopic, 209
   bypass, robot-assisted, 163
   checking on doctor for, 213

   cosmetic, <u>281</u>
   laser-activated glue vs. sutures for, 211
   spinal, with instrumentation, <u>103</u>
   stomach stapling, 27, 30
   teaching dummies for practice of, 211
   for testicular cancer, 51–52
Sweat, 288, 292
Sweetened foods, cravings for, 9–10
Sweeteners, average calories consumed
      from, <u>8</u>
Sweet Heart Vibe, 78
Swimmer's backstroke, 19, **19**
Swimming, avoiding injuries from, 23–24
Syphilis, 54

T
Talk therapy, 233–37
Tamsulosin, 200
Tanita BF662 Family Model, 35
Tanning drug, 288
Tattoo parlors, risk of infection from, <u>96</u>
Tazarotene, 163
Tea drinking to reduce risk of heart attack, <u>143</u>
Teeth, 115–16
   flossing and brushing, 165
   grinding and, 221–22
   saving costs of, 219
   sedation dentistry and, 221
   whitening, 285, <u>285</u>
Tennis, avoiding injuries from, 24–25
Testicular cancer, 49–52, <u>49</u>, <u>50</u>
Testosterone
   first impressions and, <u>267</u>
   level of, strokes and, 27
   pimples and, 282
   relation of, to prostate growth and hair
      loss, 200
Tests, medical, 217
   biopsy of testicle, 49–50
   breath, for ulcers, 212
   California Verbal Learning Test for
      predicting Alzheimer's, 247
   for cholesterol, <u>136</u>, <u>179</u>
   C6 peptide, for Lyme disease, 112
   for prostate cancer
      biopsy, 154
      complexed prostate-specific antigen,
         <u>130</u>, 156
      digital rectal exam, 152–53
      prostate specific antigen, 153–56
   self-examination for testicular cancer, <u>50</u>
   self-test for hearing loss, 221
Theobromine, for coughs and sore throats,
      113

Therapy, talk, 233–37
ThermaCare, 104
Third-helping hormone, 29–30
Thymuskin, _276_
Tinea cruris, 120
Tipping bathroom attendants, 294
Toasts, 272
Tobacco. _See_ Smoking
Toilets, infections from, 123
Tomato juice and cayenne pepper, blood
     pressure and, 87–88
Topamax, 111
Topiramate, 111
Toprol XL, _145_
Total cereal, _143_
Touching of women, recommendations for,
     64–65
TPA, _141_
Trainer, qualifications of, 31
Trancelike states, 229–30
Treadmills, 35
Treatments, drug-free, for common
     conditions, 197–201. _See also specific_
     illnesses or conditions; specific
     treatments or types of treatments
Triathlons, as alternatives to running, 22
Triceps long head, 19–20, **19**
Trichomoniasis, 55
Triglycerides, risk of arterial disease and, 151
True 540HRC, 35
Tryptophan, sleep and, 12
Tylenol, 166, _197_

U
Ulcers, breath test for, 212
Ultrasound therapy, for bone fractures,
     209–10
Ultraviolet A radiation, 281
Unprotected sex, risk of disease from, 53–55
Urine
     blood in, 94–95
     increased urination, 199–200
     postvoid dribble of, 80
UVA rays, 281

V
Vaccine for high cholesterol, 162
Vasectomy, 75
Ventolin, 200
Veuve Clicquot Yellow Label Brut NV, 74
Viagra, 73
Vibrators, 78
Vioxx, _199_
Virtual colonoscopy, 204

Viruses
     colds and flu
          drug treatment for, 117–18, _118_
          foods to combat, 121–22
          users of vitamins for, _91_
     hepatitis B, 54
     hepatitis C, 161
     herpes simplex, 120, 283
     human papillomavirus, 53
     stomach, vomiting and, 122
Vision
     correction, 211, 219
     exercises for, 91
Visualization to control fear, _239_
Vitamins, _91_
     to protect brain, 226
     supplements, 170–71
     vitamin C for rosacea, 282
     vitamin D for reducing cancer risk, 166–67
     vitamin E for protection against heart
          disease, _143_, 171
Voice and speech, in first impressions, 269
Voice mail, using, _268_
Volleyball, as alternative to basketball, 23
Vomit(ing), 107
     by animals, 108–10
     blood in, 95–96
     combating, _109_
     injuries from, 107–8
     kidney stones and, 98–99
     stomach virus and, 122
     triggers of, 107
Vulnerability, 259, 271

W
Waist size, heart disease risk and, 160
Walking, alternating, with running, 22
Warmup exercises, to avoid basketball
     injuries, 22
Water, drinking of, _143_, 150–52
Weight, body. _See_ Overweight
Weight lifting
     for back pain, 84, _85_
     boosting testosterone with, 27
     combined with running, 39–40
     for preventing softball injuries, 23
     for reducing risk of heart disease and
          diabetes, _27_
     for reducing risk of stroke, 152
     schedule for, _138_
     training to failure, 40–41
Weight loss
     bupropion for, 34, _135_
     chitosan fat blockers for, 26

controlling food cravings for, 9–12
exercise for, _13_, 15–16, **16**
gastric bypass surgery for, 27, 30
Implantable Gastric Stimulator for, 30
migraine medication and, 111
strategies, 33–37
white-kidney-bean extract for, 29
White-kidney-bean extract, 29
Wide-grip lat pulldown, 14
Wine, rosacea and, 281
Witch hazel, 282, 283
Women('s)
    attracting, 46, _47_
    flirting with, 258–59, _258_, _259_
    places to meet, 71
    reactions to male masturbation, 69–70
    romantic escapes with, 74
    seducing, 64–67, _65_

Workouts. _See_ Exercise
Workplace, masturbation in, 69
Wraps, heat, for back pain, 104, 119
Wrigley's Extra Peppermint, _109_

X
X, 254
Xopenex, _197_
X-rays, tooth, 116

Y
Yawning, erection strength and, 77
Yogurt, for weight loss, 34

Z
Zinc pyrithione, _279_
Zocor, 148
Zyban, _199_

Photo Credits

Front cover: Robert Trachtenberg
Back cover (top): Blake Little
Back cover (bottom): Wes Bell
Pages vii (top left), 1: Svend Lindbaek
Pages vii (bottom left), 43: Diego Uchitel
Pages vii (top right), 81: Stefan Nyvang
Pages vii (bottom right), 125: Sally Ullman
Pages viii (top left), 173: Augustus Butera
Pages viii (bottom left), 223: Blake Little
Pages viii (right), 255: Peter Berson
Pages 3, 4: Chris Croy
Pages 14–20: Beth Bischoff
Pages 45 (left and right), 46: Monte Isom
Pages 45 (middle), 83 (left): Deidre Dedman
Page 83 (middle): Doug Rider
Pages 83 (right), 84: Todd Bennett
Pages 127 (left), 175 (left), 176, 225 (right): Kurt Wilson
Page 127 (middle): Blair Jensen
Pages 127 (right), 128: David Deal
Page 175 (middle): Deb Porter-Hayes
Page 175 (right): Ken Love
Pages 225 (left), 226: Rex Rystreet
Page 225 (middle): Mike McCleary
Pages 257, 258: Wendy Hope